GASTROENTEROLOGY AND HEPATOLOGY

The Comprehensive Visual Reference

GASTROENTEROLOGY AND HEPATOLOGY

The Comprehensive Visual Reference

series and volume editor
Mark Feldman, MD

Southland Professor and Vice Chairman
Department of Internal Medicine
University of Texas Southwestern
  Medical Center at Dallas

Chief, Medical Service
Veterans Affairs Medical Center
Dallas, Texas

volume 3
Stomach and Duodenum

With 14 contributors

Churchill Livingstone
Developed by Current Medicine, Inc.
Philadelphia

Current Medicine

400 Market Street
Suite 700
Philadelphia, PA 19106

Managing Editor	*Lori J. Bainbridge*
Development Editors	*Kelly Streeter, Raymond Lukens, and Ira D. Smiley*
Editorial Assistants	*Jennifer Rosenblum and Scott Thomas Hurd*
Indexer	*Maria Coughlin*
Art Director	*Paul Fennessy*
Design and Layout	*Robert LeBrun*
Illustration Director	*Ann Saydlowski*
Illustrators	*Marie Dean, Wieslawa Langenfield, Beth Starkey, Larry Ward, Lisa Weischedel, and Gary Welch*
Typesetting Director	*Colleen Ward*
Production	*David Myers and Lori Holland*

Stomach and duodenum/volume editor, Mark Feldman.
     p. cm. – (Gastroenterology and hepatology; v. 3)
  Includes bibliographical references and index.
  ISBN 0-443-07843-2 (hardcover)
  1. Stomach—Diseases—Atlases. 2. Duodenum—Diseases—Atlases. I. Feldman, Mark, 1947– . II. Series.
  [DNLM: 1. Stomach Diseases—atlases. 2. Duodenal Diseases—atlases. WI 17 G257 1996 v.3]
RC807.S86 1996
616.3'3—dc20
DNLM/DLC
for Library of Congress   95-25966
                                     CIP

Library of Congress Cataloging-in-Publication Data
ISBN 0-443-07843-2

Printed in Singapore by Imago Productions (FE) Pte Ltd.

10 9 8 7 6 5 4 3 2

DISTRIBUTED WORLDWIDE BY CHURCHILL LIVINGSTONE, INC.

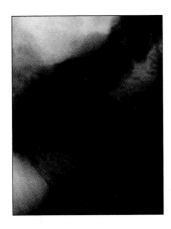

Series Preface

In recent years dramatic developments in the practice of gastroenterology have unfolded, and the specialty has become, more than ever, a visual discipline. Advances in endoscopy, radiology, or a combination of the two, such as endoscopic retrograde cholangiopancreatography and endoscopic ultrasonography, have occurred in the past 2 decades. Because of advanced imaging technology, a gastroenterologist, like a dermatologist, is often able to directly view the pathology of a patient's organs. Moreover, practicing gastroenterologists and hepatologists can frequently diagnose disease from biopsy samples examined microscopically, often aided by an increasing number of special staining techniques. As a result of these advances, gastroenterology has grown as rapidly as any subspecialty of internal medicine.

Gastroenterology and Hepatology: The Comprehensive Visual Reference is an ambitious 8-volume collection of images that pictorially displays the gastrointestinal tract, liver, biliary tree, and pancreas in health and disease, both in children and adults. The series is comprised of 89 chapters containing nearly 4000 images accompanied by legends. The images in this collection include not only traditional photographs but also charts, tables, drawings, algorithms, and diagrams, making this collection much more than an atlas in the conventional sense. Chapters are authored by experts selected by one of the eight volume editors, who carefully reviewed each chapter within their volume.

Disorders of the gastrointestinal tract, liver, biliary tree, and pancreas are common in children and adults. *Helicobacter pylori* gastritis is the most frequent bacterial infection of humans and is a risk factor for peptic ulcer disease and gastric malignancies. Colorectal carcinoma is the second leading cause of cancer mortality in the United States, with nearly 60,000 deaths in 1990. Pancreatic cancer resulted in an additional 25,000 deaths. Liver disease is also an important cause of morbidity and mortality, with more that 25,000 deaths from cirrhosis alone in 1990. Gallstone disease is also common in our society, with increasing reliance on laparoscopic cholecystectomy in symptomatic individuals. Inflammatory bowel diseases (ulcerative colitis, Crohn's disease) are also widespread in all segments of the population; their causes still elude us.

The past few decades have also witnessed striking advances in the therapy of gastrointestinal disorders. Examples include "cure" of peptic ulcer disease by eradicating *H. pylori* with antimicrobial agents, healing of erosive esophagitis with proton pump inhibitor drugs, remission of chronic viral hepatitis B or C with interferon-α2b, and hepatic transplantation for patients with fulminant hepatic failure or end-stage liver disease. Therapeutic endoscopic techniques have proliferated that ameliorate the need for surgical procedures. Endoscopic advances include placement of peroral endoscopic gastrostomy tubes for nutritional support, insertion of stents in the bile duct or esophagus to relieve malignant obstruction, and the use of injection therapy, thermal coagulation, or laser therapy to treat bleeding ulcers and other lesions, including tumors. *Gastroenterology and Hepatology: The Comprehensive Visual Reference* will cover these advances and many others in the field of gastroenterology.

I wish to thank a number of people for their contributions to this series. The dedication and expertise of the other volume editors—Willis Maddrey, Rick Boland, Paul Hyman, Nick LaRusso, Roy Orlando, Larry Schiller, and Phil Toskes—was critical and most appreciated. The nearly 100 contributing authors were both creative and generous with their time and teaching materials. Special thanks to Abe Krieger, President of Current Medicine, for recruiting me for this unique project and to his talented associates at Current Medicine, especially Kelly Streeter who served as development editor.

The images contained in this 8-volume collection are available in print as well as in slide format, and the series is soon being formatted for CD-ROM use. All of us who have participated in this ambitious project hope that each of the 8 volumes, as well as the entire collection, will be useful to physicians and health professionals throughout the world involved in the diagnosis and treatment of patients of all ages who suffer from gastrointestinal disorders.

Mark Feldman, MD

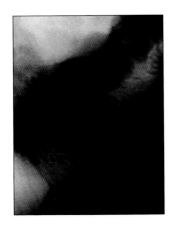

Volume Preface

The stomach and duodenum have been the heart and soul of gastroenterology during its evolution as a discipline. Gastric and duodenal ulcer disease, which have caused considerable morbidity and mortality, spawned the development of acid anti-secretory drugs and numerous ulcer operations. With the discovery of *Helicobacter pylori* infection, a treatable cause of chronic active gastritis and a major risk factor for ulcer disease, the natural history of peptic ulcer disease has changed from a chronic condition to a curable one. Other causes of ulcer diseases, such as ingestion of nonsteroidal anti-inflammatory drugs, the stress of major medical or surgical illness (stress ulcers), and gastrinoma (Zollinger-Ellison syndrome), are also recognized.

In addition to ulcer disease, gastric cancer is another concern of gastroenterologists. Once the most common cause of cancer death in the United States, gastric cancer is now less common, but is still a major cause of morbidity and mortality as most cases present in an advanced stage with a very low cure rate.

The stomach and duodenum were among the first organs of the digestive tract accessible to imaging via the endoscope. This volume contains 12 chapters, each written by experts in their respective fields. In the first chapter, Dr. Sachs reviews the current concepts of regulation of gastric acid secretion with emphasis on the hydrogen, potassium ATPase (proton pump), and drugs that inhibit this pump. Chapter 2 by Drs. Kliewer and Lechago reviews the complex endocrinology of the stomach and duodenum with emphasis on the D cell (somatostatin), enterochromaffin-like cell (histamine), and G cell (gastrin).

Chapter 3 by Dr. Walker presents a clear and erudite pictorial of the gastrointestinal immune system. This chapter illustrates the basic science of gut immunology and then uses *H. pylori* gastritis and celiac sprue as examples of immunopathic disorders of the stomach and duodenum, respectively. This chapter will also be valuable to readers of the Small Intestine volume in this series because immune function of the gut is highly relevant to understanding benign and malignant disorders of the small intestine. (Likewise, the Small Intestine volume contains a chapter on motor disorders of the small intestine and stomach, which serves as a valuable reference to readers of the Stomach and Duodenum volume.)

Chapters 4 to 8 summarize in some detail the current concepts and risk factors for ulcerative and inflammatory diseases of the stomach and duodenum. Chapter 4 by Dr. Leung begins by reviewing the many mechanisms by which the gastric and duodenal mucosae protect themselves against injury and how these protective mechanisms are interfered with by pathological processes. Chapter 5 by Drs. Lee and Cryer deals with agents, both infectious and noninfectious, that result in injury to the gastric and duodenal mucosa. Chapter 6, also by Drs. Cryer and Lee, deals with *H. pylori* gastritis and its many disease associations. Dr. Wilcox then presents in Chapter 7 a thorough and logical image collection of clinical aspects of peptic ulcer disease, including its complications. In Chapter 8, Dr. Jensen adds a scholarly review on Zollinger-Ellison syndrome, encompassing pathogenesis, clinical presentation, diagnosis, and therapy.

In Chapter 9, Drs. Fukunaga and Yang depict the panoply of bleeding lesion of the stomach and duodenum, both benign and malignant. In Chapter 10, Dr. DeMarco illustrates the many types of neoplasms of the stomach and duodenum with emphasis on gastric adenocarcinoma. Dr. Seymour then depicts in Chapter 11 the various surgical procedures on the stomach and duodenum available for the treatment of benign and malignant disorders, including morbid obesity. He also illustrates surgical procedures on the stomach to prevent gastroesophageal reflux disease, an entity discussed in greater detail in the Esophagus volume in this series.

The Stomach and Duodenum volume concludes with a well-illustrated chapter on the skin by Dr. Pandya. He reviews both dermatologic manifestations of gastrointestinal diseases as well as cutaneous lesions that, when present, are markers for diseases of the gastrointestinal tract, liver, biliary tree, or pancreas. This chapter is presented here although its contents are relevant to the entire series.

I am extremely indebted to the 14 authors who contributed to this volume on the Stomach and Duodenum, a collection which includes more than 500 separate images.

Mark Feldman, MD

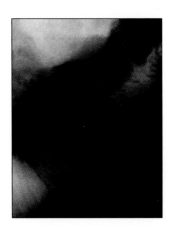

Contributors

Byron Cryer, MD
Assistant Professor
Internal Medicine
University of Texas Southwestern Medical School
Department of Digestive Disease
Dallas Veterans Affairs Medical Center
Dallas, Texas

Daniel C. DeMarco, MD
Gastroenterology Department
Baylor University Medical Center
Dallas, Texas

Karl Fukunaga, MD
Clinical Instructor
Department of Medicine
University of Southern California
    School of Medicine
Los Angeles County and University of
    Southern California Medical Center
Los Angeles, California

Robert T. Jensen, MD
Digestive Diseases Branch
National Institutes of Health
Bethesda, Maryland

Douglas Kliewer, MD
Fellow in Gastroenterology
Department of Internal Medicine
University of Texas Southwestern Medical School
Parkland Hospital/Veterans Affairs Medical Center
Dallas, Texas

Juan Lechago, MD, PhD
Professor
Department of Pathology
Baylor College of Medicine
Director, Surgical Pathology
The Methodist Hospital
Houston, Texas

Edward Lee, MD
Professor
Department of Pathology
University of Texas
    Southwestern Medical Center
Veterans Affairs Medical Center
Dallas, Texas

Felix W. Leung, MD
Professor of Medicine in Residence
University of California, Los Angeles/
   San Fernando Valley Program
University of California, Los Angeles, School of Medicine
Los Angeles, California
Sepulveda Veterans Affairs Medical Center
Sepulveda, California

Amit G. Pandya, MD
Assistant Professor
Department of Dermatology
University of Texas
   Southwestern Medical Center
Dallas, Texas

George Sachs, MD, DSc
Professor
Departments of Physiology and Medicine
University of California, Los Angeles, School of Medicine
Los Angeles, California

Neal E. Seymour, MD
Assistant Professor
Department of Surgery
Yale University School of Medicine
Veterans Affairs Medical Center
New Haven, Connecticut

W. Allan Walker, MD
Conrad Taff Professor of Pediatrics and Nutrition
Harvard Medical School
Professor of Nutrition
Harvard School of Public Health
Boston, Massachusetts
Chief, Combined Program in Pediatric
   Gastroenterology and Nutrition
Massachusetts General Hospital
Children's Hospital
Charlestown, Massachusetts

C. Mel Wilcox, MD
Associate Professor of Medicine
Department of Medicine
University of Alabama at Birmingham
Birmingham, Alabama

Russell Yang, MD, PhD
Assistant Professor
Department of Medicine
University of Southern California School of Medicine
Los Angeles County and University of
   Southern California Medical Center
Los Angeles, California

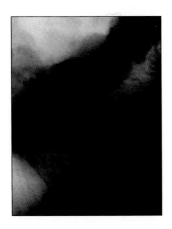

Contents

Chapter 5
Stomach and Duodenum: Injuries, Infections, and Inflammation
EDWARD LEE
BYRON CRYER

Chapter 6
Helicobacter pylori
BYRON CRYER
EDWARD LEE

Chapter 7
Peptic Ulcer Disease
C. MEL WILCOX

Chapter 12
The Skin and Gastrointestinal System
AMIT G. PANDYA

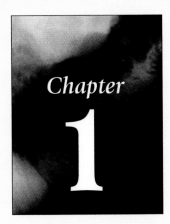

Chapter 1

Acid Secretion

GEORGE SACHS

Clinicians of the twentieth century have witnessed much change in the understanding and treating of acid-related diseases. Ulcer disease has been recognized for the past 80 years as requiring gastric acid secretion. The past 20 years have seen a revolution in the therapy of this major ailment, which is present in both acute and chronic forms.

■ REGULATION OF GASTRIC ACID SECRETION

Gastric acid secretion is a regulated, energy-expending process. A multiplicity of pathways determines the rate of acid secretion by the parietal cell. Furthermore, a multiplicity of second messenger pathways within the parietal cell and an ion motive P-type ATPase are responsible for the final step of acid secretion, the elaboration of hydrochloric acid. Advances in our understanding of these processes has led to great improvement in the treatment of acid-related disease using therapy with either receptor antagonists or pump inhibitors. Recognition that the presence of *Helicobacter pylori* in the stomach is a necessary precondition for the development of duodenal and gastric ulcers that are not related to the consumption of nonsteroidal anti-inflammatory drugs promises a further revolution in treatment of this particular type of acid-related disease (*see* Chapter 6). In the case of gastroesophageal reflux disease, where *H. pylori* infection does not appear to be involved, improvements in acid control and perhaps in the control of the lower esophageal sphincter are bringing about improvements in therapy of this disorder as well. The emphasis in this chapter is largely on the past, present, and future targets for acid control as summarized in these figures. Because this chapter is a pictorial account of the mechanisms and inhibition of acid secretion, the reader is referred to several recent reviews of the topics covered rather than to the original literature.

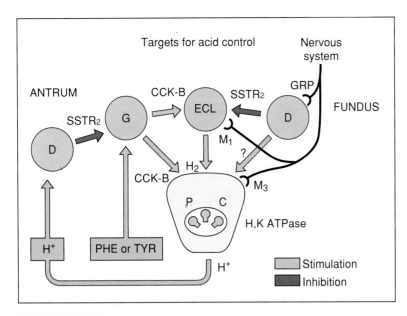

FIGURE 1-1.

Central nervous system. The central nervous system (CNS) regulates the D cell, G cell, enterochromaffin-like (ECL) cell, and the parietal cell (PC). The CNS responds to chemical and psychic factors by altering the activity of hypothalamic nuclei, which in their turn influence vagal activity. Significant sympathetic innervation of the stomach also exists, but it is less significant than vagal innervation.

The dorsal motor nucleus of the vagus appears to be the site of integration of all CNS stimulation of acid secretion; destruction of this nucleus eliminates central stimulation of acid secretion. Sensory input into the dorsal motor nucleus originates from the hypothalamus and sensory afferents from the gut. The lateral hypothalamus responds to glucose deprivation. The nucleus tractus solitarius responds to glucose deprivation as well as to sensory taste fibers and visceral afferents.

Over 95% of the vagal fibers are afferent. Although less well defined than the efferent component of the vagus, these afferents play a major role in neural regulation of acid secretion. Afferent fibers originate within smooth muscle and within the gut mucosa. Sympathetic afferents also originate within muscle and blood vessels but travel along separate (nonvagal) anatomic pathways.

Normally, the stomach is relatively insensitive to mechanical or chemical stimulation in terms of producing the sensation of pain, unless considerable distention is present. With the inflammatory response of gastritis, however, touch sensitivity is significantly increased. This activity may mean that the immune response may result in an increase of release of mediators sensitizing the mucosa to stimulation. This increase may in part be responsible for the pain associated with ulcer disease. There is almost surely a pain response to the alteration of pH within the gastric or duodenal epithelium.

Regulation of acid secretion within the gastric mucosa is the responsibility of at least three types of endocrine cells found within this epithelium. In the fundus, the enterochromaffin-like (ECL) cell releases histamine to activate the H_2 receptor on the nearby parietal cell. The fundic D cell releases somatostatin to inhibit the nearby ECL cell and possibly also the parietal cell directly. The antral D cell releases somatostatin to suppress the function of adjacent G cells. The antral G cell releases gastrin into the circulation in response to stimuli present in the antral lumen, such as tyrosine or phenylalanine, derived from dietary protein.

These cell types all use changes in intracellular calcium or cyclic adenosine monophosphate to affect alterations in release of their mediators by exocytosis. These changes in second messenger are brought about by the binding of ligands to receptors on the cell surface. These endocrine cell types are discussed in more detail subsequently. CCK—cholecystokinin; GRP—gastrin releasing peptide; H^+—hydrogen ion; H,K, ATPase—hydrogen, potassium, adenosine triphosphatase; M—muscarinic receptor; PHE—phenylalanine; $SSTR_2$—somatostatin$_2$ receptor; TYR—tyrosine.

PERIPHERAL REGULATION OF ACID SECRETION

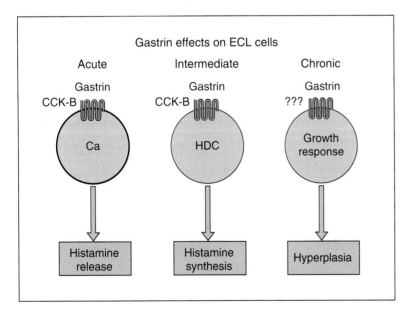

FIGURE 1-2.

Gastrin effects on ECL cells are shown. The ECL cell is probably the best understood of the endocrine cell types responsible for peripheral regulation of acid secretion. The major pathway used for acute stimulation of histamine release is activation of the cholecystokinin-B (CCK-B) receptor by gastrin. This receptor is characterized by its equal affinity to both gastrin and CCK-B. An increasing number of selective CCK-B receptor antagonists have become available. Activation of the CCK-B receptor has this acute effect, but in addition intermediate and long-term effects are present. One intermediate effect is activation of the enzyme responsible for histamine biosynthesis, histidine decarboxylase (HDC), by activation of gene transcription for this enzyme. The long-term (chronic) effect of gastrin is stimulation of ECL cell growth. Potential consequences of hypergastrinemia are therefore increased histamine release, increased HDC activity, and multiplication of ECL cells with ECL hyperplasia.

Although considerable evidence exists for a CCK-B receptor for gastrin on the parietal cell, it appears that the major action of gastrin on acid secretion is mediated by histamine release, because H_2 antagonists abolish gastrin-stimulated acid secretion.

Stimulation of histamine release

CCK-B receptor: Ligand = gastrin
Second messenger Ca ↑

Muscarinic receptor: Ligand = acetylcholine
Second messenger Ca ↑

β-Adrenergic receptor: Ligand = epinephrine
Second messenger cAMP ↑

Inhibition of histamine release

SSTR-2: Ligand = somatostatin
Second messenger Ca ↓

H_3 receptor: Ligand = histamine
Second messenger Ca ↓

FIGURE 1-3.

Enterochromaffin-like (ECL) cell receptor. In addition to the stimulatory cholecystokinin-B (CCK-B) receptor, ECL cells have other receptors that may regulate gastric secretion. The ECL cell has a stimulatory muscarinic receptor of as yet undefined subtype, possibly M_1 (*see* Fig. 1-1). Cholinergic stimulation of acid secretion is therefore mediated in part by release of histamine by the ECL cell. Although all ECL cells respond to gastrin, only about 30% respond to muscarinic stimulation, suggesting that there are subpopulations of ECL cells, perhaps defined by their anatomic location.

Both the CCK-B and the muscarinic receptors activate ECL cells by induction of an intracellular calcium ($[Ca]_i$) signal. In contrast, epinephrine stimulates histamine release from ECL cells by activation of perhaps a beta-3-adrenergic receptor, mediated by elevation of cyclic AMP (cAMP). The compound, forskolin, is a potent liberator of histamine, showing that the cAMP pathway is as effective as the $[Ca]_i$ pathway.

Inhibition of ECL cell function and histamine release is an important means of regulation of acid secretion. Somatostatin (SST) inhibits gastrin-mediated histamine release by inhibition of the $[Ca]_i$ response through a G1 subtype of G protein. The receptor on the ECL cell is of the SST receptor (SSTR)-2 subtype. It is probable that SST, which modifies ECL-cell function, is released from fundic D cells that are in relative proximity to the ECL cell. There is also a histamine-3 (H_3) subtype of receptor that acts as a negative feedback regulator or histamine release. The ligands that affect the ECL cell are shown in this figure.

The model shown in Figure 1-1 identifies the important pathways in peripheral regulation of acid secretion impinging on the ECL cell. Effective inhibition of histamine release by this cell can therefore be brought about by CCK-B receptor antagonists or agonists of the SSTR-2 receptor. Such compounds should give clinical results at least equivalent to those obtained with H_2-receptor antagonists.

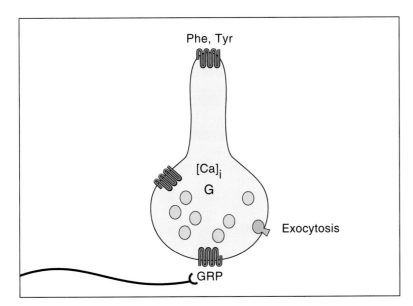

Phe, Tyr

$[Ca]_i$

G

Exocytosis

GRP

FIGURE 1-4.

The G cell. This cell is found in antral glands with processes extending to the lumen of the gland. It is considered to be the endocrine cell with major responsibility for upregulation of enterochromaffin-like cell function. Release of gastrin is stimulated by the presence of amino acids in the lumen of the gastric gland, especially phenylalanine (Phe) and tyrosine (Tyr). It seems that these amino acids induce a intracellular calcium ($[Ca]_i$) signal similar to that induced by the other receptors, and that they therefore stimulate exocytosis of gastrin by elevation of $[Ca]_i$. In addition, the neurotransmitter gastrin releasing peptide (GRP), the mammalian analog of the amphibian peptide bombesin, stimulates release of gastrin from the G cell.

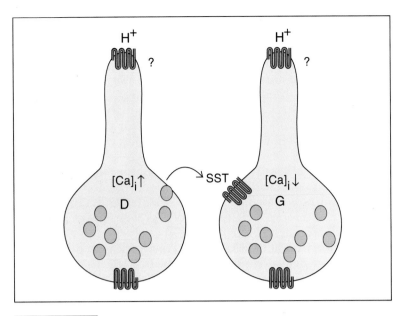

FIGURE 1-5.

Inhibition of gastrin release. The release of gastrin is inhibited by acidification of the antral lumen ("negative feedback"). Much of this inhibition appears to be mediated by acid-induced release of SST-14 from antral D cells. Some of this inhibition may depend

on acidification at the luminal surface of the G cell. SST inhibits release of gastrin from the G cell, perhaps also by stimulation of a SST receptor (SSTR)-2 subtype of receptor. The G cell therefore provides a target for acid control with the same type of SST agonist appropriate for inhibition of enterochromaffin-like (ECL) cell histamine secretion also shown in Figure 1-1.

Although both fundic D cells (*see* Fig. 1-1) and antral D cells (*see* Figs. 1-1 and 1-5) secrete SST, the receptors regulating this release may differ in these two locations. Gastrin stimulates SST release from antral D cells providing a negative feedback loop in this location. Gastrin, cholecystokinin, and many other peptides probably are involved in stimulation of SST release from the fundic D cell. Other gut hormones, such as secretin, inhibit acid secretion, also perhaps by liberation of SST or prostaglandins.

Somatostatin-14 acts as a universal inhibitor of signaling in the endocrine cells of the gastric mucosa. SSTRs may also be present on the parietal cell, enabling direct inhibition of acid secretion. In addition to its effect on preventing mediator release, this cyclic tetradecapeptide inhibits stimulation of ECL cell growth induced by gastrin. SST analogs might therefore be useful, not only in inhibition of ECL cell function, but also in regulation of growth of the gastric epithelium under conditions of severe secretory inhibition. There is already one SST analog available (octreotide [Sandostatin; Sandoz Pharmaceuticals, East Hanover, NJ]).

TABLE 1-1. NEW TARGETS FOR ACID CONTROL

CCK-B Antagonists

Somatostatin-2 receptor agonists

TABLE 1-1.

New endocrine cell receptor targets. The keys to developing a successful drug are efficacy and specificity. The cholecystokinin-B (CCK-B) receptor is expressed mainly in the stomach and brain, thus it provides a relatively specific target for inhibition of acid secretion. The somatostatin receptors have a wider distribution. Use of somatostatin agonists for acid control will therefore probably require the use of specific agonists. The next century will see the introduction of this type of receptor agonist as an alternative to the antagonists now favored for control of acid secretion.

Intense effort is being expended on development of inhibitors of the CCK-B receptor; these will have interesting applications in ulcer disease. Current antagonists based on diazepam structures are small molecules that are stable to the gastric environment and readily absorbed. Because H_2 antagonists are relatively short acting, longer acting receptor antagonists of the CCK-B type would have beneficial effects on healing rates and perhaps also in eradication of *Helicobacter pylori*. Their profile of action could be generally similar to those of the H_2-receptor antagonists, in that the gastrin-mediated component of acid secretion would be inhibited, leaving the direct cholinergic component as well as the less well-defined adrenergic component as residual stimuli of acid secretion. Somatostatin analogs that are orally bioavailable have been developed, but it is not clear that these will have the same specific applicability as a CCK-B antagonist in ulcer treatment.

The current target for receptor antagonists lies on the surface of the parietal cell, the H_2 receptor. These antagonists were the first efficacious and specific class of drug to be introduced for ulcer disease. The parietal cell and its processes may well remain as the most specific cellular target in acid-related disease.

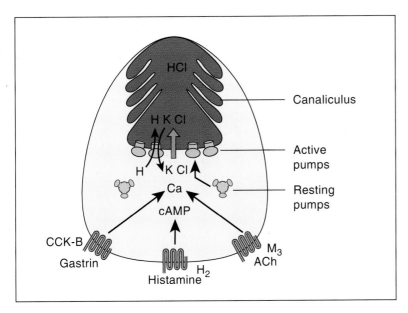

FIGURE 1-6.

The parietal cell. The parietal cell is the site of acid secretion. Stimulation of this cell involves activation of several types of receptors, activation of the gastric acid pump, the H,K, ATPase, and acid secretion by the functioning of the acid pump. The therapeutic targets present on the surface of this cell are the receptors and the pump itself. Specialized regulatory proteins such as those that regulate gene expression, membrane recycling, or the transporters associated with the pump are as yet not defined.

There are at least three known stimulatory receptors on the basolateral surface of the parietal cell. There appears to be some variation in the efficacy of the different receptors in their ability to activate acid secretion as well as variation in the distribution of the different receptors. These properties determine the efficacy and specificity of receptor antagonists.

The presence of a *muscarinic receptor* was recognized as resulting from the inhibitory action of atropine on acid secretion. The side effects of muscarinic drugs and the relatively low efficacy of even selective M_1 antagonists have prevented widespread use of this receptor as a therapeutic target. The receptor is actually an M_3 subtype of receptor; no selective M_3 antagonist is available for human use.

The *gastrin receptor* is of the cholecystokinin-B (CCK-B) subtype. The role of the CCK-B (gastrin) receptor on the parietal cell surface in stimulation of acid secretion has been controversial. One hypothesis that reconciles many of the data is to postulate that activation of the parietal cell histamine receptor is permissive for activity of the CCK-B receptor in stimulation of acid secretion. A certain level of cyclic AMP (cAMP) being necessary for gastrin, H_2 antagonists will abolish gastrin-stimulated acid secretion. Equally, abolition of histamine biosynthesis in the enterochromaffin-like (ECL) cell will also prevent gastrin stimulation of acid secretion. A gastrin (CCK-B) receptor antagonist will target mainly the ECL cell for inhibition of acid secretion. It is not known whether the trophic effect of gastrin requires activity of the H_2 receptor, but high doses of H_2-receptor antagonists also stimulate ECL cell hyperplasia, suggesting that the trophic action of gastrin on the ECL cell may not depend on H_2 receptor activity.

The most important receptor on the parietal cell for both its efficacy in stimulating acid secretion and as a therapeutic target is the H_2 receptor. This receptor elevates the production of cAMP and also elevates cell calcium. It is a member of the G_7 class of receptors, as are the CCK-B and muscarinic receptors. Binding of histamine to the receptor activates adenylate cyclase by dissociation of the Gs protein complex coupled to the receptor. There are several available H_2-receptor antagonists, such as cimetidine, ranitidine, nizatidine, and famotidine. The latter is the most potent receptor currently available clinically. The H_2 receptor is found in the heart, the uterus, and the immune system, but does not seem to play a central role in these tissues, because H_2-receptor antagonists are relatively free from side effects.

These H_2-receptor antagonists are short acting and do not inhibit the cholinergic component of acid secretion that depends on direct activation of the muscarinic receptor on the parietal cell. On twice-a-day dosage, their effect on meal-stimulated acid secretion is less than their effect on night-time acid secretion, perhaps caused by greater use of nonhistaminergic pathways during the day.

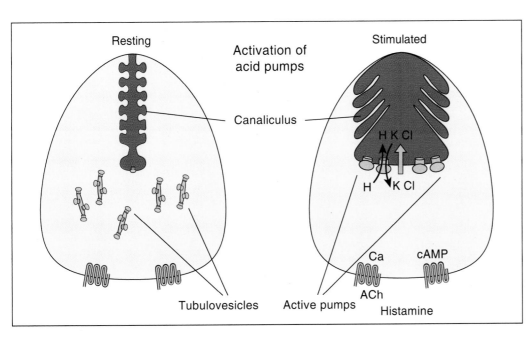

FIGURE 1-7.

Stimulation of acid secretion. The H,K,ATPase is the enzyme responsible for elaboration of hydrochloric acid. It is a member of the P-type ATPase ion-motive ATPase family. It exchanges H for K, the K being supplied to the luminal surface of the pump as a function of activation of the parietal cell. Phosphorylation of the pump is part of the enzyme cycle, with luminal K stimulating the dephosphorylation of the protein. The gastric-acid pump is present in smooth-surfaced tubules (tubulovesicles) in the resting cell, whereas it is present in microvilli lining the secretory canaliculus in the acid-secreting cell. When isolated from resting cells, the pump membrane does not conduct KCl. When isolated from stimulated cells, a KCl transport pathway is present. Stimulation of the parietal cell alters morphology and activates a KCl transport pathway in the pump membrane. All stimuli therefore converge in terms of activation of the acid pump, the final step of acid secretion. This figure shows a model for stimulation of the parietal cell. Ach–acetylcholine; cAMP—cyclic AMP.

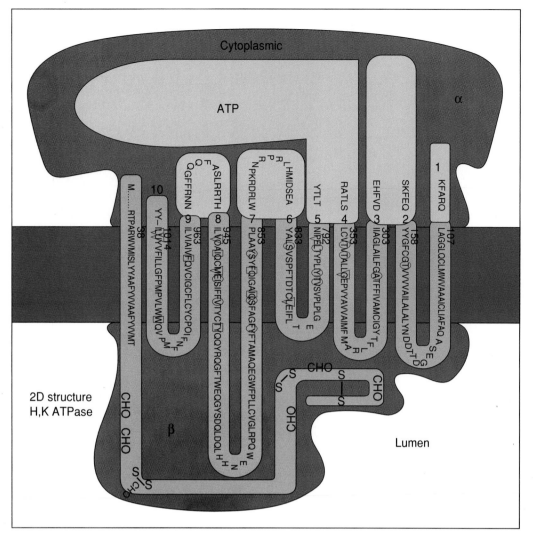

Activation of the acid pump. The structure of the pump is relevant when considering the design of pump inhibitors. It is a protein composed of two subunits. The large catalytic, or alpha, subunit is a polytopic integral membrane protein containing about 1030 amino acids. Analysis of the membrane and extracytoplasmic (luminal) domain has shown that

this region contains 10 membrane-spanning segments connected by extracytoplasmic loops. The N-terminal domain is cytoplasmic as is the C-terminal domain and the first and second cytoplasmic loops contain about 200 and 400 amino acids. The second cytoplasmic loop, located between TM4 and TM5, contains the phosphorylation site of this enzyme. This subunit carries out the transport functions of the protein and can be thought of as the pumping subunit. The smaller, or beta, subunit contains a single membrane-spanning segment, most of the protein being outside the membrane in the lumen. There are six to seven glycosylation sites, shown in this figure as "CHO" groups, in the extracytoplasmic domain of the beta subunit. There are also three disulfide bridges. This subunit is important in assembly of the complex maintenance of the structure of the enzyme and in targeting the complex to the appropriate location in the parietal cell.

From the amino acid sequence obtained from the complementary DNA (cDNA) and from analysis of the membrane domain, it is possible to construct a two-dimensional model of the enzyme, with specific postulates as to the amino acids in the membrane and extracytoplasmic domain as illustrated here. This structure allows some prediction as to the target sites or regions for selective inhibitors of this enzyme. The desired region is either in the extracytoplasmic or membrane domain, because the cytoplasmic domain coexists with many other cytoplasmic proteins. The ten transmembrane segments contain the ion transport pathway, and it is targeting to this pathway that is necessary for the design of successful drugs.

TABLE 1-2. PUMP-TARGETED DRUGS

1. PROTON PUMP INHIBITORS (PPIs)
Substituted pyridyl methylsulfinyl benzimidazoles

Omeprazole (Prilosec)

Lansoprazole (Prevacid)

Pantoprazole (Pantozole)

2. ACID PUMP ANTAGONISTS (APAs)
Imidazopyridines (SCH 28080)

Arylquinolines (SKB 96067)

Pump-targeted drugs. Two classes of pump-targeted drugs have been explored. The first, the substituted pyridyl methylsulfinyl benzimidazoles are already in worldwide clinical use, as represented by omeprazole, lansoprazole, and pantoprazole. These are known as the *proton pump inhibitor type*. The second class is still undergoing development and is based on different heterocyclic structures such as imidazopyridines or arylquinolines. They will be called *acid pump antagonists*. These two classes of drugs have the same end result, namely inhibition of acid secretion by inhibition of the H,K ATPase. They differ, however, in their mechanism of action.

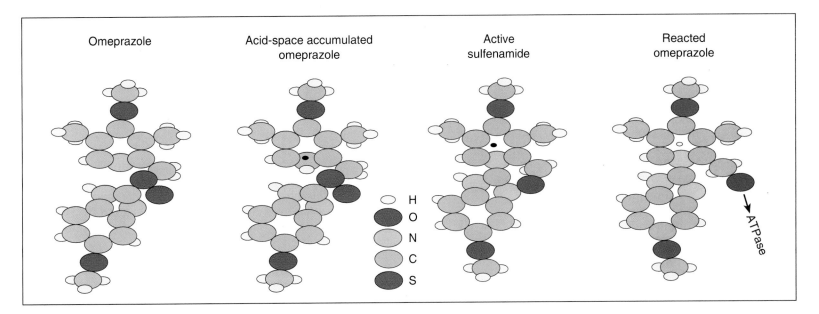

FIGURE 1-9.

The substituted benzimidazoles. This class of drug is targeted to the ATPase largely by virtue of its chemical properties. The compounds are acid-activated prodrugs. They accumulate selectively in the acid space of the parietal cell and after accumulation, undergo an acid-catalyzed rearrangement to the active drug. This cationic sulfenamide then binds covalently to the cysteines of the ATPase that are accessible from the luminal surface of the pump. The different drugs vary in the exact cysteines to which they bind. The cysteine common to all of them is within the fifth and sixth transmembrane domain region, suggesting that this cysteine is probably the critical cysteine for covalent pump inhibition by these drugs. Their general chemical mechanism of action is illustrated in Figure 1-12 showing accumulation, acid activation, and binding to the pump.

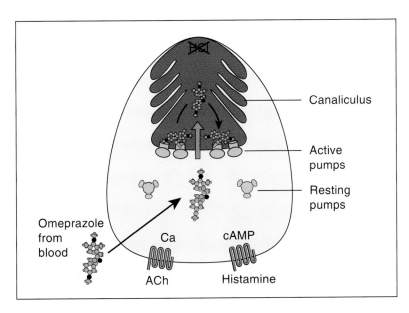

FIGURE 1-10.

Biologic mechanism of action of substituted benzimidazoles (proton pump inhibitors). The covalent inhibition of acid secretion gives these drugs a longer duration of action than their plasma half-life, which is about 60 minutes in humans. Because they require the presence of active pumps to form the acid space, and because not all pumps appear to be active at any one time, they have a cumulative effect, reaching their steady-state inhibition after about 48 to 72 hours. Restoration of acid secretion depends largely on de novo synthesis of the pump, and perhaps also on reversal of the covalent binding. In humans, their half-life of action on once-a-day dosing is about 48 hours, which means that, at steady state, about 30% acid secretory capacity is restored 24 hours after taking the drug. Because the drug is given in the morning and little stimulation of acid secretion is present during the night, these drugs are able to inhibit acid secretion more effectively than H_2-receptor antagonists. Ach–acetylcholine; cAMP—cyclic AMP.

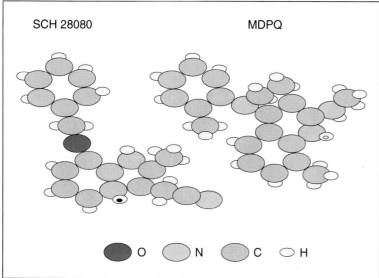

SCH 28080   MDPQ

○ O   ○ N   ○ C   ○ H

FIGURE 1-11.

Acid-pump antagonists (APAs). The APAs are reversible, generally K-competitive inhibitors of the H,K,ATPase, and do not require the presence of active pumps for their action. In contrast to the benzimidazoles, their specificity depends on their primary structure because they are not acid-activated prodrugs. They are weakly basic, however, which will allow accumulation in the active secretory canaliculus, giving them some degree of selectivity for the H,K,ATPase. Because they are not covalent inhibitors of the enzyme, it is predicted that their duration of action is related directly to their plasma concentration. If there is tight binding to the pump, however, their action might be prolonged. It is likely that these inhibitors will differ from the proton pump inhibitors by relatively immediate onset of action, with neutral pH in the stomach until the plasma level falls below threshold. They should not have a cumulative effect in gastric acidity. The degree of elevation of gastric pH would also predict greater efficacy than H2 receptor antagonists. Two representative structural classes are illustrated (SCH-28080, an imidazopyridine, and MDPQ, an arylquinoline).

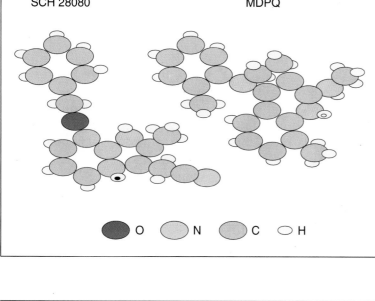

Level and duration of intragastric pH achieved for optimal treatment of:

■ Untreated
■ BID H2 Antagonist
■ OD acid pump inhibitor (once-a-day dosage)

No further improvement

Duodenal ulcer

Reflux disease

H. pylori

24 hr
16 hr
8 hr

pH>3   pH>4   pH>5

Intragastric pH

FIGURE 1-12.

Optimization of acid control. A series of meta-analyses has been performed to determine the optimization of acid control for diseases such as duodenal ulcer and gastroesophageal reflux disease. It is calculated that elevation of gastric pH above 3 for 18 hours a day is optimal for the healing of duodenal ulcer and elevation above 4 for optimal treatment of gastroesophageal reflux disease. The optimal healing of duodenal ulcer can be achieved by once-a-day dosing with pump inhibitors, but not even by twice-a-day dosing with current H2-receptor antagonists. The optimum for gastroesophageal reflux disease is almost reached by once-a-day dosing of proton pump inhibitors (PPIs), but requires at least four-times-a- day dosing with H2-receptor antagonists. In addition, preliminary analyses of the degree of acid control required for

Helicobacter pylori eradication suggests that elevation to greater than pH 5 is required if omeprazole is combined with a single, growth-dependent antibiotic. This figure compares the pH elevation obtained with H2-receptor antagonists and with PPIs as a function of percentage over a 24-hour period.

It has been suggested that PPIs result in achlorhydria. Consideration of the half-life of secretory inhibition in humans shows that achlorhydria will not be found on either once-a-day or even twice-a-day administration. If the pH of the gastric surface is important in healing of gastric ulcers or in survival of H. pylori, full elevation of the pH in this region may require alternative formulation of the PPIs or use of the acid-pump antagonist class of drug.

The data given are based on analysis of once-a-day dosage of PPIs and twice-a-day dosage of H2-receptor antagonists. It is apparent that such dosages do not reach the postulated optimum for H. pylori eradication. The synergism between PPIs and growth-dependent antibiotics is not fully explained. An attractive possibility is that H. pylori is able to survive acidic conditions but is not able to grow under acidic conditions. For growth-dependent antibiotics then, the pH has to be elevated to growth levels wherever H. pylori is found. The gastric antral wall does not secrete acid, hence it is expected to have a higher pH than the gastric fundus. Inhibition of acid secretion by the fundus will elevate pH in the antral wall sufficiently to promote growth of the organism allowing eradication in this region or any other region where the organism is growing by single antibiotics in combination with pump inhibition. Elevation of the pH in the gastric fundus requires almost full inhibition of acid secretion because any residual pumps will secrete 160 mM HCl. Because no neutralization of the acid will occur in the lumen of the gastric gland, some H. pylori will remain in an acidic environment and not grow. The H2-receptor antagonists will not be able to elevate pH sufficiently in this region and will always require use of antibiotics that are DNA targeted in addition to growth-dependent antibiotics. PPIs will have to be given with sufficient frequency to allow adequate pH elevation even in the fundus, because H. pylori is usually present in both the fundus and the antrum of the stomach.

Modern therapy of acid diseases	Inhibiton of gastric acidity	Antibiotic
Duodenal ulcer / Gastric ulcer	99%	Yes
Esophagitis	99%	No
Gastritis	99%	Yes

FIGURE 1-13.

Future trends. The finding that *Helicobacter pylori* is necessary for the development or recurrence of most cases of duodenal and gastric ulcer disease that is not related to the use of nonsteroidal anti-inflammatory drugs promises to revolutionize the treatment of these diseases. Any patient suffering from these conditions should be treated with two aims in mind, healing of the ulcer and eradication of the organism. An association between the gastritis induced by *H. pylori* and the incidence of gastric cancer probably exists. This association, if borne out, indicates that eradication of this organism may extend beyond patients presenting with symptoms of ulcer disease. Perhaps new antibiotics will be discovered that eradicate *H. pylori* without suppression of acid secretion and that allow for a simple, short protocol of treatment of the population at large. This figure postulates the protocols that will come into use in the near future for treatment of acid-related disease.

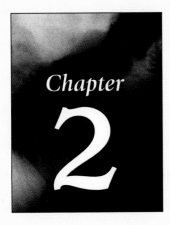

Chapter 2

Endocrinology of the Stomach

DOUGLAS KLIEWER

JUAN LECHAGO

The stomach is a muscular, sac-like organ that serves both as a reservoir for ingested foodstuffs and as a digestive organ facilitating the breakdown of foods through muscular grinding action and through the secretion of acid and proteolytic enzymes. Gastric motility and the secretion of the hydrochloric acid and enzymes necessary for the hydrolysis of dietary protein are carefully regulated through the neuroendocrine system to meet the needs of the organism in both the fasting and fed states.

The neuroendocrine system is the means by which the various cells of the body communicate with each other. Within the gastrointestinal tract, peptide hormones, secreted either from endocrine cells found scattered throughout the gastrointestinal tract or from nerves innervating the gastrointestinal tract, serve as these chemical messengers. Unlike lipophilic hormones such as the steroids, peptide hormones cannot cross plasma membranes and must interact with membrane bound receptors to effect their action. The message transmitted by the peptide hormone is not an intrinsic property of the peptide but is determined by the transduction system with which it binds. Cell to cell peptide hormone communication may be classified as:

1) Autocrine, with cells serving as both source of hormone production and as target site
2) Paracrine, with cells acting locally upon other closely associated cells
3) Neurocrine, with neurons secreting peptides at target sites
4) Endocrine, in which peptide hormones are secreted into the blood stream which then carries the hormone to distantly located effector sites

Gastric secretion is stimulated primarily by the interaction of gastrin, histamine, and acetylcholine on the parietal cell. Factors such as dietary protein, gastric distention, and the neurotransmitter gastrin-releasing peptide initiate the secretion of acid and pepsin. This secretion is in turn downregulated by a number of factors such as somatostatin, secretin, and luminal acid to prevent oversecretion. It is a finely tuned system of feedback loops that interact to provide the optimal environment needed to initiate and facilitate further digestion of food products. Occasionally, this system is interrupted in situations such as gastrin-cell and enterochromaffin-like–cell hyperplasia, which can be explained by the uninhibited action of one limb of the feedback loop.

■ GASTROINTESTINAL ENDOCRINOLOGY

Year	Substance	Discovery (ref.)
1902	Secretin	Bayliss and Starling [1]
1905	Gastrin	Edkins [2]
1910	Histamine	Dale and Laidlaw [3]
1928	Cholecystokinin (CCK)	Ivy and Oldberg {4]
1931	Substance P	von Euler and Gaddum [5]
1948	Enteric glucagon (GLI)	Sutherland and de Duve [6]
1952	Serotonin	Erspamer and Asero [7]
1962	Epidermal growth factor (EGF)*	Cohen [8], Gregory* [9]
1969	Gastric inhibitory polypeptide (GIP)	Brown [10]
1970	Gastrin-releasing peptide (GRP)	Erspamer et al [11], Walsh et al, 1979* [12]
1970	Vasoactive intestinal polypeptide (VIP #3)	Said and Mutt [13]
1971	Motilin	Brown et al [14]
1973	Neurotensin	Carraway and Leeman [15]
1973	Somatostatin	Brazeau et al [16] Arimura et al, *1975 [17]
1975	Enkephalins	Hughes et al [18] Giraud et al,* 1984 [19]
1981	Peptide YY (PYY) and Neuropeptide Y (NPY)	Tatemoto and Mutt [20]
1982	Calcintonin gene-related peptide (CGRP)	Amara et al [21] Rodrigo et al,*1985 [22]
1983	Galanin	Tatemoto et al [23]
1988	Endothelin	Yanagisawa et al [24] Inagaki et al,* 1991 [25]

Peptides and bioamines with hormonal function in the digestive system: discovery

* Discovered or localized in the gut

FIGURE 2-1.

Major developments in the history of gastrointestinal endocrinology. In 1902, Bayliss and Starling led the way into the modern era of endocrinology with the discovery of secretin. They also introduced the term *hormone* which means "I arouse" in Greek. Further advances in the field came slowly until the introduction of the radioimmunoassay in the 1960s. Assays now exist for at least 40 gastrointestinal peptides whose actions in pharmacologic doses have been defined [26].

TABLE 2-1. GUT HORMONES

Peptide	Main Active Forms	Localization	Function
Gastrin (G)	G17 and G34	Antral G cells	Regulation of gastric H+
Cholecystokinin (CCK)	CCK8, 33, 39 and 58	Intestinal I cells	Regulation of pancreatic enzyme secretion
Somatostatin	SS14 and SS28	Gastric D cells	Paracrine regulator of H+ and gastrin
Gastrin-releasing peptide (GRP)	GRP	GI nerves	Gastrin release and acid secretion
Secretin	Secretin 27	Intestinal S cells	Regulation of pancreatic HCO3
Gastric inhibitory peptide (GIP)	GIP-43	Intestinal K cells	Regulation of insulin release/inhibitor of H+
Motilin	Motilin-22	Intestinal M cells	Interdigestive intestinal motility
Glucagons	Glucagon-like peptide (GLP1)	Intestinal L cells	Regulation of insulin release
Neurotensin (N)	N14	Intestinal N cells	Mediator of ileal brake
Tachykinins	Substance P14, neurokinin A	Myenteric motoneurons	Neural stimulant of motility
Opioids	Met- and Leu-enkephalins	Myenteric neurons	Neuromodulators of motility
Calcitonin gene-related peptide (CGRP)	CGRP	Primary afferents and myenteric neurons	Neural mediator of primary afferents
Galanin (Gal)	Gal 29	Myenteric and submucosal neurons	Neural inhibitor of multiple functions
Pancreatic polypeptide (PP)-related	PP-, neuropeptide Y, protein YY-36	Enteropancreatic (PP-&L) endocrine cells, sympathetic neurons	Neural modulation of sympathetic transmission, inhibitor of pancreas
Vasoactive intestinal polypeptide (VIP)	VIP-28	Myenteric inhibitory motoneurons/ submucosal neurons	Neural inhibitor of motility/stimulant of fluid secretion
Histamine	Histamine	ECL-cells	Stimulus of gastric acid secretion
Norepinephrine	Norepinephrine	Extrinsic digestive nerves	Vascular regulation
Serotonin	Serotonin	EC cell of digestive tract	Stimulus of peristalsis
Urogastrone	Epidermal growth factor	Undefined duodenal structures	Inhibition of gastric acid
Substance P	Substance P	Digestive nerves	Neurotransmitter

TABLE 2-1.

Gut hormones: location, function, and cells of origin. Since 1902, approximately 50 substances that can be classified as candidate and established hormones have been characterized, immunolocalized, or presumed (on functional evidence) to be located in the gut. This table describes several of the established hormones identified within the gastrointestinal (GI) tract, their localization, and function. The endocrine cells are felt to be of endodermal origin and are widely distributed throughout the GI tract rather than clustered as is found in most endocrine glands. ECL—enterochromaffin-like cell.

GASTRIN

TABLE 2-2. GASTRIN: CHRONOLOGY OF DISCOVERIES

1902	Edkins	Postulated existence of a humoral substance released by digested food that stimulates gastric secretion [2].
1938	Komarov	Showed that antral mucosa extracts from which histamine had been completely extracted continued to stimulate gastric acid secretion when injected.
1948	Grossman, et al.	Showed that distention of denervated antral pouch stimulated acid secretion from transplanted gastric pouch.
1964	Gregory and Tracy	Isolated and purified two gastrins from antra mucosa (gastrin I and II).

TABLE 2-2.

Gastrin: chronology of discoveries. Soon after the description of secretin by Bayliss and Starling, Edkins postulated that gastric secretion might be influenced by a similar hormone named *gastrin*. This action was soon ascribed to histamine, until Komarov in 1938 demonstrated that histamine-free antral mucosal extracts were able to stimulate gastric secretion. In 1948, Grossman demonstrated that the action of this antral hormone persisted after the removal of the influence of acetylcholine. Finally, in the 1960s, Gregory and Tracy were able to isolate gastrin I and II from antral extracts, thus opening the door for the pharmacologic characterization and sequence analysis of this important gastric hormone.

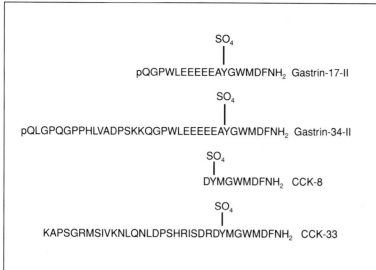

pQGPWLEEEEEAYGWMDFNH₂ Gastrin-17-II

pQLGPQGPPHLVADPSKKQGPWLEEEEEAYGWMDFNH₂ Gastrin-34-II

DYMGWMDFNH₂ CCK-8

KAPSGRMSIVKNLQNLDPSHRISDRDYMGWMDFNH₂ CCK-33

pQ–pyrogultamyl: single-letter amino acid codes are used for primary structure.

Gastrin cholecystokinin (CCK) family of peptides. Gastrin and CCK have similar C-terminal peptide sequences and probably arose from a single ancestral gene. Gastrin-17-II and gastrin-34-II have the same C-terminal pentapeptide sequence as CCK-8 and CCK-33, but the gastrins have a sulfated tyrosine (Y) at the 6 position, whereas the cholecystokinins have a sulfated tyrosine at the 7 position, with a methionine at position 6. Thus, CCK and gastrin-II can act on CCK-B receptors, but only CCK can act on CCK-A receptors in the pancreas or gallbladder at physiologic concentrations. Gastrin-17-II and gastrin-34-I are identical to gastrin-17-II and gastrin-34-II except they are not sulfated. Gastrin I and II act equally on gastrin/CCK-B receptors regulating gastric acid secretion. Not shown in the figure are other forms of gastrin and CCK, which are listed in Table 2-3. (*Modified from* Walsh and Mayer [27]; with permission.)

TABLE 2-3. GASTRIN AND CHOLECYSTOKININ FAMILY OF PEPTIDES

G cell	Gastrin 17 I (nonsulfated)*
	Gastrin 17 II (sulfated)*
	Gastrin 34 I*
	Gastrin 34 II**
	Gastrin 14 *
	Gastrin 52 *
	C-terminal hexapeptide**
	C-terminal pentapeptide†
I Cells	Cholecystokinin (CCK) 8
	CCK 33
	CCK 39
	CCK 58

*Isolated from blood
**Isolated from antral tissue
†Isolated from intestinal muscle and brain

Gastrin/cholecystokinin (CCK) family of peptides. Multiple gastrin and CCK fragments have been identified either from blood or tissue extracts. All isolated forms of gastrin contain the C-terminal tetrapeptide amide sequence needed for full gastrin activity. The various isolated forms of CCK are structurally related to gastrin in the carboxyl region with both hormones ending with an identical Gly-Trp-Met-Asp-Phe-NH₂ amino acid sequence. Differences in activity are determined by differences in sulfated residues with sulfation of tyrosine being a major determinant of CCK activity [26].

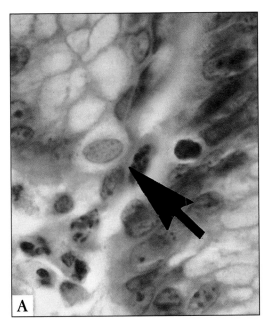 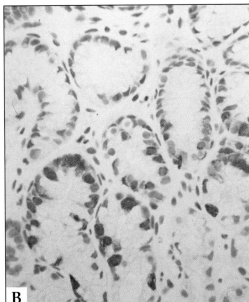 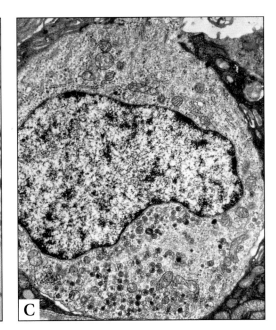

FIGURE 2-3.

Human antral gastrin-producing (G) cell: light microscopy, immunocytochemistry, and ultrastructure. **A,** Human antral mucosa stained with the routine hematoxylin and eosin (H&E) stain: an endocrine cell with the morphologic appearance of a G cell (*arrow*) is seen in one of the glands. The cell is characterized by its piriform shape, clear cytoplasm, and rounded nucleus and rests on the basal lamina. **B,** Antral gastric mucosa immunostained with an antigastrin antibody. Several brown stained G cells are seen in the neck region of the pits and in the upper portions of the glands. ABC immunoperoxidase with DAB as the chromogen. **C,** Electron micrograph of an antral G-cell. This cell type is characterized by the presence of numerous small secretory granules of variable electron density in the basal cytoplasm. The apical portion of the cell reaches the lumen of the gland, seen at the top of the figure.

TABLE 2-4. GASTRIN: GASTROINTESTINAL FUNCTIONS

Stimulation of gastric acid secretion

Stimulation of histamine release from enterchromaffin-like (ECL) cells

Regulation of mucosal growth—most pronounced in nonantral gastric mucosa, ECL-cells, and proliferative zone of mucous neck cells

Contraction of lower esophageal sphincter (pharmacologic effect)

Stimulation of smooth muscle contraction

Regulation of antral motor activity

Possible role in regulation of glucose-stimulated insulin release

Release of somatostatin from fundic endocrine cell culture

TABLE 2-4.

Gastrin has multiple physiologic effects, the most significant of which is the stimulation of gastric acid secretion. Gastrin 34, 17, and 14 all have acid-stimulating effects that are likely secondary to the ability of gastrin to stimulate histamine release from gastric enterochromaffin cells. Another important role played by gastrin is the regulation of gastric mucosal growth with the greatest trophic effects being seen in the acid-secreting portions of the stomach. Other perhaps less significant effects of gastrin include stimulation of antral motility and stimulation of somatostatin release from fundic cells resulting in feedback inhibition of further gastrin release.

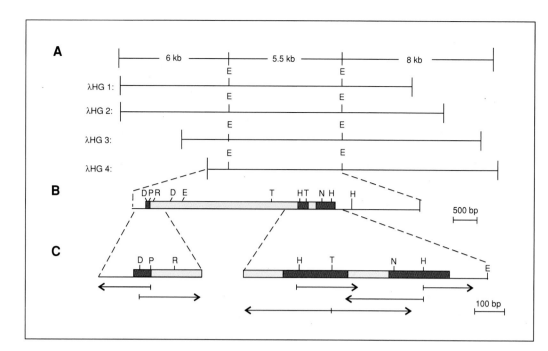

FIGURE 2-4.

Molecular structure of the gastrin gene. The human gene for gastrin is located on chromosome 17. It is 4100 base pairs long and contains two introns. Intron I is located in the 5' noncoding region, whereas intron II is located in a site separating function domains. Shown is the nucleotide sequence of the human gastrin gene, including the 5' noncoding portion. Indicated by boxes are the putative promoter sequences, presumed polyadenylation signal, splice donor, and acceptor sequences. Also shown is the 5' noncoding portion of the human gastrin messenger RNA and the amino acid sequence of the human gastrin preprohormone (*From* Wiborg *et al.* [28]; with permission.)

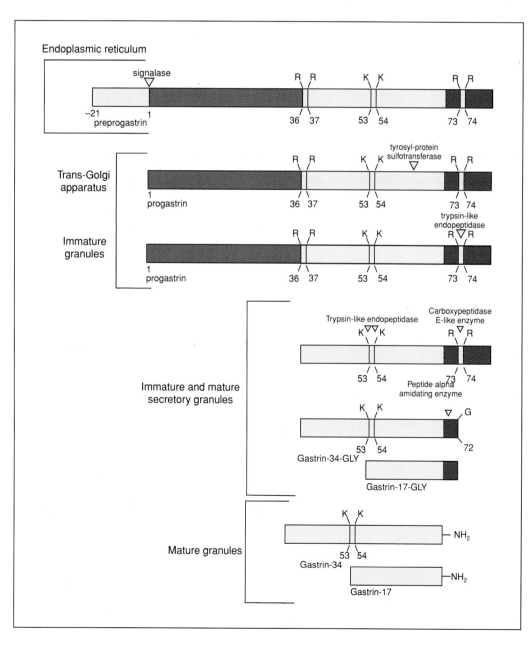

FIGURE 2-5.

Posttranslational processing of the preprogastrin. The human gastrin gene encodes a preprogastrin peptide of 101 amino acids. Posttranslational processing of the protein involves several cleavage steps and C-terminal amidation leading to production of the mature proteins gastrin-34 and gastrin-17. Shown is human preprogastrin, cleavage sites involved in the production of the mature hormone, sites of modification within the cell, and the various posttranslational products. (*From* Walsh [26]; with permission.)

Preprogastrin
→
−21   -10
Human: Met-Gln-Arg-Leu-Cys-Val-Tyr-Val-Leu-Ile-Phe-Ala-Leu-Ala-Leu-Ala-Ala-Phe-Ser-Glu-Ala

Progastrin
→
1   10   20
Human: Ser-Trp-Lys-Pro-Arg-Ser-Gln-Gln-Pro-Asp-Ala-Pro-Leu-Gly-Thr-Gly-Ala-Asn-Arg-Asp-Leu

                                                                    Gastrin-34
                                                                    ▽ →
                                        30   40
Human: Glu-Leu-Pro-Trp-Leu-Glu-Gln-Gln-Gly-Pro-Ala-Ser-His-His-Arg-Arg Gln-Leu-Gly-Pro-Gln

                                                    Gastrin-17
                                        50   ▽ →   60
Human: Gly-Pro-Pro-His-Leu-Val-Ala-Asp-Pro-Ser-Lys-Lys Gln-Gly-Pro-Trp-Leu-Glu-Glu-Glu-Glu

                            70   ☆   ▽   80
Human: Glu-Ala-Tyr-Gly-Trp-Met-Asp-Phe-Gly Arg-Arg Ser-Ala-Glu-Asp-Glu-Asn

FIGURE 2-6.

Amino acid structure of preprogastrin in the human. Demonstrated are the cleavage sites that result in the posttranslational production of biologically active gastrin. Also shown is the amidation site of the C-terminal phenylalanine residue (*). Amidation at this site is necessary for the production of the biologically active products, gastrin-34 and gastrin-17. (*From* Walsh [26]; with permission.)

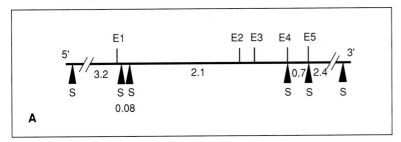

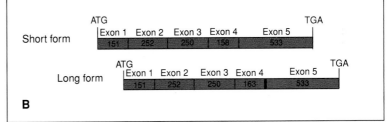

FIGURE 2-7.

Schematic of the gastrin/cholecystokinin $_B$ (CCK$_B$) receptor gene. Gastrin exerts a variety of biologic actions that are mediated through a transmembrane receptor. This receptor has been shown to be identical to the CCK$_B$ receptor. Demonstrated is the structure of the human gastrin CCK$_B$ receptor gene. **A,** Introns and exons are shown as well as the restriction sites used to create the restriction length fragments generated during sequencing of the gene. **B,** The gene encodes both short and long forms of messenger RNA. Each is composed of five exon segments; however, a region of exon four is alternatively spliced yielding two receptor isoforms, which may contribute to functional differences in gastrin and CCK-mediated signal transduction. (*From* Walsh [26]; with permission.)

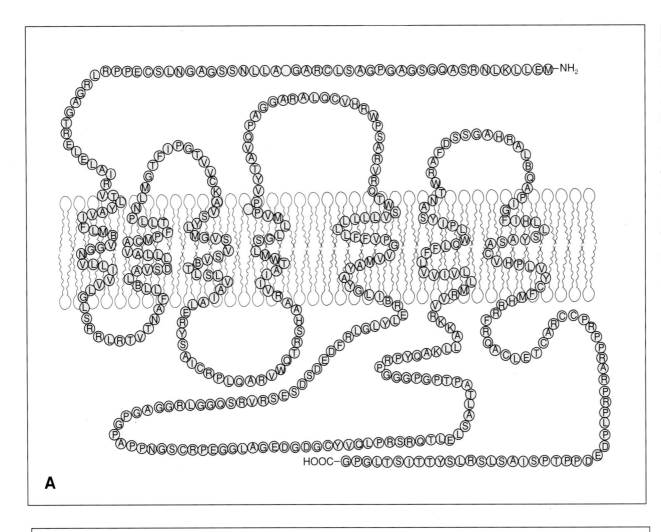

A

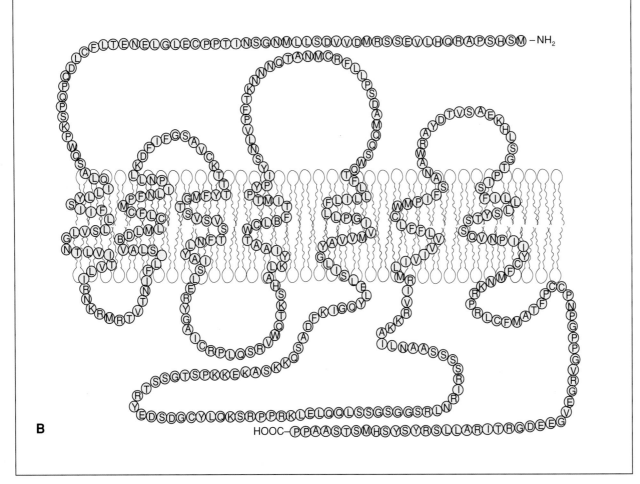

B

FIGURE 2-8.

Schematic comparison of the amino acid structure of the canine parietal cell gastrin/CCK$_B$ receptor (**A**) and the rat pancreatic acinar cell CCK$_A$ receptor (**B**). The two receptors have approximately 50% amino acid sequence homology. The seven membrane-spanning domains are typical of G-protein binding receptors. Occupation of gastrin receptors causes stimulation of inositol phosphate production, activation of protein kinase C, and increased intracellular calcium concentrations. Each of these processes is mediated via G-protein signal transduction. The CCK$_A$ receptor has about a 1000-fold lower affinity for gastrin than does the gastrin-CCK$_B$ receptor. (*From* Walsh [26]; with permission.)

TABLE 2-5. STIMULANTS OF GASTRIN RELEASE

Dietary products*	Beta-2 adrenergic agonists
proteins, peptides, amino acids, amines	Fat
Gastrin-releasing peptide (GRP)*	Sham feeding
Luminal neutralization	Truncal vagotomy
Antral distention	

*Major physiologic role

TABLE 2-5.

Stimulations of gastrin release. Gastrin secretion is stimulated by several factors. Peptides and amino acids, breakdown products of protein digestion, are potent releasing agents with the aromatic amino acids phenylalanine and tryptophan being among the most potent. Gastrin-releasing peptide, the mammalian counterpart to the amphibian peptide bombesin, is released from nerves in the antral mucosa and is a potent stimuli of gastrin release under normal conditions. Alkalinization of gastric contents and antral distention, dietary fat, adrenergic agonists, sham feeding, and truncal vagotomy also stimulate gastrin release but to a lesser degree [26].

TABLE 2-6. DEPRESSANTS OF GASTRIN RELEASE

Luminal acid*
Somatostatin*
Starvation

*Major physiologic role

TABLE 2-6.

Depressant factors of gastrin release. Release of gastrin is inhibited by acidification of luminal contents below pH 3 and by the hormone somatostatin, which acts in a paracrine fashion to inhibit gastrin release. Starvation is associated with downregulation of gastrin messenger RNA production and subsequent reduction of gastrin levels [26].

GASTRIN-RELEASING PEPTIDE

TABLE 2-7. GASTRIN RELEASING PEPTIDE CHRONOLOGY

1970	Ersparmer, et al.	Discovered bombesin in skin of amphibians (Bombina bombina and Bombina variegata)
1973/1974	Bertaccini, et al.	Showed that bombesin stimulates gastric acid secretion in dogs and rats. Showed gastrin release by bombesin in dogs.
1978	McDonald, et al.	Discovered mammalian counterpart of bombesin, gastrin-releasing peptide (GRP), in porcine stomach

TABLE 2-7.

Chronology of gastrin-releasing peptide. Bombesin, a 14 amino acid peptide, was isolated from the skin of the European amphibians Bombina bombina and Bombina variegata by Ersparmer and co-workers in 1970. By the middle 1970s, bombesin had been sequenced and shown to stimulate gastrin release and gastric acid secretion in mammals. By the late 1970s, bombesin-like activity and immunoreactivity had been found in mammalian stomach, intestine, and brain extracts. In 1978, gastrin-releasing peptide, the mammalian counterpart to bombesin, was identified from the nonantral mucosa of the porcine stomach by McDonald and co-workers [30].

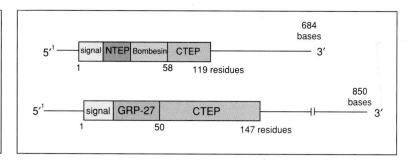

Bombesin
pQ-Q-R-L-G-N-Q-W-A-V-G-H-L-M NH₂

Porcine GRP-27
A-P-V-S-V-G-G-G-T-V-L-A-K-M-Y-P-R-G-N-H-W-A-V-G-H-L-M NH₂

FIGURE 2-9.

Amino acid sequence of bombesin and porcine gastrin-releasing peptide (GRP). Sequence analysis of bombesin and porcine GRP-27 demonstrates a great deal of homology even though GRP has little bombesin-like immunoreactivity by radioimmunoassay. The similarity of the ten carboxy-terminal residues likely accounts for similarity of biologic activity whereas differences in the amino-terminal residues likely accounts for differences in radioimmunoreactivity [30].

FIGURE 2-10.

Complementary DNA (cDNA) schematic of bombesin (*top*) and gastrin-releasing peptide (*bottom*). Bombesin cDNA codes for a messenger RNA (mRNA) approximately 684 bases in length with both 5' and 3' untranslated regions, a signal sequence, an amino-terminal extension peptide (NTEP), the bombesin sequence, and finally a carboxy-terminal extension peptide (CTEP). Translation of this mRNA produces a prohormone 119 amino acids in length, which is then processed resulting in the 14 amino acid bombesin peptide shown in Figure 2-12. The human *GRP-27* gene, located on chromosome 18 and composed of three exons and two introns, produces an mRNA 850 bases long and composed of untranslated 5' and 3' segments, an NTEP, the GRP-27 sequence, and a CTEP [30].

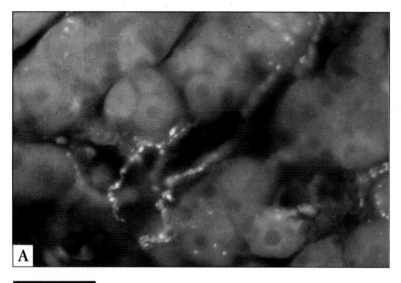

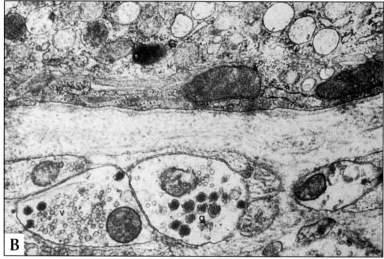

FIGURE 2-11.

Gastrin-releasing nerves in human gastric mucosa: immunocytochemistry and ultrastructure. **A,** Gastric oxyntic mucosa immunostained with an antibombesin antibody. Several thin nerve fibers surround the glands and show bright apple green fluorescence. Indirect immunofluorescence with FITC as the fluorogen. **B,** Electron micrograph of a portion of a gastric antral gland containing the basal portion of a G-cell (*top*) separated by the basal lamina and a thin strip of the lamina propria from a small nerve bundle (*bottom*). Some nerve endings contain only small clear vesicles, characteristic of cholinergic innervation, whereas others show, in addition, the presence of larger dark-cored vesicles, consistent with peptidergic (possibly GRP positive) innervation.

TABLE 2-8. DISTRIBUTION OF GASTRIN-RELEASING PEPTIDE IN THE STOMACH

Gastric mucosa
  Oxyntic (higher density)*
  Antral (lower density)**
Muscular layer[†]
  Circular (higher density)
  Longitudinal (lower density)

Plexuses
  Myenteric[†]
  Submucosal[?]*,**

*Involved n regulation of acid secretion, perhaps using somatostatin
**Involved in regulation of gastrin release
[†]Involved in regulation of motor function

TABLE 2-8.

Gastric distribution of gastrin-releasing peptide (GRP). Antibodies to bombesin and GRP have localized bombesin and GRP to nerve bodies within the digestive tract. In the stomach, the oxyntic and antral mucosa are innervated by GRP nerve fibers with antral GRP regulating gastrin release and oxyntic GRP likely participating in the control of gastric acid secretion using somatostatin. GRP-containing nerve fibers also innervate the gastric circular and longitudinal muscle layers where they participate in the regulation of gastric motility. Finally, bombesin/GRP nerve fibers have been localized within the myenteric and submucosal nerve plexuses where they likely serve as excitatory interneurons modulating control of secretion and motility (see Chapter 1) [30].

SOMATOSTATIN

TABLE 2-9. SOMATOSTATIN CHRONOLOGY

1973	Brazeau, *et al.*	Isolated peptide from hypothalamus of sheep, which inhibited secretion of growth hormone from pituitary (*growth hormone inhibitory factor*).
1975	Arimura, *et al.*	Demonstrated abundance of somatostatin in rat stomach and pancreas by immunocytochemistry.
1976	Schally, *et al.*	Isolated and determined tetradecapeptide structure of somatostatin from porcine hypothalamus.
1980	Godman, *et al.*	Isolation and closing of anglerfish islets cDNA encoding full amino acid sequence of preprosomatostatin.

TABLE 2-9.

Somatostatin chronology, chemistry, and localization. Somatostatin is a tetradecapeptide distributed throughout virtually every organ system, including the nervous and the gastrointestinal systems. It was initially isolated by Brozeau and co-workers in 1973 from sheep hypothalamic tissue and identified as an inhibitor of growth hormone release. In 1975, Arimura and co-workers localized large amounts of somatostatin-like reactivity within the stomach and pancreas of the rat. In 1976, the somatostatin tetradecapeptide (S14) was isolated from porcine hypothalamic tissue by Schally and co-workers who were then able to determine its amino acid sequence. In the 1980s, the complementary DNA encoding the full amino acid sequence of the preprosomatostatin peptide was isolated and cloned first in the anglerfish, then in the rat and human [31].

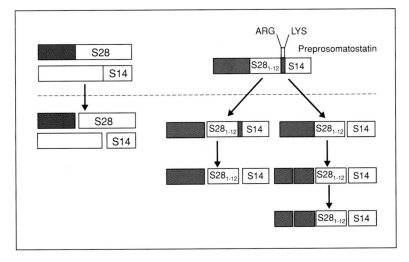

FIGURE 2-12.

The human somatostatin gene is located on chromosome 3 and contains a single intron. Translation of the messenger RNA transcribed from the complementary DNA produces preprosomatostatin that is converted into prosomatostatin by signal peptide cleavage. Prosomatostatin then undergoes posttranslational processing resulting in the formation of the two biologically active forms of somatostatin that are S-28 and S-14. Some studies have demonstrated direct processing of prosomatostatin into S-28 and S-14, whereas other studies have suggested that S-14 is produced from S-28. These two forms of somatostatin are present in differing proportions depending upon the tissue examined. S-14, for example, is the predominant form found within gastric D cells [31].

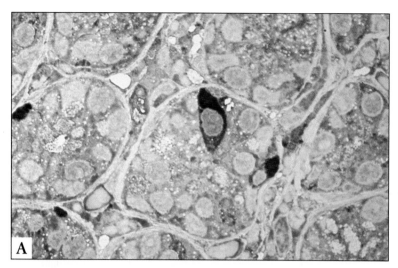

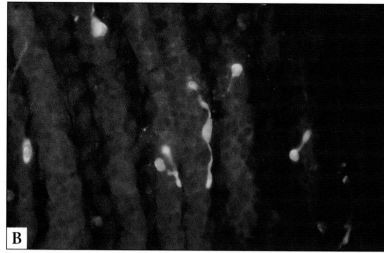

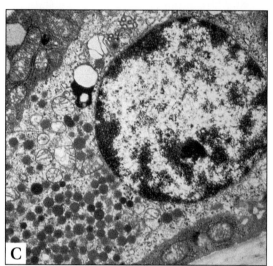

FIGURE 2-13.

Human somatostatin-producing (D) cell: immunocytochemistry and ultrastructure. **A,** Antral gastric mucosa immunostained with an antisomatostatin antibody. A brown-stained D cell is seen in the center of the picture. ABC immunoperoxidase with DAB as the chromogen. **B,** Gastric oxyntic mucosa immunostained with an antisomatostatin antibody. Several irregularly shaped brightly apple-green fluorescent D cells are seen contacting neighboring exocrine cells with their cytoplasmic extensions. Indirect immunofluorescence with FITC as the fluorogen. **C,** Electron micrograph of an antral D cell. This cell type is characterized by the presence of numerous medium-sized secretory granules of uniform, medium-electron density in the basal cytoplasm.

TABLE 2-10. ACTIONS OF SOMATOSTATIN IN THE STOMACH

Reduced exocrine secretion
    Hydrochloric acid
    Pepsin
Reduced neuroendocrine secretion
    Gastrin (from G cell)
    Histamine (from enterochromaffin-like cell)
Gastric motility
    Inhibitory
        Late phase emptying
        Migrating motor complexes (MMCs)*
    Excitatory
        Early phase emptying
Food intake
    Inhibition (in fed animals)
    Stimulation (in fasted animals)

Somatostatin has the opposite effect in the intestine and stimulates MMCs.

TABLE 2-10.

Somatostatin functions and receptors. Somatostatin may act as a neurotransmitter, as a local paracrine factor, or as a classic endocrine peptide with distribution through the circulation. It is generally recognized as a peptide that exerts a negative action on physiologic functions, including gastric function. In the stomach, somatostatin inhibits gastric acid and pepsin responses to gastrin and cholinergic stimulation as well as basal, food-stimulated, and neural-stimulated gastrin release. It also reduces the release of histamine from gastric enterochromaffin-like cells. This may be the primary mechanism by which acid secretion is inhibited. Somatostatin may also play a role in the regulation of gastric motility with both inhibitory and excitatory actions. There is also evidence that it plays a role in the regulation of food intake. In the stomach, S-14 is about 10 times more potent than S-28 [31].

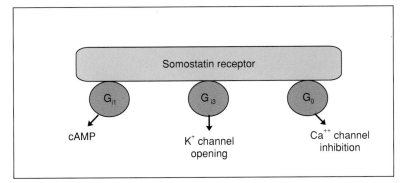

FIGURE 2-14.

Somatostatin receptors. Somatostatin receptors are members of the family of peptide receptors, like the gastrin cholecystokinin$_B$ receptors, with seven transmembrane domains coupled to various G-protein subtypes. Multiple signal transduction pathways, the result of both multiple G-protein receptor subtypes and somatostatin receptor subtypes, produce varied physiologic actions. For example, stimulation of G_{i1} decreased cyclic AMP, stimulation of G_{i3} opens potassium channels, and G_0 inhibits voltage-gated calcium channels. It appears that somatostatin receptors from different locations couple selectively to different G-protein subtypes [31].

HISTAMINE

TABLE 2-11. SOURCES OF HISTAMINE IN THE STOMACH

Enterochromaffin-like cells (ECL cells)

Mast cells

Neurons (?)

TABLE 2-11.

Sources of gastric histamine. Histamine is an endogenous stimulant of gastric acid secretion. It is synthesized from histidine, the amino acid precursor, by the action of the enzyme histidine decarboxylase. Within the gastric mucosa, histamine has been localized to enterochromaffin-like (ECL) cells, mast cells, and neurons. It appears that the ECL cell is responsible for the phasic release of histamine in response to meals and other stimulants, such as gastrin. Histamine likely acts through paracrine pathways, with its major target being the histamine-2 receptor on the parietal cell.

FIGURE 2-15.

Shown are histamine and four H_2-receptor antagonists. Histamine and cimetidine share an imidazole ring, ranitidine has a furan ring, and famotidine and nizatidine have a thiazole ring. Occupation of histamine receptors by histamine or histamine agonists on the basolateral membrane of the parietal cell activates adenylate cyclase, increasing cyclic AMP levels within the cell, whereas the H_2-receptor blocking agents shown competitively and selectively inhibit the binding of histamine to the histamine receptor [32].

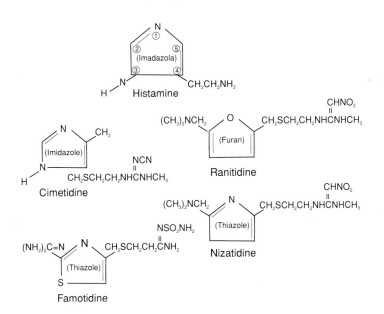

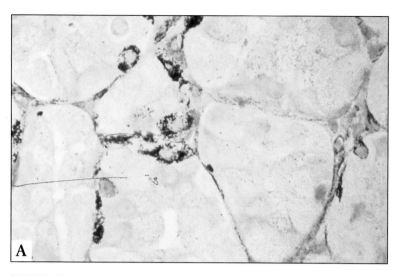

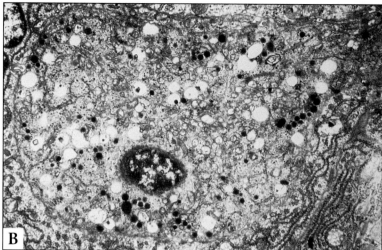

FIGURE 2-16.

Human histamine-producing (enterochromaffin-like [ECL]) cell: light microscopy and ultrastructure. **A,** Several dark staining argyrophilic cells occupy the basal portion of a few cross-sectioned gastric glands. Grimelius silver stain for argyrophilia. **B,** Electron micrograph of an ECL cell in the gastric oxyntic mucosa. This cell type is characterized by the presence of low numbers of secretory granules, composed of a small electron dense core and a wide clear halo, scattered throughout the cytoplasm.

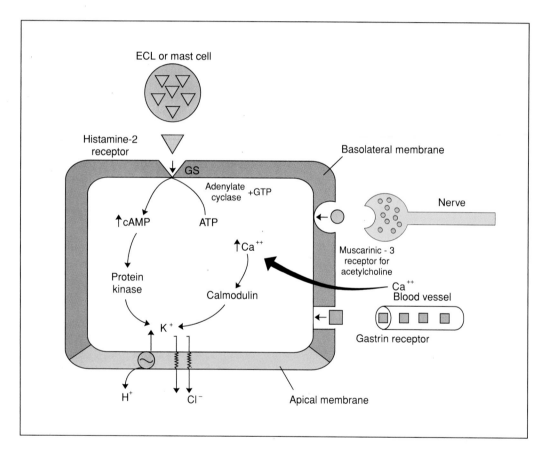

FIGURE 2-17.

Interaction between histamine and other hormones in gastric target cell. Histamine interacts in concert with gastrin and acetylcholine to activate the parietal cell proton pump, thereby increasing gastric acid secretion. This is mediated by the production of cyclic AMP within the cell following binding of histamine to the histamine (H_2) receptor on the basolateral cell membrane, binding of cytosolic guanosine triphosphate (GTP) to a GTP-regulatory protein (Gs) and subsequent activation of adenylate cyclase [33].

TABLE 2-12. PEPTIDES THAT AFFECT GASTRIC ACID SECRETION

Stimulants	Inhibitors
Gastrin	Somatostatin
Gastrin-releasing peptide (GRP)	Cholecystokinin (CCK)
	Peptide YY
	Calcitonin gene-related peptide (CGRP)
	Secretin
	Neurotensin
	Vasoactive intestinal peptide (VIP)

TABLE 2-12.

Peptides that affect gastric acid secretion. Gastric secretion is regulated in order to provide an environment favorable for the initiation of digestion. Secretion is coordinated through a series of neural, endocrine, and paracrine peptide signals originating in the stomach, intestine, and nervous systems. In addition to somatostatin, peptides such as cholecystokinin (CCK), peptide YY, calcitonin gene-related peptide (CGRP), secretin, neurotensin, and vasoactive intestinal peptide (VIP) are produced in the intestine and neural tissue and act primarily in an inhibitory fashion to decrease gastric acid secretion [34].

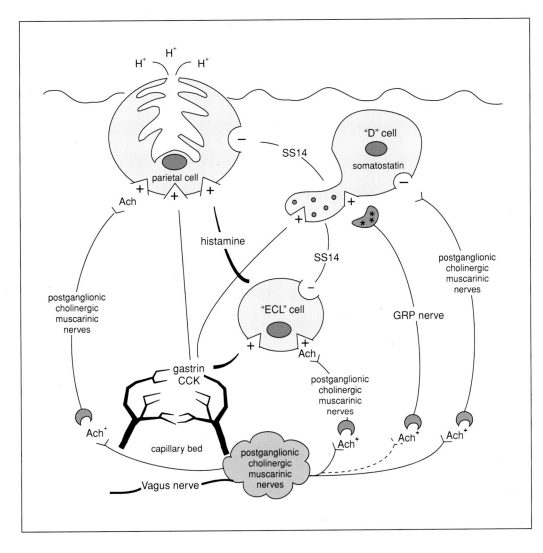

FIGURE 2-18.

Gastrin, cholecystokinin (CCK), acetylcholine (Ach), histamine, gastrin-releasing peptide (GRP), and somatostatin act together in a complex manner to regulate gastric acid secretion from parietal cells. Gastrin and CCK act in a classic endocrine fashion through the circulation whereas somatostatin and histamine act through paracrine pathways. Ach and GRP are released from neural fibers at their effector sites [34]. Although not shown, CCK also acts on the D cell to release SS14 via CCK_A receptors.

TABLE 2-13. PRIMARY G-CELL HYPERPLASIA: PRESENTATION

G-cell hyperplasia in antral and pyloric mucosa

Hypergastrinemia

Gastric acid hypersecretion

Peptic ulcer disease (often intractable)

TABLE 2-13.

Primary G-cell hyperplasia is defined as an increase in the gastrin-producing (G cell) mass for which no underlying cause can be identified. It is infrequently found, but when present, it has been associated with hypergastrinemia, gastric acid hypersecretion, and intractable peptic ulcer disease of the antropyloric mucosa. It is treated by acid antisecretory drugs, but if this is not successful, antrectomy with gastroenterostomy is curative. The role of *Helicobacter pylori* in this condition is not yet clear [35].

TABLE 2-14. G-CELL HYPERPLASIA: DIAGNOSIS

•Increased gastrin-immunoreactive cells in antral mucosa (192–239 G cells/mm vs. 41–93 G cells/mm in normals)

•Expanded G-cell compartments with antral glands

•Clusters, clones of G cells in antral mucosa

•Enlarged G cells seen with electromicroscopy

•G cells found to contain electron lucent secretory granules in cytoplasm evident with electromicroscopy

Whether primary or secondary, G-cell hyperplasias may be characterized morphologically by the criteria shown in this table.

TABLE 2-14.

Digestive endocrine cell hyperplasias are often difficult to document because the different cell types are often dispersed throughout the gastrointestinal tract and mucosa containing the cell types in question often undergo hypertrophy or atrophy, making it difficult to establish a reliable reference point. The morphometric methodologies used by various authors also often vary widely. G-cell hyperplasia, whether primary or secondary in origin, has been characterized morphologically by the criteria listed in this table [35].

TABLE 2-15. SECONDARY G-CELL HYPERPLASIA: CAUSES*

Achlorhydria

Hypochlorhydria

    Atrophic gastritis (especially pernicious anemia)

    Helicobacter pylori—associated chronic superficial gastritis

    Vagotomy (without antrectomy)

    H_2-blocker therapy

    Proton pump inhibitor therapy

Chronic antral-pump inhibitor therapy

Hypercalcemia (of multiple causes including hyperparathyroidism)

Acromegaly

Uremia

*Secondary G-cell hyperplasia is much more common than the primary form.

TABLE 2-15.

When a cause can be ascertained that produces G-cell hyperplasia, the condition is called *secondary G-cell hyperplasia*. Achlorhydria and hypochlorhydria (of any cause but especially when associated with pernicious anemia) may result in G-cell hyperplasia. The cell population expands with the lack of physiologic negative feedback normally provided by gastric acid. Chronic antropyloric distention, often associated with posttruncal vagotomy, may also be a cause. Hypercalcemia, uremia, or acromegaly may also cause G-cell hyperplasia; however, the mechanism by which this occurs is unknown. *Helicobacter pylori* gastritis is also associated with elevated gastrin levels, which decreased after eradication [35].

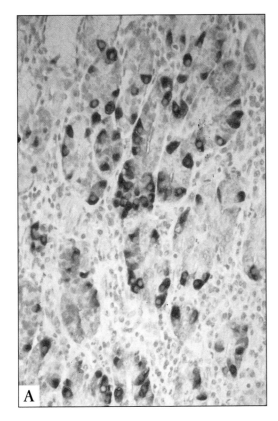

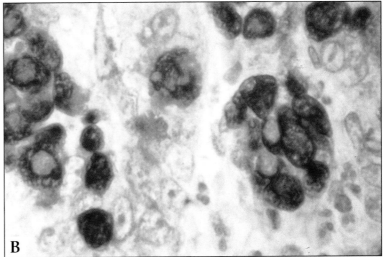

G-cell hyperplasia: morphologic characteristics. **A**, Gastric antral mucosa of a patient with pernicious anemia, immunostained with an antigastrin antibody. Increased numbers of brown-staining G cells occupy most of the length of the glands. **B**, High-power view of the G-cell hyperplasia (shown in panel **A**), illustrating the characteristic clustering or *cloning* of the hyperplastic G cells. ABC immunoperoxidase with DAB as the chromogen.

TABLE 2-16. ECL-CELL HYPERPLASIA: CAUSES

Marked
   Chronic atrophic gastritis with
   pernicious anemia
   Zollinger-Ellison syndrome
Limited
   Proton pump inhibitory therapy
   (*eg*, omeprazole)

Enterochromaffin-like (ECL)—cell hyperplasia represents an expansion of the argyrophilic cells within the glands of the gastric oxyntic mucosa. Zollinger-Ellison syndrome and chronic atrophic gastritis associated with pernicious anemia, two conditions which are functionally different but which share an underlying hypergastrinemia, are associated with marked ECL-cell hyperplasia. Proton pump inhibitor therapy, also associated with elevated gastrin levels, is also associated with mild ECL-cell hyperplasia [35].

TABLE 2-17. ECL-CELL HYPERPLASIA

Stage I:	Increased numbers of enterochromaffin-like (ECL) cells appear in the mucosa.
Stage II:	Cells show piling up of the nuclei with formation of clusters and cellular buds.
Stage III:	Small clusters of proliferating ECL cells, called *microcarcinoids*, appear to violate the basement membrane of the gastric glands.
Stage IV:	The microcarcinoids evolve into larger masses that invade the other layers of the gastric wall and eventually show the ability to metastasize.

Enterochromaffin-like (ECL)–cell hyperplasia may be classified into one of four stages based upon morphologic patterns. These stages are shown. In pernicious anemia of long-standing duration, one may find examples of stage III/IV ECL–cell hyperplasia. In Zollinger-Ellison syndrome, carcinoid tumors (Stage IV) are rare except when the syndrome is part of the multiple endocrine neoplasia type I syndrome (MEN I). Thus, hypergastrinemia plus a genetic alteration (deletion) are required for tumor (carcinoid) formation [36].

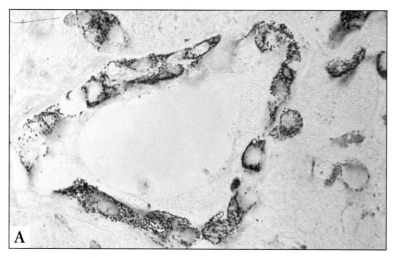
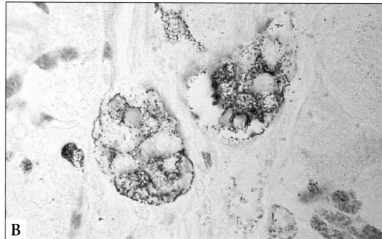

FIGURE 2-20.

FIGURE 2-20.

Enterochromaffin-like (ECL) cell-hyperplasia: morphologic characteristics. **A,** Gastric oxyntic mucosa of a patient with pernicious anemia demonstrating the linear disposition of the hyperplastic argyrophilic ECL cells that encircle the exocrine cells of the gland.

B, A different area of the same antral mucosa, in this instance, showing micronodular ECL-cell hyperplasia. The hyperplastic argyrophilic cells are seemingly detached from glandular structures. Grimelius silver stain for argyrophilia.

TABLE 2-18. CLASSIFICATION OF GASTRIC (FOREGUT) CARCINOID TUMORS*

Silver affinity	
Argentaffinity	- (+)*
Argyrophilia	+ (-) **
Secretion	Gastrin
	Somatostatin
	Others
Functional	Zollinger-Ellison syndrome
expression	Atypical carcinoid

*Gastric carcinoid tumors may be associated with hypergastrinemia or be sporadic.
**Usually positive, but some tumors are negative.

TABLE 2-18.

Classification of gastric carcinoid tumors. Carcinoid tumors are endocrine neoplasias of the gastrointestinal tract that are commonly classified into three groups: 1) foregut, 2) midgut, and 3) hindgut. Foregut carcinoids, which include gastric carcinoids, represent a variable group of lesions detectable based on silver stains and immunocytochemical investigations. They may be sporadic or associated with progression of enterochromaffin-like (ECL)–cell hyperplasia in hypergastrinemic conditions such as Zollinger-Ellison syndrome and gastric atrophy with pernicious anemia. Gastric and duodenal carcinoids generally secrete gastrin or somatostatin and are rarely associated with the carcinoid syndrome. Those associated with hypergastrinemic states are generally benign, whereas sporadic carcinoids behave more aggressively [36].

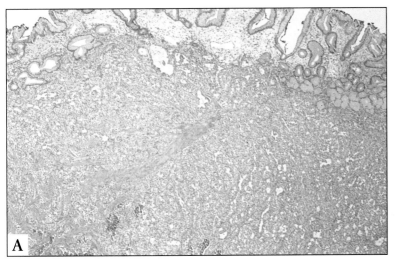

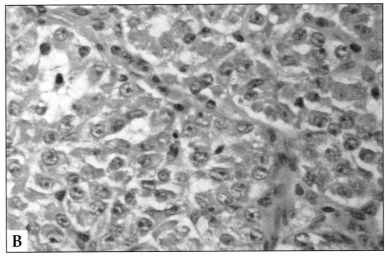

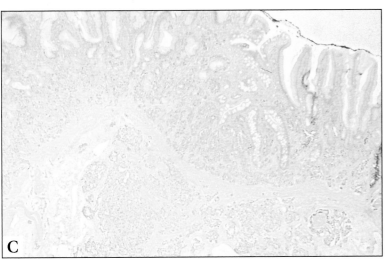

FIGURE 2-21.

Gastric carcinoid: morphologic aspects. **A,** Low-power view of a gastric carcinoid arising in the corpus of the stomach in a patient with pernicious anemia. The neoplasm replaces the lower mucosa and extends into the submucosa (hematoxylin and eosin stain). **B,** High-power view of the carcinoid tumor depicted in *A*. The tumor cells, arranged in large clusters and sheets, show little atypia and negligible mitotic activity (hematoxylin and eosin stain). **C,** Low-power view of the same lesion depicted in *A* and *B*, this time stained with Grimelius silver stain for argyrophilia.

TABLE 2-19. GASTRIC CARCINOIDS: TREATMENT

Hypergastrinemia-associated	Sporadic
Observation only	Resection
Antrectomy	? Endoscopic
Resection of tumor(s)	Surgical
? Endoscopic	
Surgical	

TABLE 2-19.

Gastric carcinoid tumors (more appropriately called *neuroendocrine tumors* or *ECLomas* in the stomach) usually follow an indolent course and were at one time felt to be entirely benign. Histologically and cytologically, they appear indolent with a low mitotic rate and little atypia. Despite this, 20% of carcinoids will have metastasized when surgery is performed. In general, carcinoids greater than 2 cm in size follow a malignant course, whereas those smaller than 1 cm in size rarely metastasize. Multiple approaches for treatment have been proposed including observation, antrectomy, or endoscopic removal for small tumors smaller than 1 cm, and wide excision including regional node metastasizes for those greater than 2 cm. Chemotherapy has been used for those with metastasis who are deemed unsuitable for surgery with mild success [36].

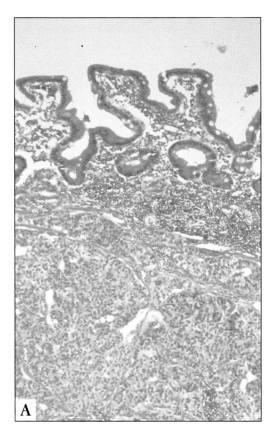

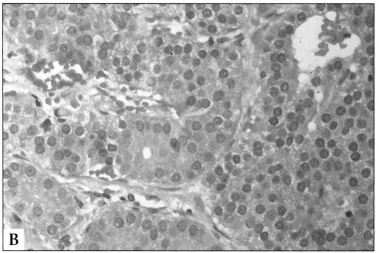

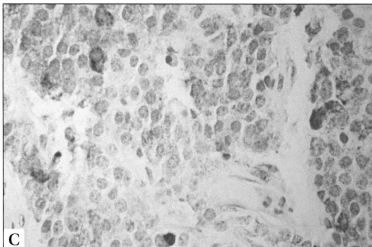

FIGURE 2-22.

Duodenal gastrinoma: morphologic aspects. **A**, Low-power view of a gastrinoma, arising in the first portion of the duodenum, in a patient with the Zollinger-Ellison syndrome. The tumor appears to originate in the mucosa and extends into the submucosa (hematoxylin and eosin stain). **B**, High-power view of the same neoplasm, the tumor cells, arranged in a mixture of solid and rosettelike patterns, display negligible cytologic atypia and mitotic activity (hematoxylin and eosin stain). **C**, The same gastrinoma depicted in *A&B*, immunostained with an antigastrin antibody. All tumor cells exhibit brown immunoreactivity, although to a highly variable extent (ABC immunoperoxidase with DAB as the chromogen).

■ REFERENCES AND RECOMMENDED READING

1. Bayliss WM, Starling EH: The mechanism of pancreatic secretion. *J Physiol (London)* 1902, 28:325–353.

2. Edkins JS: On the chemical mechanism of gastric secretion. *Proc R. Soc Lond (Biol)* 1905, 76:376.

3. Dale HH, Laidlaw PP: The physiological action of beta-imidazolyl-ethylamine. *J Physiol* 1910–1911, 41:318–344.

4. Ivy AC, Oldberg E: A hormone mechanism for gallbladder contraction and evacuation. *Am J Physiol* 1928, 65:599–613.

5. von Euler US, Gaddum JH: An unidentified depressor substance in certain tissue extracts. *J Physiol* 1931, 72:74–87.

6. Sutherland EW, de Duve C: Origin and distribution of the hyperglycemic-glycogenolytic factor of the pancreas. *J Biol Chem* 1948, 175:663–674.

7. Erspamer V, Asero B: Identification of enteramine, the specific hormone of the enterochromaffin cell system, as 5-hydroxytryptamine. *Nature (London)* 1952, 169:800–801.

8. Cohen S: Isolation of mouse submaxillary gland protein accelerating incisor eruption and eyelid opening in the new-born animal. *J Biol Chem* 1962, 237:1555–1562.

9. Gregory H: Isolation and structure of urogastrone and its relationship to epidermal growth factor. *Nature (London)* 1975, 257:325–327.

10. Brown JC, Pederson RA, Jorpes JE, Mutt V: Preparation of a highly active enterogastrone. *Can J Physiol Pharmacol* 1969, 47:113–114.

11. Erspamer V, Falconieri–Erspamer G, Inselvini M: Some pharmacological actions of alytesin and bombesin. *J Pharm Pharmacol* 1970, 22:875.

12. Walsh JH, Wong HC, Dockray GJ: Bombesin-like peptides in mammals. *Federation Proc* 1979, 38:2315–2319.

13. Said SI, Mutt V: Potent peripheral and splanchnic vasodilator peptide from normal gut. *Nature (London)* 1970, 225:863–864.

14. Brown JC, Mutt V, Dryburg JR: The further purification of motilin, a gastric motor activity stimulating polypeptide from the mucosa of the small intestine of hogs. *Can J Physiol Pharmacol* 1971, 49:399–405.

15. Carraway R, Leeman SE: The isolation of a new hypotensive peptide, neurotensin, from bovine hypothalami. *J Biol Chem* 1973, 248:6854–6861.

16. Brazeau P, Vale W, Burgus R, *et al.*: Hypothalamic polypeptide that inhibits the secretion of immunoreactive pituitary growth hormone. *Science* 1973, 179:77–79.

17. Arimura A, Sato H, Dupont A, *et al.*: Somatostatin: abundance of immunoreactive hormone in rat stomach and pancreas. *Science* 1975, 189:1007–1009.

18. Hughes J, Smith TW, Kosterlitz HW, *et al.*: Identification of two related pentapeptides from the brain with potent opiate agonist activity. *Nature* 1975, 258:577–579.

19. Giraud AS, Dockray GJ, Williams RG: Immunoreactive Metenkephalin, Arg [6] in rat brain, and bovine brain, gut and adrenal. *J Neurochem* 1984, 43:1236–1242.

20. Tatamoto K, Mutt V: Isolation of two novel candidate hormones using a chemical method for finding natural occurring polypeptides. *Nature* 1981, 285:417–418.

21. Amara SG, Jonas V, Rosenfeld MG, *et al.*: Alternative RNA processing in calcitonin gene expression generates mRNAs encoding different polypeptide products. *Nature* 1982, 298:240–244.

22. Rodrigo J, Polak JM, Fernandez L, *et al.*: Calcitonin gene-related peptide immunoreactive sensory and motor nerves of the rat, cat, and monkey esophagus. *Gastroenterology* 1985, 88:444–451.

23. Tatomoto K, Rökaeus Å, Jörnvall H, *et al.*: Galanin—a novel biologically active peptide from porcine intestine. *FEBS Lett* 1983, 164:124–128.

24. Yanagisawa M, Kirihara H, Kimura S: A novel potent vasoconstrictor peptide produced by vascular endothelial cells. *Nature* 1988, 332:411–415.

25. Inagaki H, Bishop AE, Escrig C, *et al.*: Localization of endothelinlike immunoreactivity and endothelin binding sites in human colon. *Gastroenterology* 1991, 101:47–54.

26. Walsh JH, Gastrin. In *Gut Peptides and Physiology*. Edited by Walsh JH and Dockray GJ. New York: Raven Press, 1994:75–121.

27. Walsh JH, Mayer EA. Gastrointestinal hormones. In *Gastrointestinal Diseases*. Edited by Sleisenger M and Fordtran JS. Philadelphia: W.B. Saunders, 1994, Vol 1., pg 22.

28. Wiborg O, Berglund L, Boel E, *et al.*: Structure of a human gastrin gene. *Proc Natl Acad Sci* 1984, 81:1067–1069.

29. Song I, *et al.*: The human gastrin/cholecystokinin type B receptor gene: alternative splice donor site in exon 4 generates two variant mRNAs. *Proc Natl Acad Sci* 1993, 90:9085–9089.

30. Bunnett N: Gastrin-releasing peptide. In *Gut Peptides and Physiology*. Edited by Walsh JH and Dockray GJ. New York: Raven Press, 1994:423–445.

31. Chiba T, Yamada T: Gut somatostatin. In *Gut Peptides and Physiology*. Edited by Walsh JH and Dockray GJ. New York: Raven Press, 1994:123–145.

32. Feldman M. Bruton M: Drug therapy: histamine$_2$-receptor antagonists. *N Engl J Med* 1990, 323:1672–1680.

33. Goldschmiedt M, Feldman M: Gastric secretion in health and disease. In *Gastrointestinal Diseases*, 5th ed. Edited by Sleisenger M and Fordtran JS. Philadelphia: W.B. Saunders, 1993, Vol 1, pg 526.

34. Lloyd KC, Walsh JH: Gastric secretion. In *Gut Peptides and Physiology*. Edited by Walsh JH and Dockray GJ. New York: Raven Press, 1994:633–654.

35. Lechago J: Gastrointestinal neuroendocrine cell proliferations. *Human Pathology* 1994, 25:1114–1122.

36. Lechago J: Neuroendocrine cells of the gut and their disorders. In *Gastrointestinal Pathology*. Edited by Goldman H, Appelman HR. Baltimore, MD: Williams & Wilkins, 1990:181–219.

Chapter 3

Mucosal Immunology of the Stomach and Duodenum

W. ALLAN WALKER

The gastrointestinal tract is the largest lymphoid organ in the body. Isolated lymphocytes and aggregates of lymphoid cells in Peyer's patches, which line the interstitial and intraepithelial spaces of the stomach and duodenum, are uniquely programmed to handle antigens and microorganisms crossing the mucosal barrier [1,2]. As research efforts in mucosal immunology have entered a *log* phase during the past decade and as the field of molecular and cell biology has blossomed, we now recognize the importance of immunologic reactions in the pathogenesis of many gastrointestinal disease states [3,4]. A thorough understanding of gut immunology is necessary for the clinical gastroenterologist to approach the diagnosis and management of many disease states involving the stomach and duodenum [5]. Establishing such a background is helpful in selecting new, more specific treatment modalities for inflammatory, allergic, and infectious gastrointestinal disease states [6–8].

In this pictorial review of gut immunology involving the stomach and duodenum, a concept of immunophysiology of the gut is described [8,9]. This concept takes in the dynamic interaction of intestinal flora on the intestinal epithelium with gut lymphoid elements and the respective influences of the epithelial, mesenchyme, and enteric nervous system on mucosal immune function [10,11], as well as the role of lymphocytes and their cytokines on epithelial secretion [12] and peristalsis [13]. The term *immunophysiology of the gut* was first used by Dr. Gil Castro [14] in a review that appeared in the *American Journal of Physiology*. Since then the field has expanded enormously to become the subject of two major international symposia during the past 3 years [15,16]. Enteric stimuli, whether bacterial colonization, antigen uptake, or nutrient or trophic factor interaction, must first cross the epithelium to interact with lymphoid tissues in the intestine [17]. The nature of this interaction may influence the type of immune response evoked, *ie*, antibody production, T-cell cytotoxicity, or immune tolerance. In addition, interaction of bacterial lipopolysaccharide with enterocytes can stimulate the expression and secretion of cytokines and defensins, which further influence the immune response [18]. In like manner, factors released from lymphoid cells, such as histamine from mast cells or cytokines from T cells, may act to stimulate active secretion of fluid into the lumen through a receptor-mediated, signal-transduction stimulus to chloride channels in the enterocyte [19] or by a two-step process involving fibroblasts. These same cytokines may influence intestinal connective tissue and leukocytes to release leukotrienes or stimulate an activation of the enteric nervous system, resulting in increased peristalsis or release of neuromediators such as substance P/vasoactive intestinal peptide released from neurons, thereby having secondary effects on lymphoid cells [20]. These interrelating processes are termed *immunophysiologic responses* because they mobilize multiple components of the gut (epithelial, mesenchyme, and lymphoid) to protect the human collectively against noxious stimuli attempting to cross the mucosal barrier to cause systemic infection or inflammation.

As mentioned, the mucosal immune system is distinct from the systemic immune system and produces a unique response to foreign stimuli. Antigens crossing the epithelial surface through a specialized epithelium (the microfold cell) are processed in such a way that polymeric immunoglobulin A (pIgA)-producing plasma cells in the submucosa secrete antigen-specific IgA antibody, which is shuttled across the epithelium by a specific pIgA receptor and released onto the mucosal surface as secretory IgA. The latter's presence on the mucosal surface modulates bacterial or viral adherence and antigen uptake in a controlled fashion [21]. In addition to stimulating a pIgA response, lymphoid elements responding to antigen or microbial uptake produce a downregulation of the system's cellular and humoral response (oral tolerance) [22]. The mechanism of this response is the subject of extensive research efforts and to date is not completely understood.

Mucosal immune response in newborn infants is underdeveloped and requires several months to years for fully protective secretory IgA levels to be attained [22]. In addition, antigens or microbes crossing immature intestinal mucosal surfaces stimulate, rather than downregulate, systemic responsiveness. These inappropriate mucosal immune responses, such as stimulation of the systemic immune response rather than downregulation or tolerance, has been suggested as a possible pathogenic mechanism for age-related diseases occurring in this patient population (*eg*, food allergy and necrotizing enterocolitis). Complete development of a normal intestinal mucosal immune response requires bacterial colonization of the neonatal gut, introduction of enteric nutrients, and exposure to intestinal growth factors such as epidermal trophic factor [23]. Breast milk contains large quantities of active trophic factors and exposes the newborn infant to stimuli that accelerate the normal developmental process.

A generalized concept of a mucosal barrier to protect against luminal factors that can cause immune-mediated gastrointestinal diseases has evolved over the past several decades [24]. This barrier includes factors in the intestinal lumen, on the epithelial surface of enterocytes, and in the mucosal immune system. These factors work collectively to control microbial and pathologic quantities of antigen penetration of the gut. For example, gastric acidity in the stomach helps prevent swallowed bacteria from entering the duodenum where they may lead to colonization and bacterial overgrowth [25]. In addition, peptic activity and mucin released into the stomach help to degrade proteins and trap microorganisms and antigens. In addition, the surface glycoconjugates of epithelial cells may express adhesion molecules which also help to control bacterial attachment and colonization. Because bacterial attachment molecules depend on epithelial glycoconjugates for adherence, the glycosylation of epithelial surfaces can control the nature of bacterial attachment [26]. Finally, when the mucosal barrier is operational, the controlled uptake of antigens and microorganisms can elicit appropriate protective immune response. Genetic factors and environmental circumstances may contribute to a modification of the mucosal barrier that could result in an increased incidence of infection, inflammation, or immune responses leading to gastrointestinal disease states [27]. Two examples of such disease states, which are discussed in Figures 3-10 and 3-11, are *Helicobacter pylori* infection leading to gastritis and ulcer disease and gluten-sensitive enteropathy.

Of importance to the gastroenterologist is a complete knowledge of those derangements in the host defense or immunologic processes that may result in gastrointestinal disease states. Three prototypic diseases involving the stomach and duodenum are considered as examples of immune-mediated gastrointestinal disease. *H. pylori* has been implicated in both gastritis and ulcer disease and may lead to gastric carcinoma and lymphoma. Each of these mucosal injuries are mediated in part through an aberrant immune system. For example, cytokines released by either gastric epithelial cells or mucosal lymphoid cells in the stomach may stimulate increased acid secretion and mediate recruitment of neutrophil with a resultant increased release of inflammatory cytokines such as interleukin-1 and tumor necrosis factor-α among others [28]. In like manner, patients with gluten-sensitive enteropathy appear to have a subtle defect in gliadin interaction with the mucosal immune system [29]. The specific mechanism of celiac disease is not completely understood but appears to relate to a specific HLA expression that could result in abnormal presentation of gliadin peptides to lymphocytes leading to increased numbers of intraepithelial lymphocytes and increased T-cell cytotoxicity against enterocytes [30]. In addition, the diagnosis of celiac disease is made in part by a specific immunoglobulin G/IgA mucosal antibody response to gliadin fragments [31]. In like manner, food allergies resulting in gastritis and enteropathies occur predominantly in young infants and are presumed to relate to an altered response of the stomach or duodenum to food-antigen handling [32].

A major area of active investigation among mucosal immunologists is the induction of oral tolerance to antigens or microbes crossing the mucosa [33]. As mentioned, antigens fed orally result in a downregulation of systemic humoral and cellular immune responsiveness. An absence of this normal component of the immune mucosal response may lead to the expression of organ-specific autoimmune diseases (arthritis, encephalitis, gastritis, and colitis). If the specific mechanism of oral tolerance induction is determined, the pathogenesis of autoimmune disease with regard to defective antigen handling and responsiveness can be determined. In addition, exciting new studies involving treatment of autoimmune disease states by oral inges-tion of the *putative* antigen may represent a breakthrough in the management of this debilitating group of diseases [34].

Finally, we consider future directions in the mucosal immunology of the stomach and duodenum in gastroin-testinal disease. Future approaches to management of gastrointestinal disease will require a better understanding of the normal mucosal immune response in the stomach and its relationship to gastric immunophysiology. With the advent of cellular and molecular approaches in the study of gastric and duodenal immunology, we can more carefully determine the contribution of epithelial cells to mucosal immune function

and the mechanisms of immunologic mediation of epithelial function, such as secretion of acid and mucus and altered regulation of mucosal blood flow. With this information, new drug therapies can be specifically devised to treat inflamma-tion, bacterial infection, and mucosal ulceration. This treat-ment is done by specifically interfering with a known immune-mediated inflammatory pathway, so that reliable vaccines can be produced to prevent intestinal infections. A classic example of what these future studies can provide would be specific vaccines to the high incidence of *H. pylori* infection of the stomach thereby affecting the incidence of gastritis, peptic ulcer disease, and gastric malignancy.

■ CONCEPT OF IMMUNOPHYSIOLOGY OF THE GUT

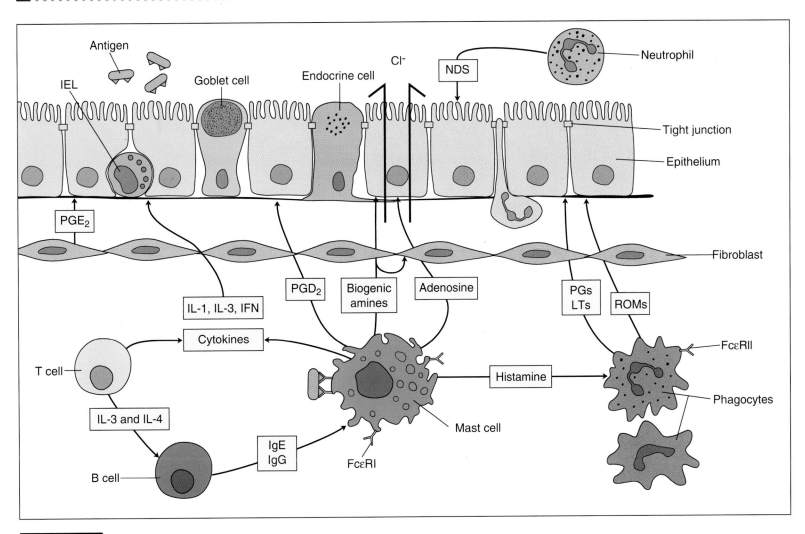

FIGURE 3-1.

Diagram of a potential immunophysiologic response in which lymphoid tissues within the intraepithelium or submucosal com-partments of the gut affect the physiologic function of epithelial cells. Antigens, allergens, or microorganisms within the intestinal lumen or on the mucosal surface can cross the mucosal barrier and be presented to lymphoid elements underlying the intestinal mucosa. These lymphoid cells can in turn produce cytokines that directly affect the epithelium or modulate B-cell responsiveness. Antibodies produced by this stimulation, particularly immuno-globulin E (IgE) and immunoglobulin G (IgG), can interact with other mucosal cells, *ie*, mast cells or fibroblasts, to release media-tors (histamine, prostaglandins) that also may stimulate epithelial

cells to express IgE receptors or lead to increased expression of chloride channels, resulting in increased secretion. This immuno-physiologic process is part of the collective host defense of the gut. For example, secretion of intestinal fluid washes away IgA immune complexes formed with bacteria or antigens on the luminal surface as an adjunctive protective process to keep the gut free from potential noxious agents. Cl—chloride; FcεRI—Fc receptor for IgE Fc antibody; FcεRII—Phagocyte Fc position of the immunoglobulin G molecule receptor; IEL—intraepithelial leukocyte; IFN—interferon; IL—inter-leukin; LT—leukotriene; NDS—neutrophil-derived secretagogue; PG—prostaglandin; ROM—reactive oxygen metabolite; not to scale. (*Adapted from* McKay and Perdue [6]; with permission.)

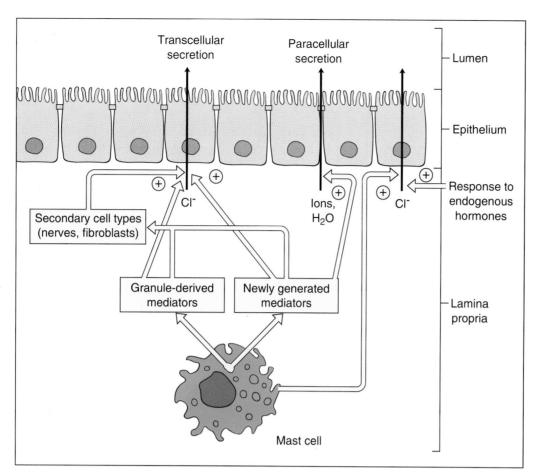

FIGURE 3-2.

Proposed specific mechanism of mast cell–epithelial interactions in immune-mediated intestinal secretion leading to diarrhea. Mast cells in the lamina propria of the gut can be stimulated through immunoglobulin E receptors to release mediators that may have either a primary effect (histamine) on enterocytes and goblet cells or through secondary pathways (*ie*, fibroblast activation) that may stimulate transcellular and paracellular secretion of fluid and electrolytes. This diagram is presumed to depict the pathophysiologic mechanism for inflammatory diarrhea of the stomach (allergy) and duodenum (parasitic infestations). (*Adapted from* Barrett [35]; with permission.)

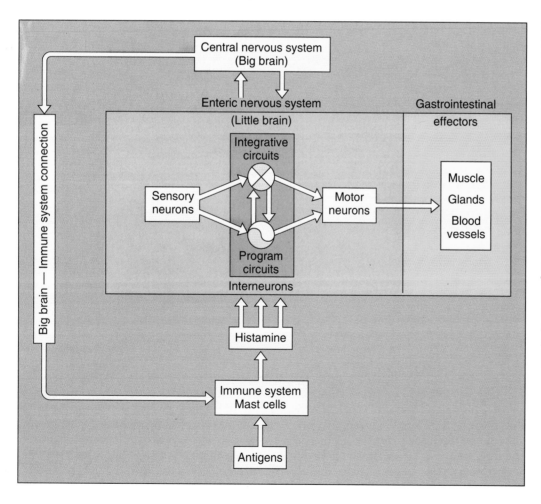

FIGURE 3-3.

Diagram of coordinated neuroimmune system depicts interactions between the enteric nervous system and mucosal immunologic elements resulting in secondary effects on intestinal smooth muscle (increased peristalsis) and enterocytes (fluid secretion and goblet-cell mucus release). The sequence of events includes antigen stimulation of the mucosal immune system causing release of mediators (paracrines), which may stimulate enteric neurons to release mediators (neurocrines) that interact directly with smooth muscle cells and enterocytes or goblet cells through specific receptors located on their surface. This process can move in multiple directions (neuroimmunoepithelial vs immuno-neuroepithelial) making discovery of a specific mechanism of secretion difficult to sort out. (*Adapted from* Castro and Arntzen [7]; with permission.)

TABLE 3-1. SOURCE AND EFFECTS OF CYTOKINES IN THE HUMAN INTESTINE

CYTOKINE	SOURCE	EFFECTS
Interleukin 1	Macrophages Epithelial cells Endothelial cells Fibroblasts Mast cells Eosinophils	Proinflammatory Activates CD4+ cells, natural killer cells Attracts neutrophils and macrophages Increases expression of intracellular adhesion molecules fever
Interleukin 2	T cells (lipoprotein lipase and intraepithelial leukocyte	Induces proliferation and differentiation of antigen-stimulated T cells Induces proliferation and immunoglobulin (Ig) secretion of activated B cells Activates natural killer cells
Interleukin 3	CD4+ T cells Mast cells	Induces growth and differentiation of basophils
Interleukin 4	T cells Mast cells B cells Macrophages Basophils	Induces differentiation of IgA committed B cells Induces isotype switching to IgG- and IgE-producing cells in uncommitted B cells
Interleukin 5	T cells Mast cells Eosinophils	Stimulates growth, differentiation, and activation of eosinophils
Interleukin 6	T cells Macrophages Fibroblasts Endothelial cells Mast cells	Induces growth and differentiation of B cells and T cells
Interleukin 7	Unknown in gut	Activates γ-δ T cells
Interleukin 8	T cells Fibroblasts Endothelial cells Epithelial cells Neutrophils Mast cells	Induces adhesion of neutrophils to endothelial cells Activates neutrophils to secrete lysosomal enzymes
Interleukin 10	T cells B cells Macrophages	Suppresses macrophages including production of inflammatory cytokines Enhances B-cell proliferation and Ig secretion
Interleukin 12	B cells Macrophages	Stimulates the differentiation of TH1 cells from uncommitted T cells Stimulates growth of T and natural killer cells
Interleukin 13	T cells	Inhibits inflammatory cytokine production by macrophages Stimulates B-cell growth and differentiation
Stem cell factor	Endothelial cells Fibroblasts	Stimulates the proliferation and maturation of mast cells
Transforming growth factor–α	Macrophages Epithelial cells Eosinophils	Induces angiogenesis and epithelial development Induces proliferation of fibroblasts
Transforming growth factor–β	T cells Fibroblasts Epithelial cells Mast cells Eosinophils	Promotes epithelial repair Induces IgA production by uncommitted B cells Inhibits growth of mature cells Stimulates extracellular matrix production May mediate oral tolerance
Tumor necrosis factor–α	Neutrophils Lymphocytes Endothelial cells NK cells Smooth muscle cells Mast cells Eosinophils	Proinflammatory Activates neutrophils and macrohpages, mesenchymal, and epithelial cells
Interferon–γ	T cells Natural killer cells	Modulates class II major histocompatibility complex expression Antiviral activity Stimulates macrophages

TABLE 3-1.

Source and effects of cytokines in the human intestine. Many cytokines produced by enterocytes or intestinal lymphoid cells can have direct or indirect effects on intestinal function. (*From* Mannick and Udall [36]; with permission.)

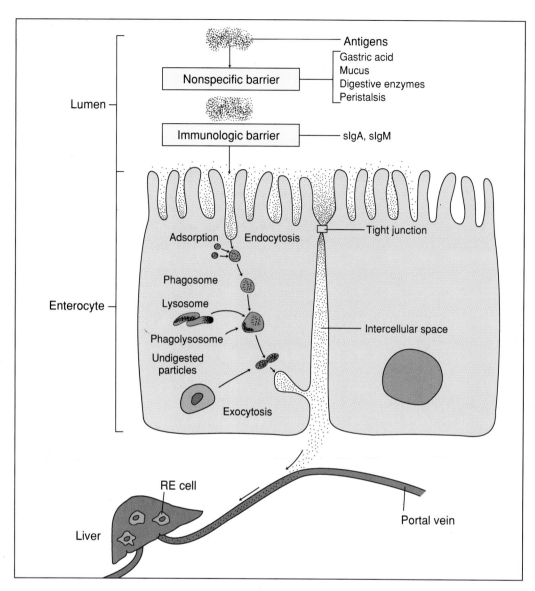

FIGURE 3-4.

Diagrammatic representation of components of the mucosal barrier of the gastrointestinal tract. Multiple barriers exist to control the uptake of antigens and microorganisms in the gut. These include nonspecific luminal factors such as gastric acidity, mucus, digestive enzymes, which alter bacterial colonization and antigen proteolysis, and nonspecific intestinal factors such as peristalsis, which help expel microorganisms and antigens trapped in mucus from the intestine. In addition, an immunologic barrier unique to mucosal surfaces (polymeric immunoglobulin A [pIgA]) acts to agglutinate antigens or microorganisms to prevent their attachment to the mucosal surface. Furthermore, the microvillous surface and epithelial cells control antigen uptake through endocytosis and the migration across tight junctions between cells. Enterocytes also contribute to the breakdown of potential antigens in the lysosomal compartment. Transport of antigen or peptic fragments and microorganisms after uptake across the epithelial surface are filtered through the fixed phagocytes in the reticuloendothelial (RE) system (Kupffer's cells) in the liver before entering the circulation. sIgA—secretory IgA; sIgM—secretory immunoglobulin M. (*Adapted from* Iyngkarm [37]; with permission.)

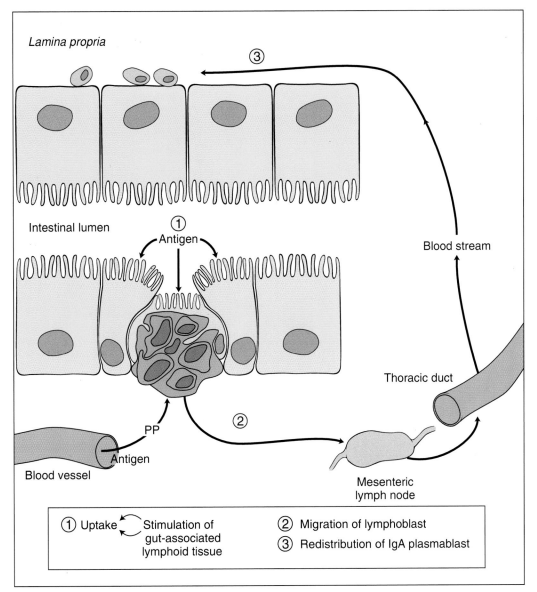

Lamina propria

Intestinal lumen

①
Antigen

Blood stream

Thoracic duct

PP
Antigen

Blood vessel

Mesenteric
lymph node

②

③

① Uptake ⇄ Stimulation of
gut-associated
lymphoid tissue

② Migration of lymphoblast
③ Redistribution of IgA plasmablast

FIGURE 3-5.

Immunoglobulin A (IgA) response to antigens crossing the mucosal surface. Physiologic quantities of antigens in the lumen preferentially cross microvilli or follicular epithelial cells (M cells) overlying Peyer's patches and are presented by macrophage to lymphoblasts. These cells release cytokines that begin a multistep process toward the maturation of the lymphoblast into an IgA-producing plasma cell. These cells mature sequentially in Peyer's patches and mesenteric lymph nodes and home to sites in the lamina propria as IgA-producing plasma cells specifically available to respond to the original antigen stimulus. (*Adapted from* Walker and Isselbacher [21]; with permission.)

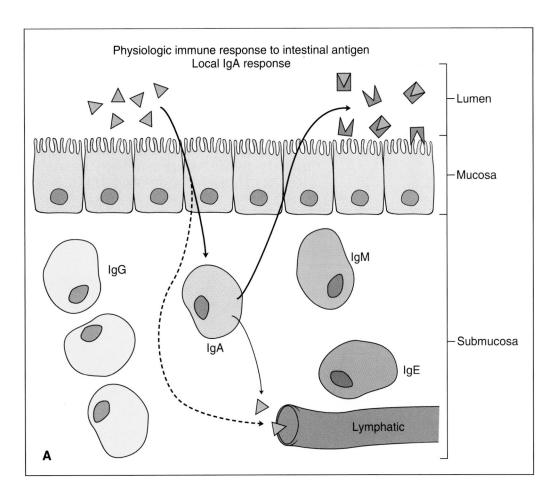

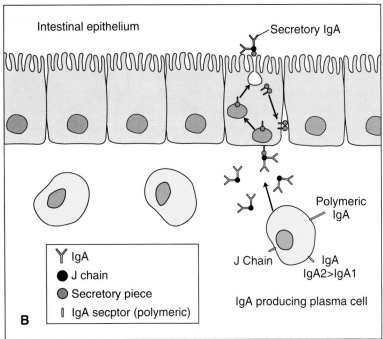

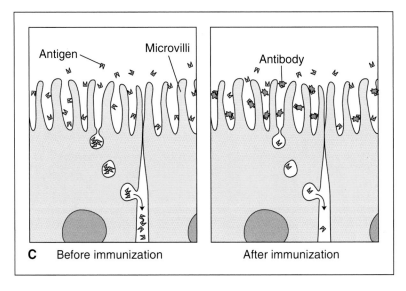

FIGURE 3-6.

Physiologic immune response to intestinal antigens—local immuno-globulin A (IgA) response. **A,** The response of IgA-producing plasma cells to specific antigens crossing the mucosal barrier. **B,** Antigens presented to these plasma cells trigger a dimeric IgA response. Dimeric IgA is then transported across the epithelium by a receptor-mediated process, which deposits secretory IgA onto the mucosal surfaces. **C,** They function there to agglutinate luminal antigens to protect against excessive (pathologic) antigen uptake. IgE—immuno-globulin E; IgG—immunoglobulin G; IgM— immunoglobulin M. (*From* Walker [38]; with permission.)

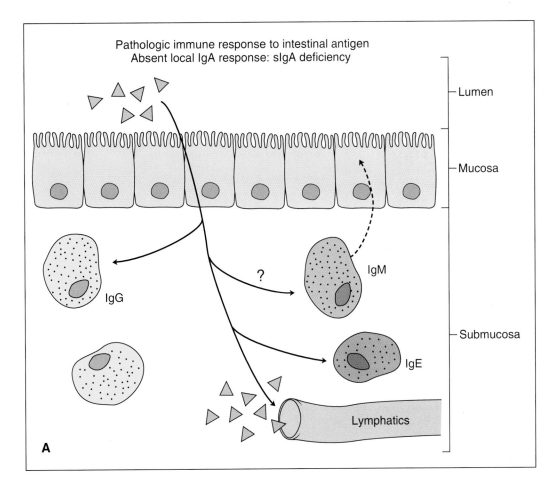

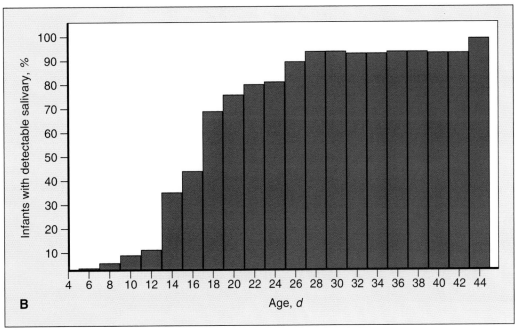

Pathologic immune response to intestinal antigen—absence of or decreased secretory immunoglobulin A (sIgA) response. **A,** In the absence of, or with a decreased capacity for, a sIgA response to antigens crossing the mucosa, excessive antigen crosses the mucosal barrier and is available to produce an adverse local or systemic immune response. With the absence of protective sIgA antibodies to luminal antigens, excessive quantities cross the mucosal barrier. **B,** In all full-term infants, production of protective levels of sIgA is delayed because of an immature local immune response. The period of delay in protective levels is extended in premature or sick newborns. These infants are susceptible to the same illnesses as genetically deficient sIgA deficient patients (giardiasis, bacterial or viral gastro-enteritis) during the transient period of deficiency. (*From* Walker [39]; with permission.)

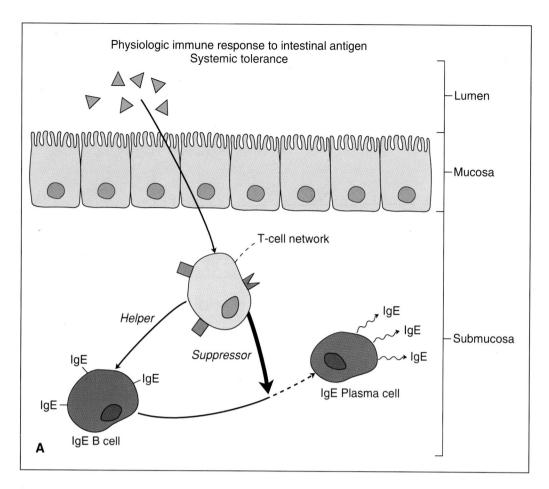

Physiologic immune response to intestinal antigen
Systemic tolerance

Lumen

Mucosa

T-cell network

Helper

Suppressor

Submucosa

IgE

IgE

IgE

IgE Plasma cell

IgE

IgE

IgE

IgE B cell

A

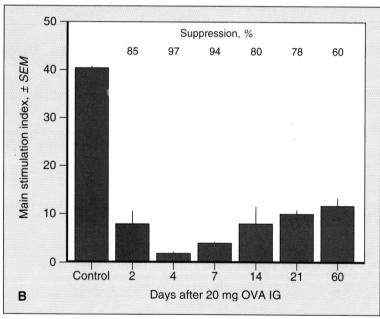

B

Suppression, %

85 97 94 80 78 60

Main stimulation index, ± SEM

Control 2 4 7 14 21 60

Days after 20 mg OVA IG

FIGURE 3-8.

Physiologic immune response to intestinal antigen—oral tolerance. **A,** Antigens crossing mucosal surfaces not only evoke a specific secretory immunoglobulin A response but also by virtue of their presentation stimulate suppressor subsets of T cells to release cytokines that downregulate systemic humoral and cellular immune responsiveness. This process is termed *oral tolerance* and is an important mechanism in downregulating the intestinal immune response and controlling autoimmunity. **B,** This figure, taken from a classic study, depicts animals who were systemically injected with ovalbumin (OVA) in both the presence and absence of previous intragastric (IG) exposure to the same OVA antigen. Those animals that were not orally exposed to the antigen had a normal systemic immune response (Control). Those animals previously exposed to OVA orally and systemically challenged had a marked suppression of systemic responsiveness for at least 60 days. The normal response of oral tolerance to foreign antigen is important in the prevention of allergic disease and autoimmune states. IgE—immunoglobulin E. (*From* Challacombe and Tomasi [40]; with permission.)

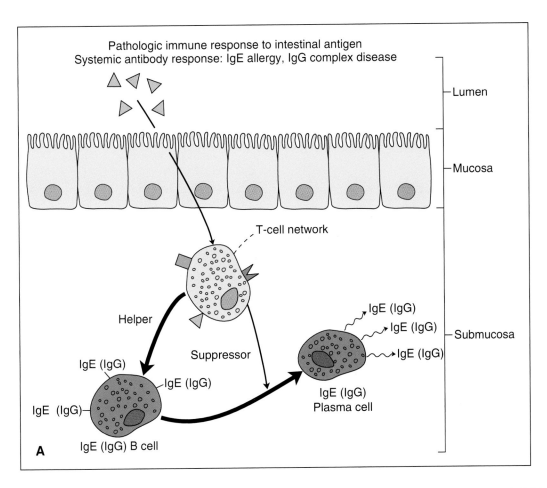

Pathologic immune response to intestinal antigen
Systemic antibody response: IgE allergy, IgG complex disease

Lumen

Mucosa

T-cell network

Helper

Suppressor

IgE (IgG)
IgE (IgG)
IgE (IgG)

Submucosa

IgE (IgG)
IgE (IgG)
IgE (IgG)
Plasma cell

IgE (IgG)
IgE (IgG)
IgE (IgG)

A IgE (IgG) B cell

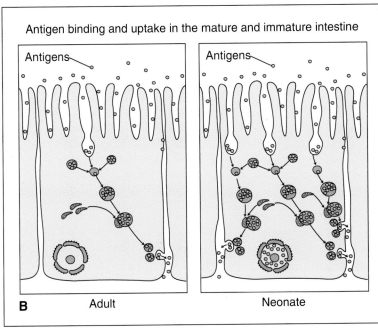

Antigen binding and uptake in the mature and immature intestine

Antigens

Antigens

B Adult   Neonate

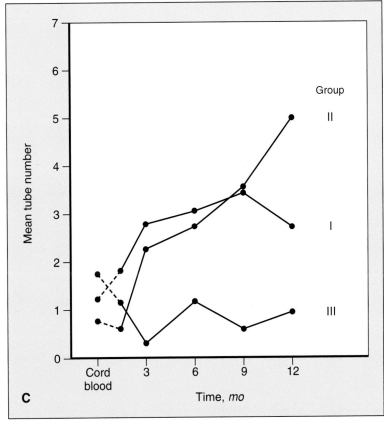

FIGURE 3-9.

Pathologic response to intestinal antigen—systemic priming resulting
in immunoglobulin E (IgE) allergy and immunoglobulin G (IgG)
immune complex disease (Arthus reaction). **A,** When excessive antigens
cross the mucosal barrier or when antigens are handled or presented
improperly, the systemic humoral or cellular immune response favors
stimulation (priming) rather than tolerance. This figure depicts the
priming of antibody-producing lymphocytes resulting in a systemic IgE
or IgG response. The presence of systemic antibodies to foreign antigens can result in allergic (IgE) or Arthus-type (IgG complex) reactions,
resulting in allergic enteropathy or celiac disease states. **B,** Because of
the absence of secretory immunoglobulin A antibodies to prevent
excessive uptake of intestinal antigens or the immaturity of endocytosis
in the neonatal gut, excessive quantities of antigen cross the mucosal

barrier. **C,** This excessive uptake of ingested food antigens provokes
a systemic immune response. This figure shows the mean titer of
milk agglutinins in infants fed formula (I), cow's milk (II), and
breast milk (III) for 3 months followed by formula feeding. In the
presence of foreign antigen exposure from birth on, the systemic
immune response is greater than after breast feeding. (**A** and **B,**
From Walker [39]; with permission.) (**C,** *From* Eastham and Walker
[41]; with permission.)

CONCEPT OF THE INTESTINAL MUCOSAL BARRIER AS A DETERRENT TO CLINICAL DISEASE

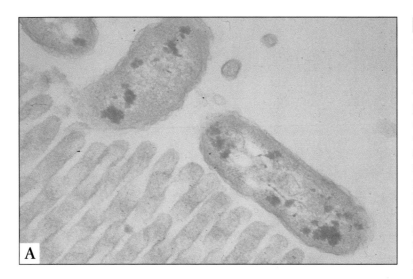

A

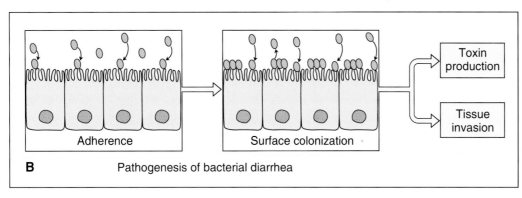

B   Pathogenesis of bacterial diarrhea

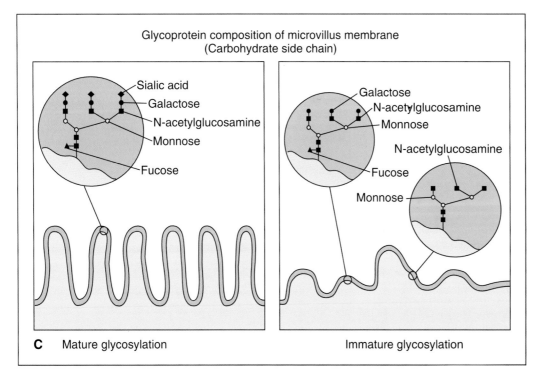

Glycoprotein composition of microvillus membrane
(Carbohydrate side chain)

C   Mature glycosylation   Immature glycosylation

FIGURE 3-10.

Bacterial colonization and maturation of the mucosal immune response. **A,** This electron microscopic photograph of bacteria adhering to the intestinal or gastric microvillus surface underscores the need for intestinal colonization in order to stimulate maturation of the infant's mucosal immune system. **B,** Bacteria adhere to specific glycoconjugates on the microvillus membrane for colonization to occur. Colonization with pathogenic bacteria may result in toxin-induced diarrhea or in invasive or inflammatory gastroenteritis. Lipopolysaccharide and toxins from bacteria are important stimuli for the normal maturation of mucosal immune responses. **C,** This diagram depicts developmental differences in microvillus glycoprotein composition in newborn versus adult intestinal cells. These developmental differences may help explain the increased incidence of pathologic bacterial infestation of the stomach and small intestine in young infants.

DISEASE CONSEQUENCES OF IMMUNE DYSFUNCTION

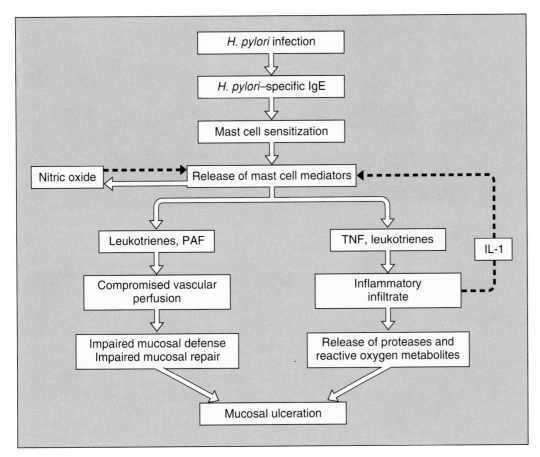

FIGURE 3-11.

This diagram depicts a possible immune mechanism by which *Helicobacter pylori* causes gastritis and mucosal ulceration in patients. The mechanism may involve mast cells and an immunoglobulin E (IgE) immune response. *H. pylori* adheres to gastric mucosa and causes gastric infection which may include an IgE-anti–*Helicobacter* response. As infection persists, *Helicobacter* antigen-IgE antibody complexes form and adhere to IgE receptors on mast cells, causing a release of mast-cell mediators including platelet activating factor (PAF) and tumor necrosis factor (TNF). Other factors such as leukotrienes and nitric oxide also participate in the inflammatory response and in cell necrosis. This process includes a disruption of vascular perfusion and chemotactic stimulus for neutrophil infiltration leading to tissue damage and mucosal ulceration. IL—interleukin. (*From* Wallace [42]; with permission.)

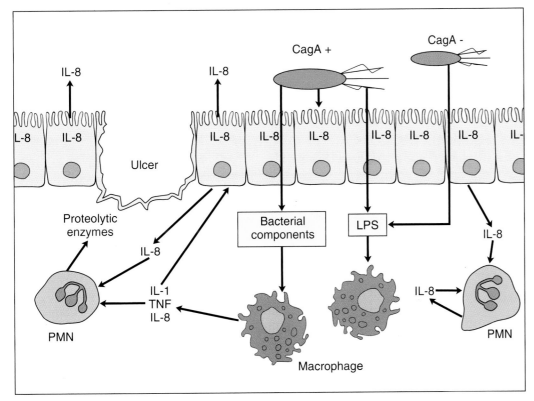

FIGURE 3-12.

Pathway of *Helicobacter pylori* induction of the cytokine interleukin (IL)-8 by gastric epithelial cells. Bacteria may attach to or translocate across the surface molecule and their cell wall components (lipopolysaccharides [LPS]) stimulate macrophages which in turn release cytokines including IL-8, tumor necrosis factor (TNF), and IL-1. These cytokines stimulate gastric epithelium to express and release IL-8 which in turn stimulates neutrophils (polymorphonuclear [PMN] leukocyte) to release proteolytic enzymes leading to epithelial destruction and gastric ulceration. (*From* Crabtree *et al.* [43]; with permission.)

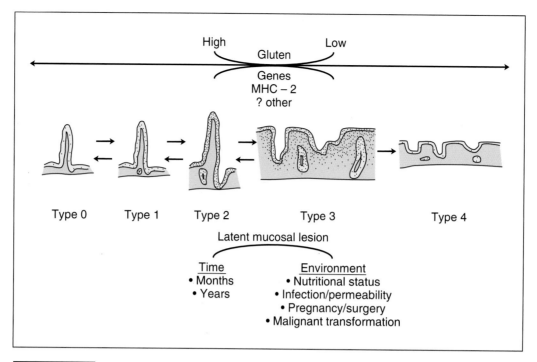

FIGURE 3-13.

Immunogenetic basis for celiac disease. A very close association exists between HLA typing in patient groups and expression of celiac disease. It has been hypothesized that the HLA type-specific relationship to disease may represent an example of an immunogenetic basis of disease. This figure shows the association between HLA genetic predisposition and gluten exposure in gluten sensitivity. Essential ingredients in the production of each of the defined mucosal responses are shown. Genes, other than those encoded by the major histo-compatibility complex (MHC) class 2D subloci, are also likely to play an important role. In becoming flat, it has been shown, both from clinical and experimental observation, that the mucosa progresses through each phase in a sequential manner, although it does not neces-sarily follow that all gluten-sensitized individuals inevitably develop flat mucosal lesions. What is certain, however, is that the majority of individuals regardless of the type of lesion, are asymptomatic. Those developing a symptomatic sprue-like malabsorption illness usually are found to have a flat, type 3 lesion. This lesion may be precipitated by a variety of environ-mental stimuli or stresses. (*From* Marsh [44]; with permission.)

TABLE 3-2. SUGGESTED IMMUNOLOGIC CAUSES OF END-STAGE (IRREVERSIBLE) INTESTINAL FAILURE

Presumptive immune-mediated

    Unresponsive gluten sensitivity

    Protracted diarrhea of infancy (immunologic variant)

    Scleroderma

    Diffuse intestinal lymphomas

    Graft-versus-host disease

    Marasmus/kwashiorkor/persistent diarrhea

TABLE 3-2.

Suggested immunologic causes of end-stage (irreversible) intestinal failure. This list is representative of possible immunologic mechanisms of celiac disease.

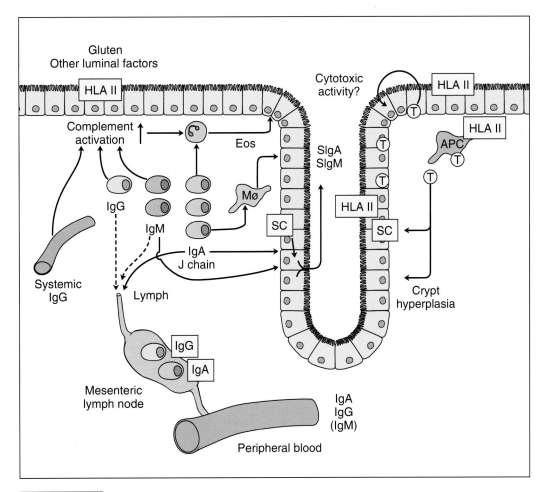

FIGURE 3-14.

Hypothetical scheme for immunopathologic mechanisms in celiac disease. Gluten, other (unidentified) luminal factors, and HLA class II molecules or enterocytes determine the initiation of the disease. Cell-mediated immunity is stimulated, and release of cytokines from activated T cells (T), antigen presenting cells (APC), and macrophages (Mϕ) induces crypt hyperplasia and enhances the expression of secretory component (SC) and epithelial class II molecules. Humoral immunity is also stimulated along with enhanced external transport of secretory immunoglobulin A (sIgA) and M (sIgM). Excess of locally produced IgA (and IgM?) antibodies will reach peripheral blood and reflect the severity of the mucosal lesions. The immunoglobulin G (IgG) antibodies are mainly produced in mesenteric lymph nodes and are a proper indicator of the activity in the lesion. Mucosal IgG and IgM antibodies activate complement and may thus harm the surface epithelium. Toxic proteins from eosinophilic granulocyte (Eos) also have deleterious effects, and these cells may be degranulated by polymeric IgA or immune complexes. Polymeric IgA also stimulates Mϕ to produce cytokines with effects on the epithelium, which in addition may be harmed by cytotoxic T cells, perhaps of the TCRγ or δ+ subset. (*From* Brandtzaeg [45]; with permission.)

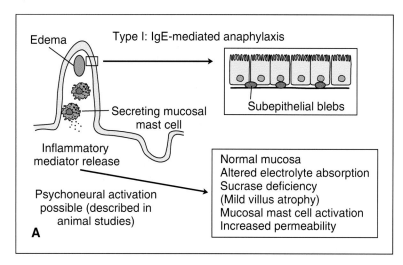

A

Type I: IgE-mediated anaphylaxis

Edema

Secreting mucosal mast cell

Inflammatory mediator release

Psychoneural activation possible (described in animal studies)

Subepithelial blebs

Normal mucosa
Altered electrolyte absorption
Sucrase deficiency
(Mild villus atrophy)
Mucosal mast cell activation
Increased permeability

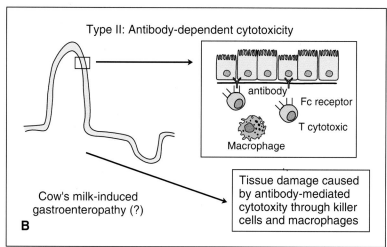

B

Type II: Antibody-dependent cytotoxicity

antibody

Fc receptor

T cytotoxic

Macrophage

Cow's milk-induced gastroenteropathy (?)

Tissue damage caused by antibody-mediated cytotoxity through killer cells and macrophages

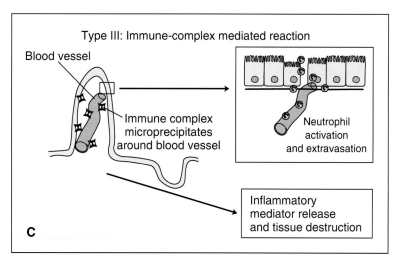

C

Type III: Immune-complex mediated reaction

Blood vessel

Immune complex microprecipitates around blood vessel

Neutrophil activation and extravasation

Inflammatory mediator release and tissue destruction

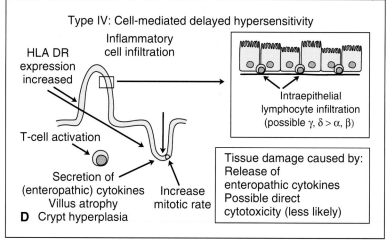

D

Type IV: Cell-mediated delayed hypersensitivity

Inflammatory cell infiltration

HLA DR expression increased

T-cell activation

Secretion of (enteropathic) cytokines
Villus atrophy
Crypt hyperplasia

Increase mitotic rate

Intraepithelial lymphocyte infiltration (possible γ, δ > α, β)

Tissue damage caused by:
Release of enteropathic cytokines
Possible direct cytotoxicity (less likely)

FIGURE 3-15.

Summary of the basic mechanisms of immunologically mediated damage to the gastrointestinal tract according to the Gell and Coombs classification. A, Type I: immunoglobulin E (IgE)-mediated anaphylaxis. B, Type II: antibody-dependent cytotoxicity. C, Type III: immune complex mediated. D, Type IV: cell-mediated immunity. (*From* Strobel [46]; with permission.)

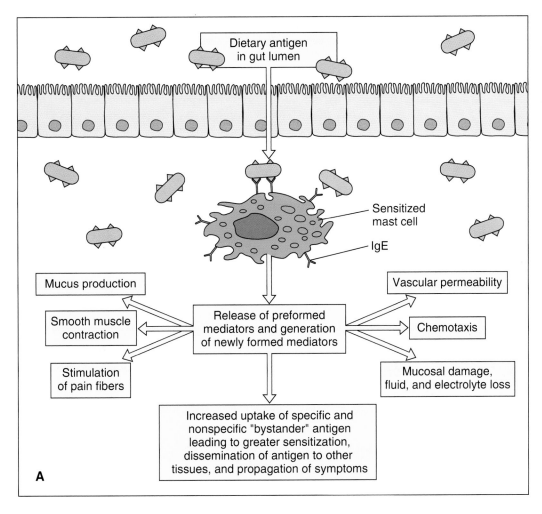

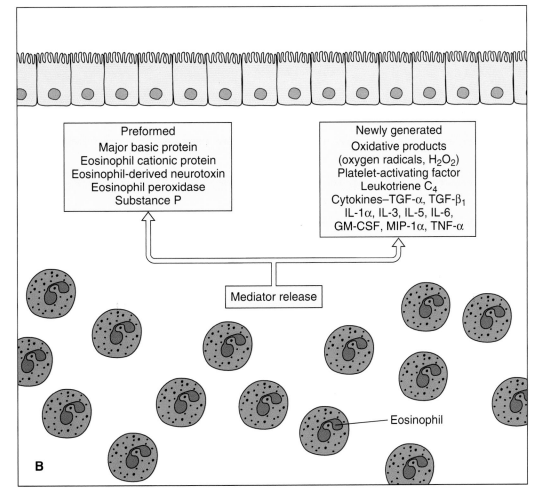

FIGURE 3-16.

A and B, Mechanisms of type I immunoglobulin E (IgE)–mediated hypersensitivity in food allergy. This diagram depicts the presumed mechanism of food allergy in young infants. Intact undigested antigens cross the mucosal barrier in large quantities. In the absence of an immune tolerogenic response, these antigens stimulate T-cell and B-cell responses. In this case, IgE antibodies are produced that form IgE-food protein complexes and interact with mast cells leading to mediator release and the symptoms of intestinal and systemic allergy and to a broadening of the allergic response to other antigens. GM-CSF—granulocyte macrophage-colony stimulating factor; IL—interleukin; MIP—macrophage inflammatory protein; TGF–transforming growth factor; TNF—tumor necrosis factor. (*From* Durr [47]; with permission.)

TABLE 3-3. MECHANISMS OF ORAL TOLERANCE

Antigenic peptides

Antigen presentation

Nature of intestinal lymphocytes suppressor vs helper

TABLE 3-3.

Mechanisms of oral tolerance. The precise mechanisms of oral tolerance are not established. The process may depend on the nature of the presenting peptide, *ie*, the degree of breakdown of proteins within the intestinal lumen or within the lysosomal compartment of the enterocytes. Some evidence suggest that intact nonhydrolyzed peptides are more likely to prompt a systemic immune process than to cause tolerance. In addition, the manner in which antigens are presented to T cells may influence the T-cell response. As the molecular biology of HLA class II antigens is established, it is apparent that multiple ancillary molecules are necessary before an antigen peptide can appropriately interact with T cells. In the absence of these ancillary molecules, an inappropriate T-cell response can occur. Finally, the nature of intestinal T cells may be the major deterrent of oral tolerance. Specific clones of T cells that preferentially suppress immune function might dominate over those that enhance immune responsiveness.

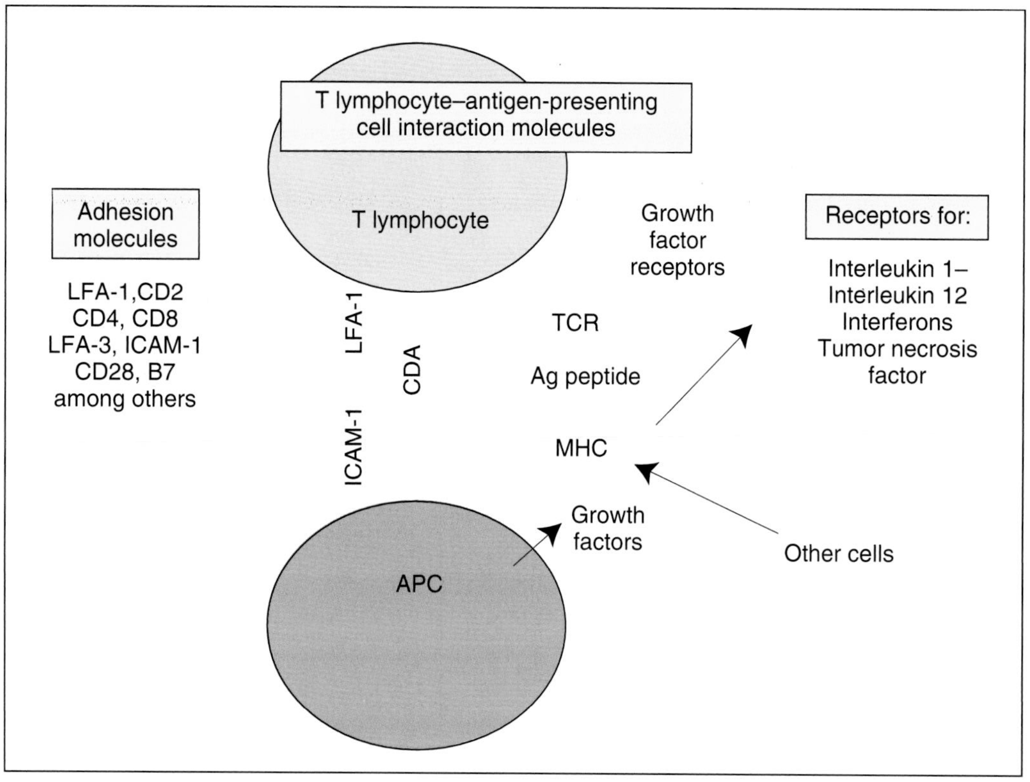

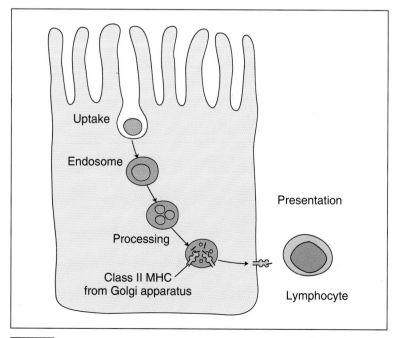

FIGURE 3-17.

This diagram depicts the complex interaction of antigen-presenting cell (APC) with a T lymphocyte. There are three types of molecular interactions between a T cell and an APC. First, the specific T-cell receptor recognizes the foreign antigen, in the form of a processed peptide (the antigen [Ag] peptide), bound in the cleft of the major histocompatibility complex (MHC) molecules of the APC. Second, a series of adhesion molecules on the T cell bind to their ligands on the APC. These include CD4 and CD8, which are coreceptors for the MHC molecules, and CD28, which interacts with the APC ligand B7 to provide "costimulation". Third, the T cell expresses receptors for various factors that regulate growth and differentiation (cytokines), such as interleukin 2, some of which are produced by other activated T cells and form the basis of "help" and collaboration. Although the T-cell receptor binding provides the primary signal to trigger the T cell, the outcome, which can be either a proliferate response or the induction of a nonresponsive state, depends on further signals from these adhesion molecules and growth factor receptors in order to put the antigen recognition "in context." (*From* Waldmann [48]; with permission.)

FIGURE 3-18.

Model of antigen presentation by an intestinal epithelial cell. Class II antigen expression occurs constitutively on villus cells in the small intestine and can be upregulated in crypt cells by inflammatory cytokines such as γ-interferon (γ-INF). Experimentally, enterocytes have been shown to present soluble protein antigen fragments to lymphocytes. One theory of oral tolerance is that enterocyte presentation to intestinal lymphocytes may cause a downregulation of the systemic immune response. One accessory antigen-presenting molecule, B7, is absent on enterocytes of preweaned neonates. Oral tolerance does not occur in the preweaned animal and the B7 molecule has been shown to be necessary for the induction of oral tolerance. This observation supports but does not conclusively prove the enterocyte's contribution to antigen presentation in oral tolerance. MHC—major histocompatibility complex. (*From* Sanderson and Walker [49]; with permission.)

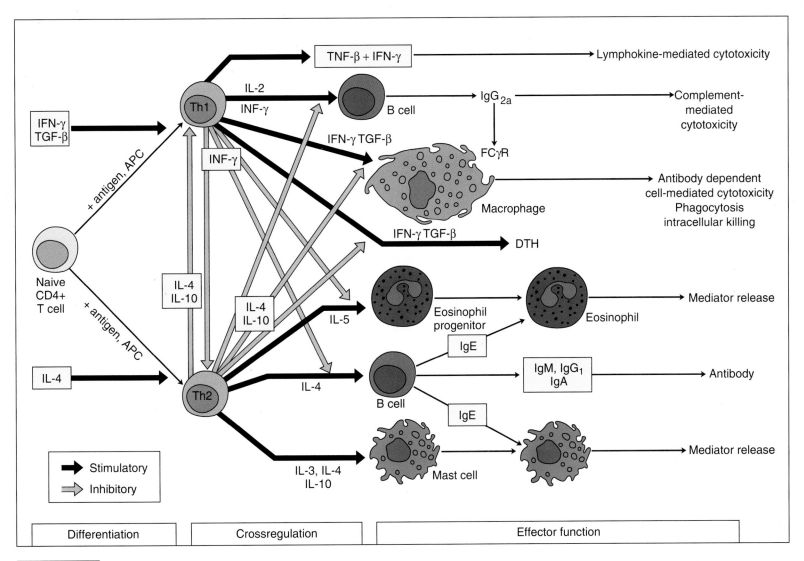

| Differentiation | Crossregulation | Effector function |

Legend:
- ➡ Stimulatory
- ⇨ Inhibitory

FIGURE 3-19.

Mechanisms of T-cell nonresponsiveness. Some possible mechanisms whereby the lymphocyte may contribute to oral tolerance include T-cell clonal deletion leading to cell death, clonal anergy, and suppressive cytokines produced by T-cell activation of suppressor T cells. This complex diagram illustrates the possible processes of T-cell suppression (inhibition). Under appropriate antigen presentation conditions, T helper cell 2 (Th2) subclass of T cells are stimulated to release cytokines (*ie*, interleukin (IL)-4, IL-10, among others) which act to *inhibit* or suppress T-cell and B-cell responsiveness. Many laboratories are actively defining these suppressive mechanisms which may determine new approaches to inducing oral tolerance in allergic and autoimmune patients. APC—antigen presenting cell; DTH—delayed type hypersensitivity; IFN—interferon; IgA—immunoglobulin A; IgE—immunologloblulin E; IgG—immunoglobulin G; IgM—immunoglobulin M; IL—interleukin; TGF—transforming growth factor; Th—T helper cells; TNF—tumor necrosis factor.

TABLE 3-4. USE OF ORAL TOLERANCE TO PREVENT ANTIGEN-SPECIFIC IMMUNOPATHOLOGY*

IMMUNOPATHOLOGY	ANTIGEN
Arthritis	Collagen
Encephalomyelitis	Myelin basic protein
Uveoretinitis	Uveal S antigen
Glomerulonephritis	Various proteins
Allograft rejection	Allogenic leukocytes

*Feeding a range of antigens of pathologic significance has been found to prevent induction of associated immunopathologic disease *·*

TABLE 3-4.

Practical application to the use of oral tolerance induction to prevent autoimmune disease states. Several recent studies have shown that oral feeding of a specific tolerogens in models of autoimmunity (arthritis, uveitis, encephalitis, etc) results in a decrease in symptoms and in immunopathy. This table illustrates the practical importance of understanding oral tolerance in the treatment of clinical disease.

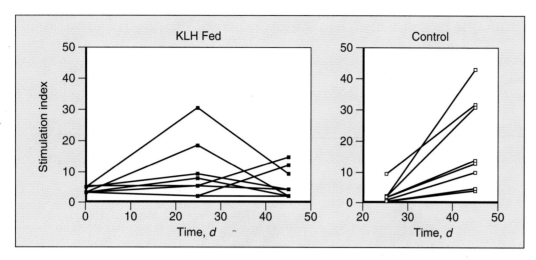

FIGURE 3-20.

Primary data from a recent clinical study show that oral ingestion of an antigen in humans can result in systemic tolerance. This general observation is the first evidence of this phenomenon occurring in normal human subjects and underscores its potential usefulness as a basis of treatment for immunopathologic conditions. Keyhole limpet hemocyanin (KLH)-induced prolif- eration of peripheral blood T cells. Data from each individual shown at day 0 before the study, at day 25 of oral feeding, and at day 44 after subcutaneous immunization. (From Husky [50]; with permission.)

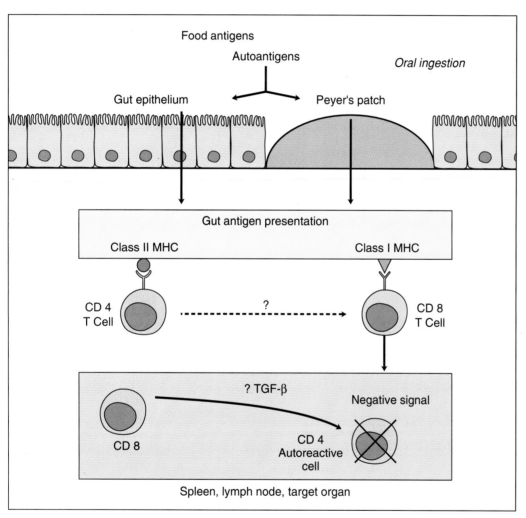

FIGURE 3-21.

Role of oral tolerance as a means of preventing or treating allergy and autoim- munity. This figure depicts a possible mechanism for this process. Oral antigen administration and subsequent specific suppression as a therapeutic option for the treatment of autoimmune diseases. After passage (processing?) through the mucosa and processing by the gut-associated lymphoid tissue (including enterocytes), antigen is presented in connection with class I or class II molecules. Preferential presentation in association with class I anti- gens will lead to activation of specific CD8+ T suppressor cells. Presentation in associa- tion with class II antigens will activate CD4+ T cells. A possible regulatory interac- tion between CD4+ and CD8+ T cells in this context is conceivable. Activated CD8+ T cells can provide a negative signal to (auto)reactive cells in affected target organs. A negative signal could be provided by transforming growth factor (TGF)-β. MHC—major histocompatibility complex (*From* Strobel [46]; with permission.)

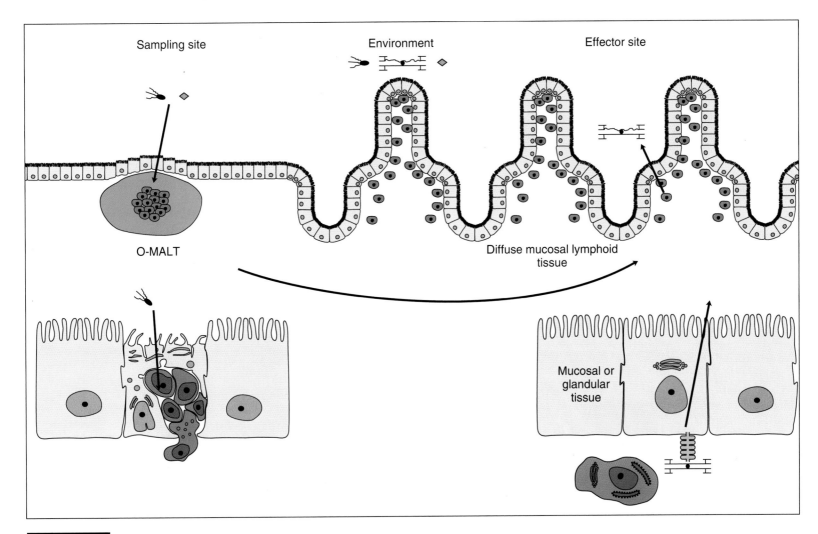

FIGURE 3-22.

Possible mechanisms of oral vaccine production. This figure depicts the known mechanism of bacterial stimulation of a mucosal immune response. A better understanding of this process may lead to an effective vaccine program against life-threatening enteric pathogens such as shigella and salmonella. The mucosal immune system is separated from environmental antigens by a tight epithelial barrier. Antigens are transported into mucus by specialized cells, M-cells found in epithelia over organized mucosa-associated lymphoid tissue (O-MALT) of intestinal, bronchial, nasal, and oral cavities. Following antigen stimulation in O-MALT, effector B cells leave O-MALT and migrate to distant glandular and mucosal sites where they differentiate into polymeric immunoglobulin A (pIgA)-producing plasma cells. Polymeric IgA is transported across mucosal and glandular epithelial cells by receptor-mediated transcytosis. During transport pIgA is cleaved and secretory IgA (sIgA) antibodies are released into secretion where they can interact with and eventually neutralize the antigens. (*From* Kraehenbuhl and Neutra [1]; with permission.)

■ REFERENCES AND RECOMMENDING READING

1. Kraehenbuhl JP, Neutra MR: Molecular and cellular basis for immune protection of mucosal surfaces. *Physiol Rev* 1992, 72:853–879.

2. Mestecky J, McGhee JR: Immunoglobulin A (IgA): Molecular and cellular interactions involved in IgA biosynthesis and immune response. *Adv Immunol* 1987, 40:153–245.

3. Elson CO, Kagnoff MF, Fiocchi C, *et al.*: Intestinal immunity and inflammation: Recent progress. *Gastroenterology* 1986, 91:746–748.

4. Walker-Smith JA, Jones RP, Phillips RD: The spectrum of gastrointestinal allergies to food. *Ann Allergy* 1984, 53:629–636.

5. Blaser MJ: Hypothesis on the pathogenesis and natural history of Helicobacter pylori–induced inflammation. *Gastroenterology* 1992, 102:720–727.

6. McKay DM, Perdue MH: Intestinal epithelial function: The case for immunophysiologic regulation implications for disease (part II). *Dig Dis Sci* 1993, 36:1735–1745.

7. Castro GA, Arntzen CJ: Immunophysiology of the gut: A research frontier for integrative studies of the common mucosal immune system. *Am J Physiol* 1993, 265:G599–G610.

8. Wick MJ, Madara JL, Fields BN, Normark SJ: Molecular crosstalk between epithelial cells and pathologic microorganisms. *Cell* 1991, 67:651–659.

9. Cooke HJ: Neuroimmune signaling in regulation of intestinal transport. *Am J Physiol* 1991, 226:G167–G178.

10. Crowe SE, Perdue MH: Gastrointestinal food hypersensitivity: Basic mechanism of pathophysiology. *Gastroenterology* 1992, 103:1075–1095.

11. Perdue MH, Gelbratti R, Davidson J: Evidence for substance P as a functional neurotransmitter in guinea pig small intestinal mucosal. *Regul Pept* 1987, 18:63–74.

12. Reichlin S: Neuroendocrine-immune interactions. *N Engl J Med* 1993, 329:1246–1253.

13. Hiribarren A, Heyman M, Desjeuz JF: Effect of cytokines on epithelial function of the human colon carcinoma cell line HT29. *Gut* 1993, 34:616–620.

14. Castro GA: Immunological regulation of epithelial function. *Am J Physiol* 1982, 243:G321–G329.

15. Stead P, Perdue M, Cooke H, *et al.*: Neuro-immuno-physiology of the gastrointestinal mucosal: Implications for inflammatory disease (Editorial). *Ann N Y Acad Sci* 1992, 321:654.

16. Walker WA, Harmatz P, Wershil B: *Immunophysiology of the Gut.* San Diego: Academic Press; 1993.

17. Kagnoff MF: Immunology and disease of the gastrointestinal tract. In *Gastrointestinal Disease.* Edited by Sleisenger JH, Fordtram JS. Philadelphia: WB Saunders; 1983:1001–1020.

18. Stenson WK, Alpers DH: A parable on the dangers of over classification: can an enterocytes assume immune functions? *Curr Opin Gastroenterol* 1994, 10:121–124.

19. Calderaro V, Giovane A, De Simone B, *et al.*: Arachidonic acid metabolites and chloride secretions in rabbit distal colonic mucosa. *Am J Physiol* 1991, 24:G443–G450.

20. Borivant M, Fais S, Annibale B, *et al.*: Vasoactive intestinal polypeptide modulates the *in vitro* immunoglobulin A production by intestinal lamina propria lymphocytes. *Gastroenterology* 1994, 106:576–582.

21. Walker WA, Isselbacher KD: Intestinal antibodies. *N Engl J Med* 1977, 296:767–773.

22. Bousvaros A, Walker WA: The development of the intestinal mucosal barrier. In *Ontogeny of the Immune Response of the Gut.* Edited by MacDonald T. Miami: CRC Press; 1990:1–21.

23. Israel EJ, Armentz P, Walker WA: Structural and functional maturation of rat gastrointestinal barrier with thyroxine. *Am J Physiol* 1987, 252:762–767.

24. Sanderson IR, Walker WA: Mucosal barrier. In *Handbook of Mucosal Immunology.* Edited by Ogra R, Mestecky J, Lamm ME, *et al.* San Diego: Academic Press; 1994:41–51.

25. Elson CO: Intestinal immunity and inflammation: Recent progress. *Gastroenterology* 1986, 91:746–768.

26. Freter R: Mechanisms of association of bacteria with mucosal surfaces. *Ciba Found Symp* 1981, 80:36–55.

27. Nadal D, Braegger CP, Knoflach P, *et al.*: Malabsorption syndromes and intestinal protein loss. In *Handbook of Mucosal Immunology.* Edited by Ogra R, Mestecky J, Lamm ME, *et al.* San Diego: Academic Press; 1994:457–480.

28. Blaser MJ: *Helicobacter pylori* and the pathogenesis of gastrointestinal inflammation. *J Infect Dis* 1990, 161:626–633.

29. Kagnoff M: Understanding the molecular basis of coeliac disease. *Gut* 1990, 31:497–499.

30. Dawoud AM, Mowat A: Immunohistochemical analysis of mucosal gamma-interferon production in celiac disease. *Gut* 1992, 33:1482–1486.

31. Marsh MW: Celiac disease. In *Immunopathology of the Small Intestine.* Edited by Marsh MN. Chichester: John Wiley; 1987:371–399.

32. Robey E, Urban A: Tolerance and immune regulation. *Immunology Today* 1991, 12:175–178.

33. Mowat A: The regulation of immune responses to dietary antigens. *Immunology Today* 1987, 8:93–98.

34. Husby S, Mestecky J, Moldoveanu Z, *et al.*: Oral tolerance in humans. *J Immunol* 1994, 152:4663–4669.

35. Barrett K: Acute and chronic chloride secretion by mast cell mediators. In *Immunophysiology of the Gut.* Edited by Walker WA, Harmatz PR, Wershil BK. San Diego: Academic Press; 1993:71–81.

36. Mannick E, Udall J: Nutrition and immunophysiology of the gut. In *Nutrition in Pediatrics: Basic Science and Clinical Application*, edn. 2. Edited by Walker WA, Watkins J. Toronto: Dekker 1996.

37. Iyingkarm: In *Clinical Diseases of Pediatric Nutrition.* New York: Marcell Dekker; 1981:453.

38. Walker WA: Antigen handling by the small intestine. *Clin Gastroenterol* 1986, 15:1–20.

39. Walker WA: Pathophysiology of intestinal uptake and absorption of antigens in food allergy. *Ann Allergy* 1987, 59:7–16.

40. Challacombe SJ, Tomasi TB. Systemic tolerance and secretory immunity after oral immunization. *J Exp Med* 1980, 132:1459–1472.

41. Eastham EJ, Lichauco T, Grady MI, Walker WA: Antigenicity of infant formulas: Role of immature intestine on protein permeability. *J Pediatr* 1978, 93:561–564.

42. Wallace JK: The role of inflammation in acid secretion and ulceration. *Mucosal Immunology Update* 1994, 2:3–5.

43. Crabtree JE, Lindley IJ: Mucosal interleukin-8 and *Helicobacter pylori*-associated gastroduodenal disease. *Eur J Gastroenterology Hepatol,* 1994, 6(suppl 1):S33–S38.

44. Marsh MN: Gluten, major histocompatibility complex, and the small intestine: A molecular and immunobiologic approach to the spectrum of gluten sensitivity (celiac sprue). *Gastroenterology* 1992, 102:330–354.

45. Brandtzaeg P: The serologic and mucosal immunologic basis of celiac disease. In *Immunology of the Gut.* Edited by Walker WA, Harmatz PR, Wershil BK. San Diego: Academic Press; 1993:295–333.

46. Strobel S: Food allergy: Role of mucosal immune regulation and oral tolerance: Facts, fiction and hypotheses. In *Immunology of the Gut.* Edited by Walker WA, Harmatz PR, Wershil BK. San Diego: Academic Press; 1993:336–375.

47. Duerr R, Fergus S: In *Immunology and Immunopathology of the Liver and Gastrointestinal Tract*, edn 1. Edited by Targen SR, Shanahan F. New York: Igaku Shoin; 1990:507–533.

48. Waldmann H: *Immunol Today* 1993, 2:15–21.

49. Sanderson IR, Walker WA: Uptake and transport of macromolecules by the intestine: Possible role in clinical disorders. (An update). *Gastroenterology* 1993, 104:622–639.

50. Husky: *Immunology* 1994, 152:4663.

Chapter 4

Mucosal Defense

FELIX W. LEUNG

The classic concept of ulcer formation is based on the premise that ulcers develop as a result of an imbalance between luminal aggressive and mucosal protective mechanisms. This chapter focuses on recent developments in concepts related to the defense mechanisms. Data based on human as well as animal studies in the stomach and duodenum are used to illustrate these concepts.

A hydrophobic surface (phospholipids and their bound fatty acids) is thought to provide the physical barrier to repel aqueous solutions, including acid. The hydrophobicity of tissue is measured by the plateau-advancing contact angle of a drop of saline (*see* Fig. 4-1). Evidence indicates that pathologic conditions are associated with decreased contact angles in the stomach and duodenum. Subjects with gastric or duodenal ulcers have significantly lower contact angles than controls (*see* Fig. 4-2) [1]. In subjects without ulcers, those with *Helicobacter pylori* in the gastric mucosa have a significantly lower contact angle compared with those without *H. pylori* (*see* Fig. 4-3) [1]. Surface active phospholipids constitute an important factor in determining tissue hydrophobicity. Decrease in the normal amount of surface active phospholipids presumably has adverse effects on mucosal protection. *H. pylori* infection significantly reduces (about 30%) the absolute amount of total phospholipids (*see* Fig. 4-4) [2]. In human gastric epithelium, *H. pylori* has been demonstrated by electron microscopy to damage the surface phospholipid zone (*see* Fig. 4-5) [3]. Ingestion of gastric mucosal surfactant by *H. pylori* (*see* Fig. 4-6A) and coating themselves with the surfactant (*see* Fig. 4-6B) have been demonstrated by electron microscopy [4]. These observations suggest that *H. pylori* may overcome one of the defense mechanisms by ingesting the gastric mucosal barrier of gastric surfactant, exposing the surface to attack by acid while simultaneously rendering the mucosa less hydrophobic. A detergent (Brij 35; Sigma, St. Louis, MO) attenuates protection conferred by dilute acid and prostaglandin against duodenal mucosal damage induced by concentrated acid (*see* Fig. 4-7), suggesting that surface active phospholipids are critical for adaptive cytoprotection against acid-induced injury in the rat duodenum [5].

The mucous layer maintains a pH gradient between the lumen and the epithelial surface (see Fig. 4-8A). The epithelial cell surface pH is higher than luminal pH during stimulated acid secretion (see Fig. 4-8A) [6]. The significantly higher surface pH in acid-secreting stomach (see Fig. 4-8B) probably reflects better availability of interstitial mucosal bicarbonate during stimulated acid secretion. Bulk transport of secreted acid in channels created by the gland luminal hydrostatic pressure may additionally act to limit acidification of the mucus gel. Recent in vitro studies showed that hydrochloric acid (HCl) secreted by the gastric glands can penetrate the mucus gel layer (pH 5 to 7) only through narrow fingers, whereas HCl in the lumen (pH 2) is prevented from diffusing back to the epithelium by the high viscosity of gastric mucus gel on the luminal side (see Figs. 4-9 and 4-10) [6]. These observations are consistent with the notion derived from in vivo microscopic study that acid is transported through mucus layer only at restricted sites (see Fig. 4-11) [7]. In experimental animals, intragastric nicotine protects the gastric mucosa against 40% ethanol-induced gastric mucosal injury. The protection is associated with an increase in gastric mucus and is related to activation of the α_2-adrenoceptors (see Fig. 4-12) [8]. Nitric oxide and guanosine 3',5'-cyclic monophosphate (cGMP) may play an effector role in mucus release from isolated gastric cells (see Fig. 4-13) [9]. In the proximal duodenum of duodenal ulcer patients, HCl-stimulated bicarbonate response is impaired (see Fig. 4-14) [10]. Carbonic anhydrase modulates basal and prostaglandin-stimulated, but not HCl-stimulated, duodenal bicarbonate secretions in humans (see Fig. 4-15) [11].

In vivo measurement of rat gastric surface cell intracellular pH (pH_i) indicates that these cells have the ability to regulate pH_i when pH in the luminal fluid is altered (see Fig. 4-16) [12]. Heat treatment induces heat shock protein and significantly reduces ethanol-induced damage in cultured guinea pig gastric mucosal cells (see Fig. 4-17) [13]. Endogenous glutathione in isolated rabbit gastric mucosal cells participates in protection against cellular damage (see Fig. 4-18) [14]. In humans, exogenous glutathione preserves gastric mucosal glutathione level and reduces ethanol-induced gastric mucosal lesions (see Fig. 4-19) [15].

Architectural arrangement of the mucosal capillaries facilitates delivery of bicarbonate from parietal cells to surface epithelial cells during acid secretion (see Fig. 4-20) [16]. Considerable evidence exists to indicate that mucosal blood flow plays an important role as a mucosal defensive factor. Tactile stimulation of the gastric mucosa leads to a prostaglandin-dependent increase in mucosal blood flow, which may play a role in protecting mucosa against contact damage with gastric content (see Fig. 4-21) [17]. Endogenous nitric oxide is a defensive factor (see Fig. 4-22A) and acts by preserving mucosal blood flow in the presence of a damaging agent (see Fig. 4-22B) [18]. Chronic normovolemic anemia increases gastric mucosal blood flow and enhances resistance of the gastric mucosa to ethanol-induced damage (see Fig. 4-23) [19]. Afferent nerve-mediated gastric mucosal hyperemia plays an important role in modulating the gastric mucosal injury associated with acid-back diffusion (see Fig. 4-24). Two hypotheses exist concerning the neural pathway that mediates the protective hyperemia supported by the afferent nerves (see Fig. 4-25) [20]. Studies in rats have shown that tobacco cigarette smoke aggravates a gastric ulcer by attenuation of ulcer margin hyperemia (see Figs. 4-26A and 4-26B) [21]. Such attenuation is reversed by prostaglandin treatment, which also reduces the aggravation of ulcer size (see Figs. 4-26C and 4-26D) [21]. Reduction in blood flow at the margin of duodenal ulcer is a factor associated with delayed ulcer healing (see Fig. 4-27) [22,23]. Afferent nerves mediate in part the protective mesenteric hyperemia after intraduodenal acidification in rats (see Fig. 4-28) [24].

Hypertonicity of gastric luminal fluid up to 1 mol/L (1000 mM) NaCl protects the gastric mucosa (see Fig. 4-29) [25]. Gastric mucosal hyperemia induced by 2 mol/L NaCl is blocked by indomethacin, suggesting that endogenous prostaglandin mediates the hyperemia (see Fig. 4-30) [26]. The gastric surface mucous cells contain the apparatus to respond to prostaglandin stimulation to induce an increase in the volume of iodoplatinate reactivity (a measure of phospholipids) of a family of lipid-containing organelles, which may underlie the ability of prostaglandin to increase the hydrophobic surface properties of the stomach (see Fig. 4-31) [27]. Cirrhosis is associated with a reduction in gastric mucosal prostaglandin and increased susceptibility to ethanol damage. The increased susceptibility is reversed by exogenous prostaglandin (see Fig. 4-32) [28]. Active and passive immunization against prostaglandins led to the development of gastric and duodenal ulcerations in rabbits (see Fig. 4-33), further confirming the important role played by prostaglandins in mucosal defense [29]. Bicarbonate in the blood is the mechanism of protection of increased blood flow after mucosal injury is induced by 2 mol/L NaCl (see Fig.4-34) [30]. Removal of serosal (extracellular) bicarbonate lowers pH_i in a gastric preparation (see Fig. 4-35) [31]. In an animal model of acid-induced duodenal villous damage, 16,16-dimethyl prostaglandin E_2–induced increase in basal alkaline secretion appeared to be a better predictor of protection against exogenous acid-induced deep villous damage than increased duodenal blood flow (see Fig. 4-36), because corticotropin-releasing factor similarly increases blood flow but does not enhance alkaline secretion nor reduce acid-induced villous damage (data not shown) [23]. In defense of the gastric mucosa during acid secretion, the increase in gastric mucosal blood flow is more important than the change in mucus secretion (see Fig. 4-37). Intravenous infusion of pentagastrin in a dose associated with maximal acid secretion increased mucus gel thickness, pH_i, and mucosal blood flow during superfusion with a neutral solution. Cimetidine abolished the increase in blood flow associated with pentagastrin, thus impairing pH_i homeostasis, although cimetidine increased mucus gel thickness in the absence of pentagastrin [32]. Evidence to support the hypothesis that endogenous nitric oxide mediates gastric mucosal protection continues to accumulate. Stimulation of endogenous nitric oxide synthesis by acetylcholine significantly reduces ischemia-reperfusion injury, and inhibition of nitric oxide synthesis by N^G-methyl-L-arginine abolishes the protective effect of acetylcholine (see Fig. 4-38) [33]. Inhibition of endogenous nitric oxide synthesis by N^G-nitro-L-arginine methyl ester attenuates alkaline response to 1 mol/L NaCl (see Fig. 4-39) [34].

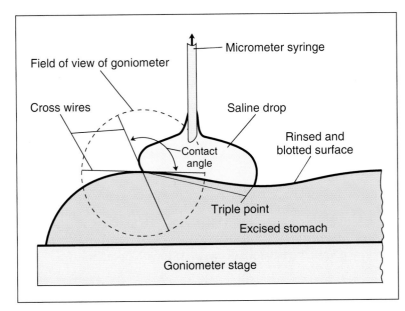

FIGURE 4-1.

Hydrophobicity of a surface is the tendency of a liquid to form beads on the surface rather than to spread evenly. The contact angle measures hydrophobicity and is defined as the angle between the solid-liquid and liquid-air interfaces at the triple point where solid, liquid, and air meet. The larger the angle, the more hydrophobic the surface. The schematic diagram demonstrates the ex vivo measurement of the contact angle of a drop of saline on a gastric mucosal surface. (*From* Hills *et al.* [35]; with permission.)

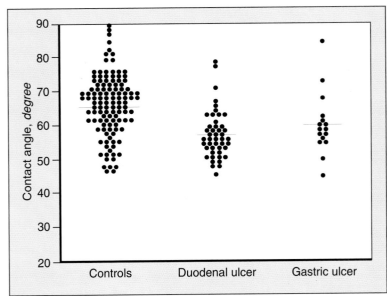

FIGURE 4-2.

Endoscopic biopsies of nonulcerated mucosa in the antrum and body of the stomach were obtained. The contact angle of a drop of saline on the fresh specimen was determined by an observer without knowledge of the endoscopic or histologic findings. Patients with duodenal ulcers (*n*=49) or gastric ulcers (*n*=17) had significantly lower mean contact angles than controls (*n*=124) without ulcers (57° in duodenal ulcer and 59° in gastric ulcer versus 66° in controls; *P* < 0.0001). (*From* Spychal *et al.* [1]; with permission.)

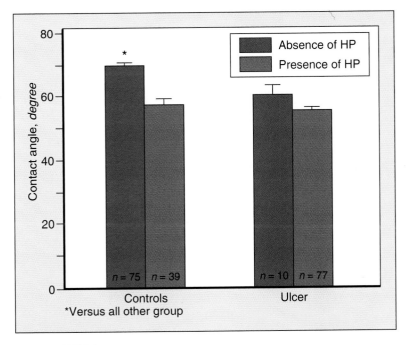

FIGURE 4-3.

Diagnosis of ulcer and *Helicobacter pylori* (HP) status are associated with significantly reduced contact angle (*P* < 0.001). (*From* Spychal *et al.* [1]; with permission.)

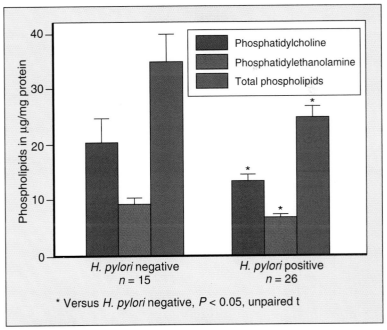

FIGURE 4-4.

Forty-one patients with chronic gastritis were endoscopically examined. Antral biopsies were obtained. Phospholipids were extracted from homogenates of mucosal samples, purified, and separated by thin layer chromatography, whereas bound fatty acids were analyzed by gas liquid chromatography. *Helicobacter pylori*-positive status is associated with a significant reduction in phosphatidylcholine, phosphatidylethanolamine, and total phospholipids. (*From* Nardone *et al.* [2]; with permission.)

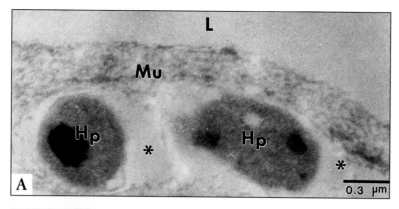
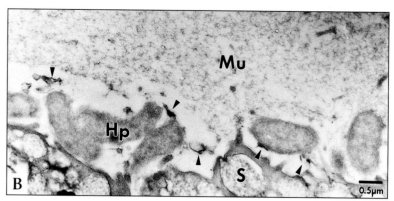

FIGURE 4-5.

In five patients with *Helicobacter pylori* (Hp) infection of the gastric antrum, endoscopic biopsies were prepared for iodoplatinate (a phospholipid-selective stain) staining and examination by electron microscopy. **A**, Electron micrograph showing Hp in the mucous layer (Mu). In the vicinity of the bacteria, there is a dramatic reduction in mucus (*asterisks*). **B**, Electron micrograph showing material reactive to iodoplatinate in Hp-infected surface mucous cells. Only residual surfactant-like material (*arrowheads*) is recognizable, adhering to the cell wall of the bacteria. L—lumen; S—secretory granules. (*From* Mauch *et al.* [3]; with permission.)

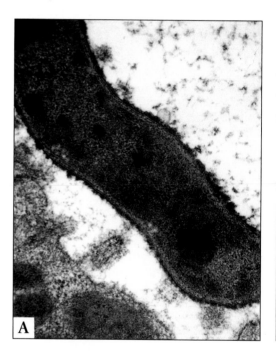
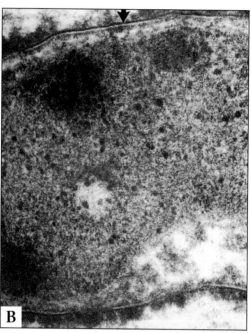

FIGURE 4-6.

In subjects whose *Helicobacter pylori* status was determined by *Campylobacter*-like–organism (CLO) test, Delta West Pty. Ltd, Bentley, Western Australia, endoscopic biopsies were processed for examination by electron microscopy. **A**, *H. pylori* is identified by its characteristic spiral configuration. Osmiophilic inclusions are demonstrated. *Bar* represents 100 μm. **B**, Enlargement of the cell wall of the bacterium shown in *A* reveals that the outer rail (*arrows*) of the tramlines representing the cell membrane is much denser than that on the cisternal side. *Bar* represents 25 μm. These observations suggest that *H. pylori* ingests gastric mucosal surfactant and coat themselves with the surfactant (*From* Hills [4]; with permission.)

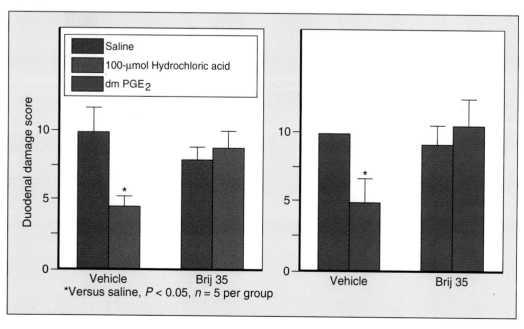

FIGURE 4-7.

Rats were treated intraduodenally with saline, 100-μmol HCl, or 16,16-dimethyl prostaglandin E$_2$ (dmPGE$_2$). They were given either vehicle or 5% Brij 35 (Sigma, St. Louis, MO) (a detergent) to solubilize and remove phospholipid layer from the luminal surface of the duodenal mucosa, followed by 500-μmol HCl. Duodenal damage scores (composite of gross and histologic evaluations) revealed that the protection conferred by acid or dmPGE$_2$ pretreatment were abolished by Brij 35 (analysis of variance with contrasts). (*From* Lugea *et al.* [5]; with permission.)

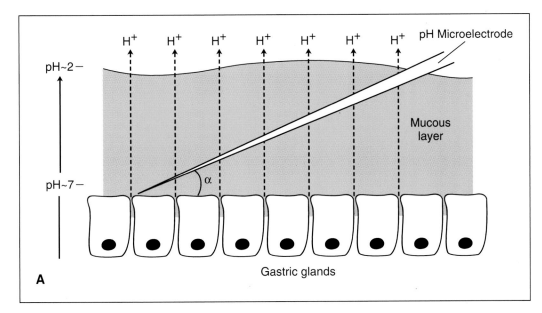

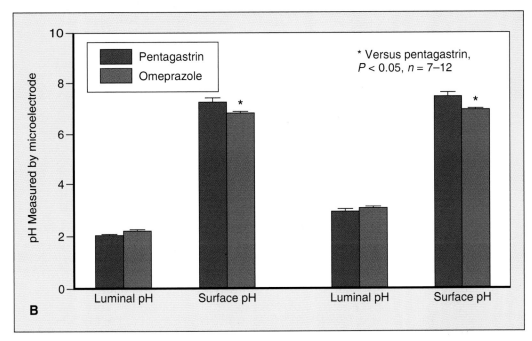

FIGURE 4-8.

A, Schematic of the continuous mucus gel adherent to the gastric mucosa. Epithelial and luminal pH were assessed by microelectrode. *Arrows* represent the suggested bulk transport of secreted acid. The distance between the two adjacent gland openings is approximately 45 μm. **B**, During pentagastrin stimulation, epithelial surface pH is significantly higher than that achieved with exogenous acid and inhibition of endogenous acid secretion by omeprazole (40 μg/kg/h of pentagastrin; 10 μmol/kg of omeprazole). (*From* Schade *et al.* [36]; with permission.)

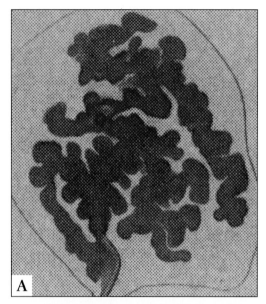

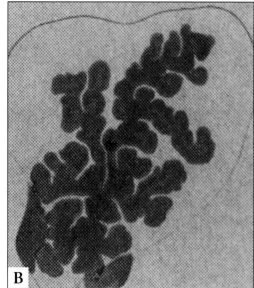

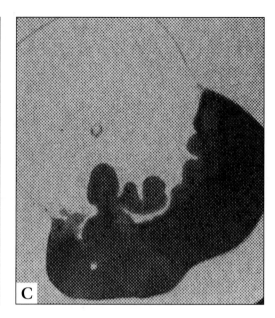

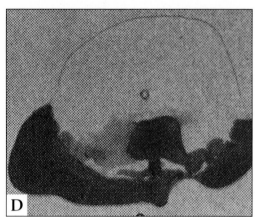

FIGURE 4-9.

Pig gastric mucin in a concentration of 10 mg/mL in 10 mM phosphate buffer was prepared (*white*). HCl (*dark*) (0.1 mol/L) containing 0.04% trypan blue was injected into the mucin solution from the periphery. At pH levels of 7 and 5, viscous fingering patterns developed (**A** and **B**). At pH 4, the bulk of the injected HCl remained on the periphery of the mucin preparation and only small, poorly formed fingers were observed (**C**). At pH 2, the acid did not enter the mucin at all (**D**) but instead flowed around the sample. (*From* Bhaskar *et al.* [6]; with permission.)

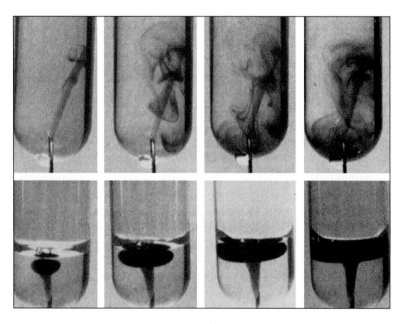

FIGURE 4-10.

To simulate the in vivo situation wherein secreted HCl travels toward the lumen through a layer of mucus, HCl was injected through a column of mucin solution in a test tube. When HCl (0.1 mol/L) containing trypan blue (0.04%) was injected into water solution alone, it diffused irregularly throughout the tube (*upper panels*). When HCl was injected into a solution of gastric mucin, the acid traveled in a discrete channel to the top, where it then layered horizontally on top of the mucus layer and did not diffuse downward into the solution (*lower panels*). (*From* Bhaskar *et al.* [6]; with permission.)

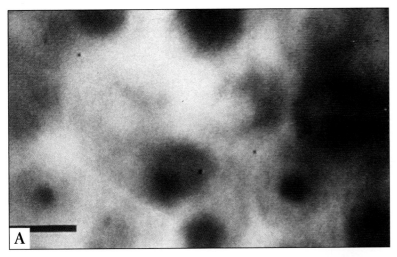

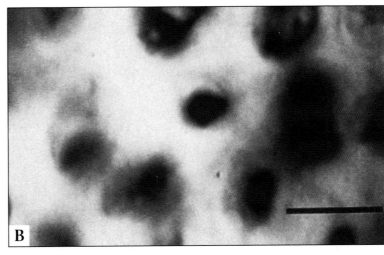

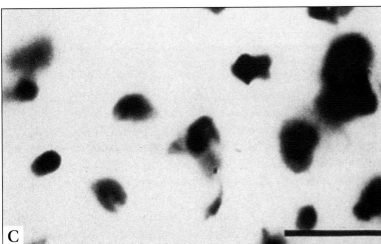

FIGURE 4-11.

In vivo microscopy of rat gastric mucosa and pH-sensitive dyes were used to study movement of acid formed in the gastric crypts across the mucus layer. Images of the gastric mucosa of a pentagastrin-stimulated rat were photographed. The surface mucus gel was stained with congo red. The dark areas correspond to areas of pH less than 3 in an actively secreting stomach. Each *bar* represents 50 μm. **A**, Focus is on the mucus gel closest to the epithelial surface. **B**, Focus is on a more superficial region of the mucus gel. **C**, Focus is on the luminal surface of the mucus gel. The images suggest that acid is transported across the mucus gel only at restricted sites. (*From* Holm and Flemstrom [7]; with permission.)

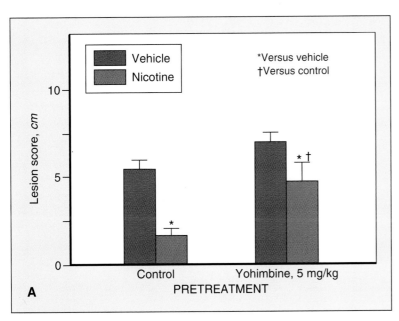

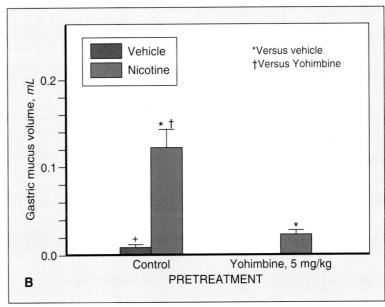

FIGURE 4-12.

A, Gastric mucosal injury was induced by intragastric 40% ethanol in rats. The lesions were significantly reduced by 4 mg/kg of intragastric nicotine. The protection was attenuated by yohimbine, an α_2-adrenoceptor antagonists ($P < 0.05$, $n=16$ per group). **B**, Intragastric nicotine significantly increased gastric mucus volume, but the increase is significantly attenuated by yohimbine ($P < 0.05$, $n=12$ per group). Data suggest that an endogenous protective mechanism involving increase in mucus secretion and mediated by α_2-adrenoceptor can be induced by intragastric nicotine. (*From* Endoh *et al.* [8]; with permission.)

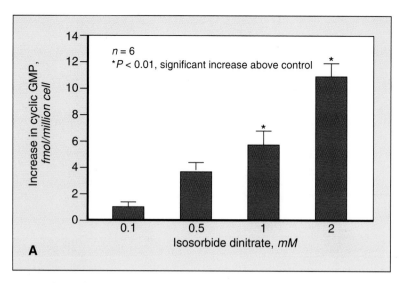

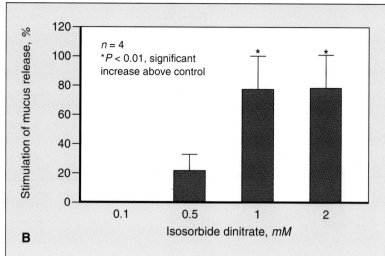

FIGURE 4-13.

In enriched suspension of isolated rat gastric mucous cells, mucin was assessed by an enzyme-linked immunosorbent assay. Isosorbide dinitrate significantly increased cyclic GMP content (**A**) and mucous release (**B**) (Mean ± SEM). (*From* Brown *et al.* [9]; with permission.)

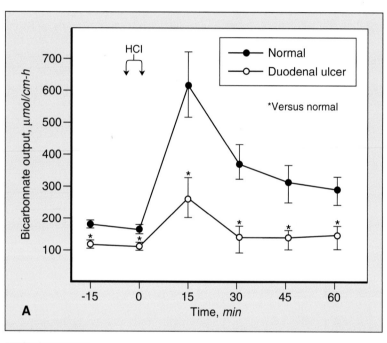

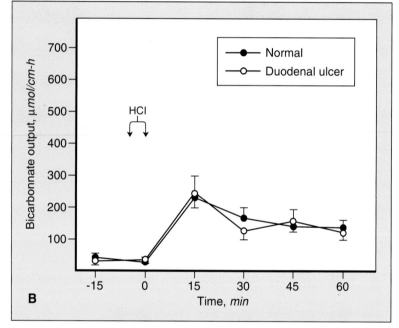

FIGURE 4-14.

A, Proximal duodenal bicarbonate output was measured in 16 normal subjects and 12 duodenal ulcer patients. **B,** Distal duodenal bicarbonate output was measured in nine normal subjects and nine duodenal ulcer patients. After basal measurements, 100 mmol/L HCl was infused for 5 minutes and bicarbonate production was measured ($P < 0.05$). Data indicate that in duodenal ulcer patients basal as well as acid-stimulated bicarbonate output in the proximal duodenum are significantly reduced. (*From* Isenberg *et al.* [10]; with permission.)

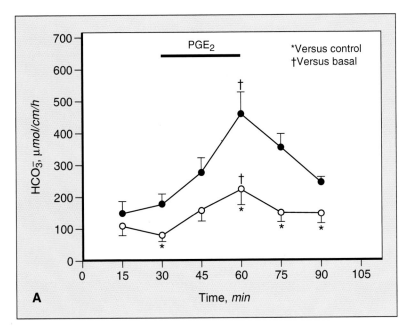

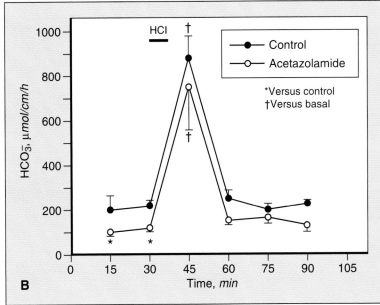

FIGURE 4-15.

Proximal duodenal mucosal bicarbonate secretion was assessed in seven human subjects. **A,** Luminal prostaglandin E$_2$ (PGE$_2$) increased duodenal bicarbonate secretion that was attenuated by the carbonic anhydrase inhibitor acetazolamide. ($P < 0.05$). **B,** Luminal HCl increased duodenal bicarbonate secretion, but the increase was not attenuated by acetazolamide ($P < 0.05$). Data suggest that duodenal mucosal carbonic anhydrase activity plays an important role in regulation of basal and PGE$_2$-stimulated duodenal mucosal bicarbonate secretion in humans. (*From* Knutson *et al.* [11]; with permission.)

EPITHELIAL CELLS

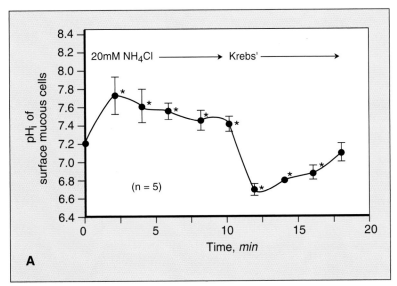

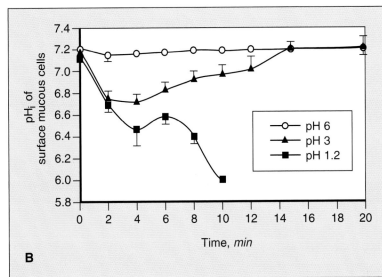

FIGURE 4-16.

Intracellular pH (pH$_i$) of the surface mucous cells of the rat stomach was measured by an in vivo fluorescent microscopic technique. **A,** NH$_4$Cl alkalinized surface mucous cells to pH$_i$ of approximately 7.7, with slow return of pH$_i$ to baseline. After replacement with Krebs' buffer, pH$_i$ dropped to 6.7 and then gradually returned toward baseline. **B,** Krebs' solution at pH 6 did not alter pH$_i$. At pH 3, there was transient decrease of pH$_i$ that gradually returned to baseline. At pH 1.2, pH$_i$ dropped quickly and did not return to baseline (Mean ± SEM). (*From* Kaneko *et al.* [12]; with permission.)

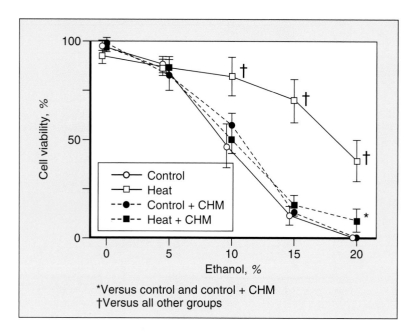

FIGURE 4-17.

Cultured guinea pig gastric mucosal cells were exposed to ethanol, and damage was assessed by trypan blue exclusion. Heat pretreatment that induced the synthesis of heat-shock protein in these cells (data not shown) significantly enhanced cell viability. The enhancement is diminished by cycloheximide (CHM), a protein synthesis inhibitor ($P < 0.05$, $n=4–5$ per group). Data support the hypothesis that production of heat-shock protein is an intracellular mechanism of gastric protection against ethanol damage. (*From* Nakamura *et al.* [13]; with permission.)

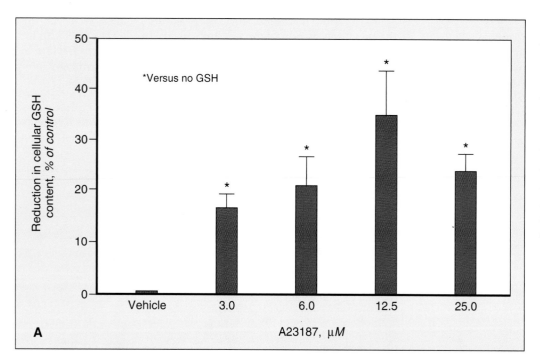

FIGURE 4-18.

Trypan blue exclusion was used as an index of viability of rabbit isolated gastric mucosal cells exposed to the calcium ionophore A23187. **A**, A23187 significantly reduced cellular glutathione (GSH) content ($P < 0.05$, $n=10$). **B**, A23187 decreased cell viability evidenced by the increased uptake of trypan blue. Exogenous GSH attenuated the uptake of trypan blue ($P < 0.05$, $n=6$). Data suggest that endogenous GSH plays a role in resisting damage induced by excessive increase in cellular calcium. (*From* Wong and Tepperman [14]; with permission.)

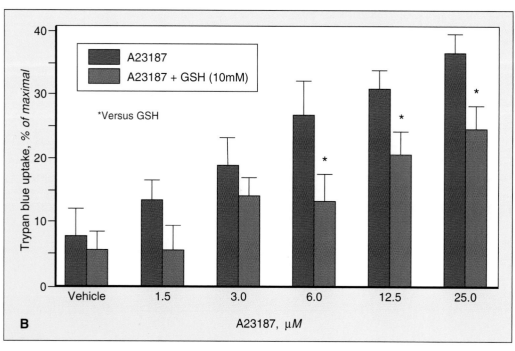

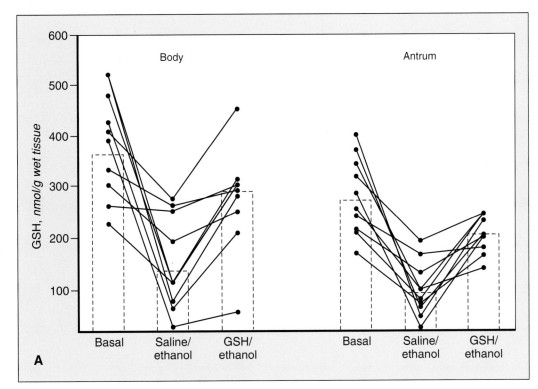

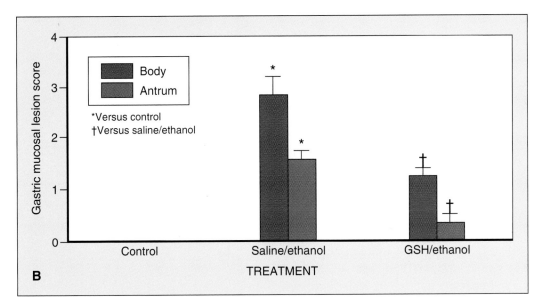

FIGURE 4-19.

In 10 healthy volunteers, gastric mucosal damage was induced by spraying 80% ethanol onto the mucosa. Endoscopic gastric mucosal biopsies were obtained. **A**, The ethanol significantly reduced glutathione (GSH) level, and the reduction was attenuated by exogenous GSH. **B**, The increase in gastric mucosal damage was also attenuated by exogenous GSH ($P < 0.05$). Data indicate that mucosal GSH plays a role in defending against ethanol-induced damage. (*From* Loguercio *et al.* [15]; with permission.)

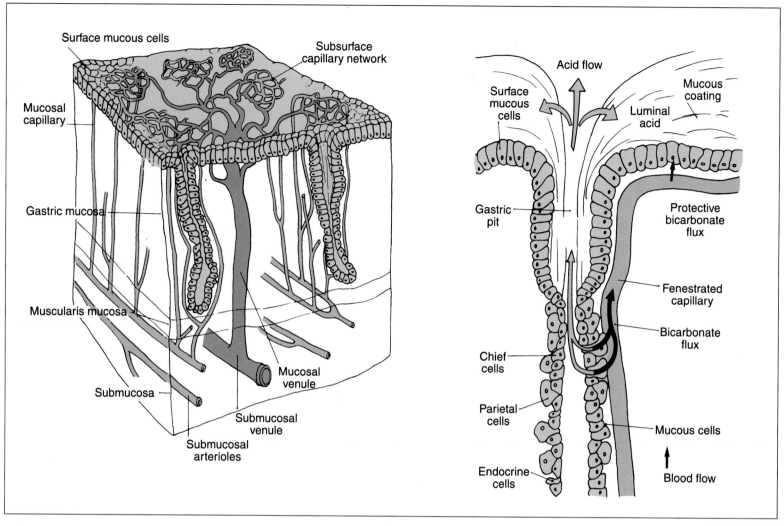

FIGURE 4-20.

Vascular casts of human oxyntic mucosa, examined by scanning electron microscopy, revealed an intimate association between the fenestrated mucosal capillaries and parietal cells. Capillaries drain into venules only in the most luminal aspect of the lamina propria immediately underlying the surface mucous cells. These architectural relationships support the hypothesis of vascular transport of bicarbonate released interstitially by secreting parietal cells from deep within the mucosa toward the surface epithelium to assist in defending the gastric mucosa against luminal acid. (*From* Gannon *et al.* [16]; with permission.)

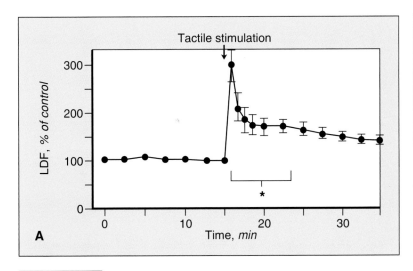

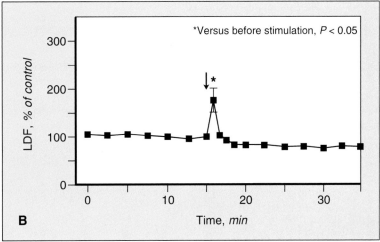

FIGURE 4-21.

Gastric mucosal blood flow monitored by laser Doppler flowmetry (LDF). Tactile stimulation led to a significant increase in blood flow (**A**) that was inhibited by indomethacin pretreatment (**B**) (analysis of variance with contrasts; *n*=6; Mean±SEM). Data suggest mechan-ical contact between the mucosa and food may increase mucosal prostaglandin, which can mediate amongst other protective events an increase in gastric mucosal blood flow. (*From* Holm and Jagare [17]; with permission.)

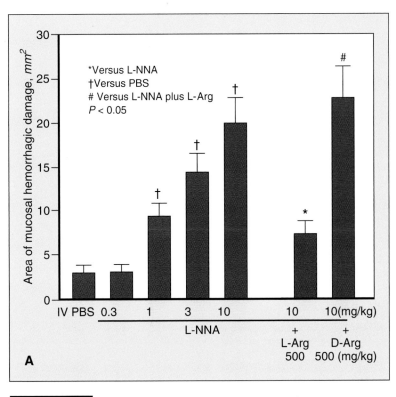

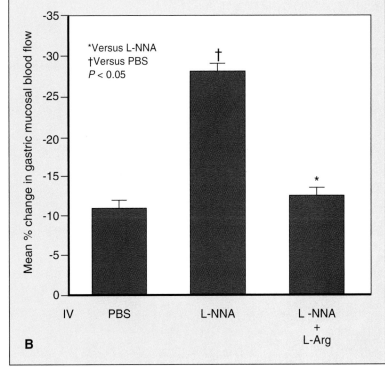

FIGURE 4-22.

A, Gastric mucosal injury was induced in anesthetized rats using 30% ethanol. N Omega-nitro-L-arginine (L-NNA), which blocks nitric oxide synthesis, significantly enhanced these lesions. L-Arginine (L-Arg) (a nitric oxide donor), but not D-arginine (D-Arg), significantly attenu-ated exacerbation in damage (*n*=5 per group; Mean ± SEM). **B,** Gastric mucosal blood flow was measured by laser Doppler flowmetry. L-NNA significantly decreased blood flow. Decrease was attenuated by L-Arg (*n*=5 per group; Mean ± SEM). The observations suggest that endo-genous nitric oxide is a defense in preserving gastric mucosal blood flow. (*From* Masuda *et al.* [18]; with permission.)

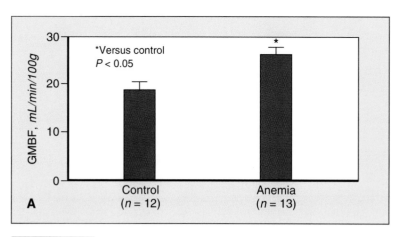
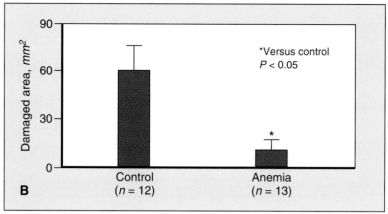

FIGURE 4-23.

Chronic normovolemic anemia was induced by withdrawing blood and replacing volume by plasma expander. Gastric mucosal blood flow (GMBF) was assessed by hydrogen gas clearance. Gastric mucosal damage was induced by 100% ethanol. Ethanol decreased gastric mucosal blood flow in control and anemic animals, although the final value was significantly higher in the anemic animals (**A**). Mucosal injury was also reduced in the anemic animals (**B**). Data suggest that chronic normovolemic anemia induces a protective mechanism associated with preservation of mucosal blood flow. (*From* Marroni *et al.* [19]; with permission.)

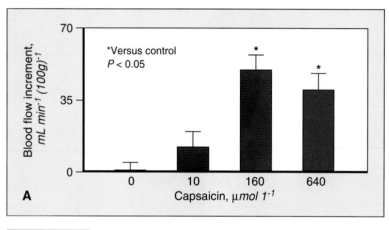
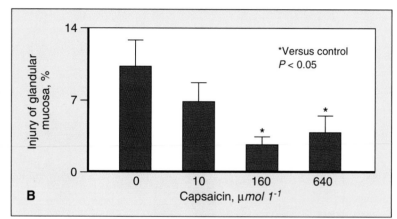

FIGURE 4-24.

A, Intragastric perfusion of the afferent nerve stimulant, capsaicin, significantly increased gastric mucosal blood flow in anesthetized rats. **B**, When capsaicin was perfused simultaneously with 25% ethanol, gross mucosal damage induced by the ethanol was significantly attenuated (*n*=8 per group). (*From* Holzer [20]; with permission.)

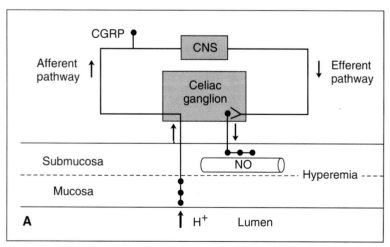
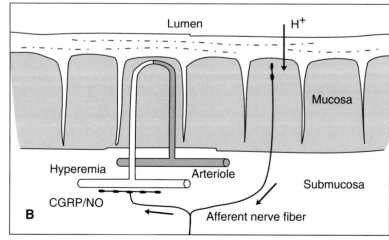

FIGURE 4-25.

A, Schematic representation of afferent nerve-mediated gastric mucosal hyperemia. Back diffusion of acid (H⁺) into the mucosa initiates an autonomic reflex involving afferent as well as pre- and postganglionic efferent neurons. Calcitonin gene-related peptide (CGRP) mediates the afferent neuron function. The efferent vasodilator involves in part activation of the nitric oxide (NO) system. **B**, An alternative hypothesis invokes an axon reflex between mucosal and submucosal collateral of an afferent nerve fiber. Back diffusion of H⁺ in the superficial mucosa activates the mucosal branch. Nerve activity is transmitted to the submucosal branch that releases CGRP to activate the NO system causing arteriolar dilatation. CNS—central nervous system. (*From* Holzer [20]; with permission.)

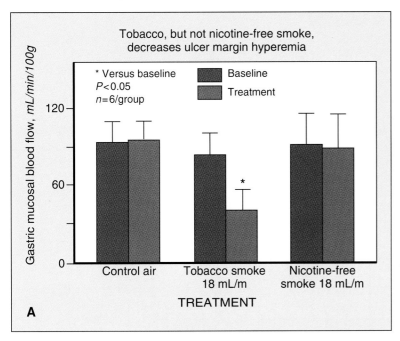

A

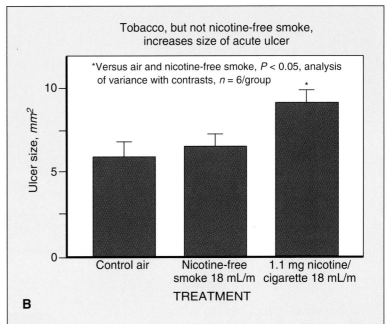

B

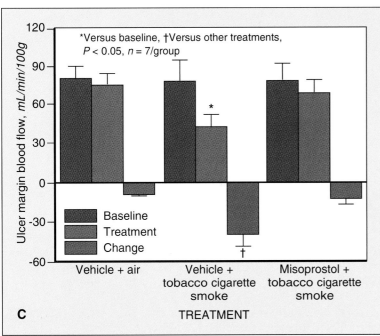

C

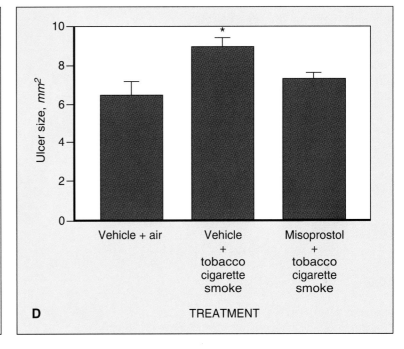

D

FIGURE 4-26.

Gastric ulcers were induced by application of acetic acid to the serosal surface of rat stomach. Blood flow at the ulcer margin was assessed by hydrogen gas clearance. Blood flow at the ulcer margin was higher than that of the adjacent nonulcerated mucosa (ulcer margin hyperemia). **A,** Acute exposure for 30 minutes to tobacco cigarette smoke, but not nicotine-free smoke, significantly reduced the blood flow at the margin of the ulcer. **B,** Repeated exposure to the former, but not the latter, three times a day for 5 days led to a significant increase in the size of the ulcer. Subcutaneous nicotine also produced similar effects (data not shown). **C,** The inhibitory

effect of tobacco cigarette smoke on ulcer margin hyperemia was attenuated by misoprostol (a prostaglandin E_1 analogue). **D,** The exacerbation of ulcer size was also attenuated by misoprostol. These findings suggest tobacco cigarette smoke exacerbates ulcers by weakening the protective mechanism of ulcer margin hyperemia, possibly by a nicotine-dependent pathway, which also involves an inhibitory effect on mucosal prostaglandin synthesis. (**A** and **B,** *Data from* Iwata and Leung [37]; with permission.) (**C,** *Data from* Iwata and Leung [21]; with permission.) (**D,** *From* Iwata and Leung [21]; with permission.)

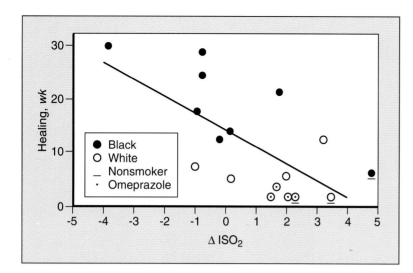

FIGURE 4-27.

The index of oxygen saturation (ISO_2), which is a measure of mucosal perfusion at the margin of duodenal ulcer and adjacent mucosa, was measured by endoscopic reflectance spectrophotometry. A higher value at the ulcer margin than at the adjacent mucosa represents increased blood flow at the ulcer margin. The difference in these values (ΔISO_2) was significantly correlated with rate of ulcer healing ($r=-0.6$, $P < 0.05$). Data suggest that increased blood flow at the ulcer margin compared with that at the adjacent mucosa is associated with faster healing. (*From* Leung *et al.* [22]; with permission.)

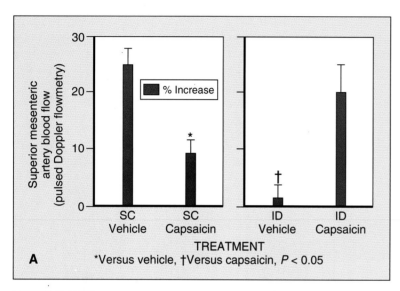

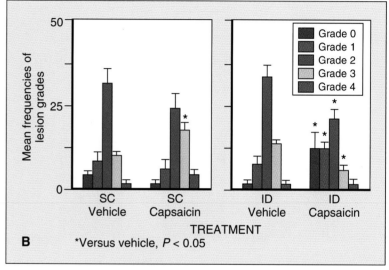

FIGURE 4-28.

Rats were given subcutaneous (SC) capsaicin to induce functional ablation of the afferent nerves or intraduodenal (ID) capsaicin to stimulate the mucosal afferent nerves. **A,** Functional ablation of the afferent nerves by SC capsaicin significantly reduced ID acid-induced increase in superior mesenteric artery (SMA) blood flow (t test; $n=8$ per group), whereas stimulation of the mucosal afferent nerves by ID capsaicin significantly enhanced SMA blood flow (t test; $n=6-7$ per group). **B,** These manipulations also enhanced or diminished deep (grade 3 or 4) duodenal villous damage, respectively (t test). Data are consistent with the hypothesis that the mucosal afferent nerves mediate protection against acid-induced deep villous damage. (*From* Leung [24]; with permission.)

■ INTERACTIONS AMONG PROTECTIVE FACTORS

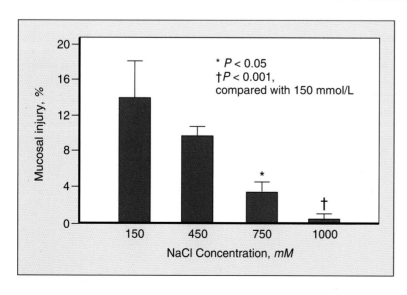

FIGURE 4-29.

Rats were treated with NaCl solutions. Thirty minutes later, the gastric epithelium was exposed to 100% ethanol ($n=6$ rats per group). A significant protective effect was observed with increasing tonicity. (*From* Barreto *et al.* [25]; with permission.)

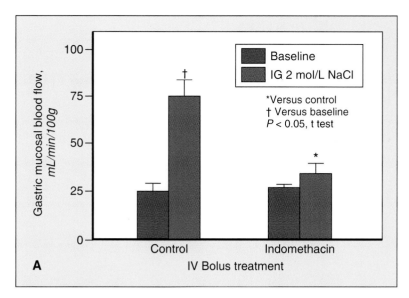

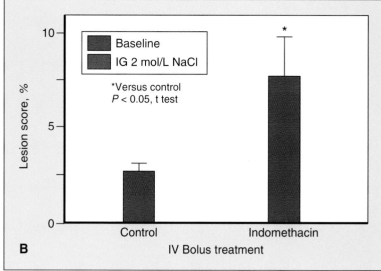

Anesthetized rats were prepared for gastric mucosal blood flow measurement by hydrogen gas clearance. After baseline measurement, rats were given intravenous (IV) control or indomethacin treatment, followed by 2 mol/L NaCl administered intragastrically (n=6 per group). Inhibition of endogenous prostaglandin by indomethacin significantly attenuated the gastric mucosal hyperemia (**A**) and increased gastric mucosal damage induced by 2 mol/L NaCl (**B**) (n=12 per group). (*From* Endoh *et al.* [26]; with permission.)

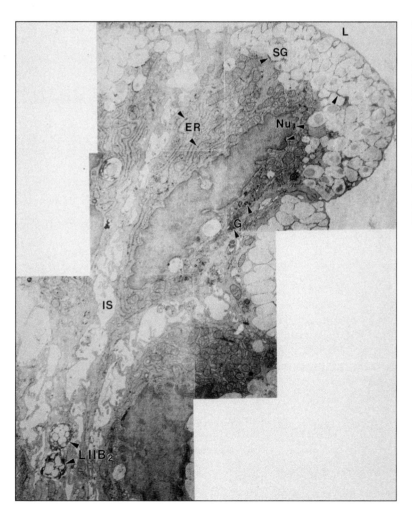

Rats were given 16, 16-dimethyl prostaglandin E_2 (2 μg/kg). Electron micrograph of the gastric mucosa revealed increased electron-dense iodoplatinate (a selective stain for phospholipids) reaction products in association with nuclear envelope (Nu), endoplasmic reticulum (ER), Golgi apparatus and its carrier vesicles (G), and mucus secretory granules (SG). The observation provides plausible explanation for the ability of prostaglandin to increase the hydrophobic surface properties of the stomach. $LIIB_2$ contained vesicular internal structures with intense iodoplatinate reactivity. $LIIB_2$ were located between the infranuclear region and cell membrane of the surface mucous cells. IS—intercellular space; L—lumen; $LIIB_2$—intranuclear inclusion body. (*From* Kao and Lichtenberger [27]; with permission.)

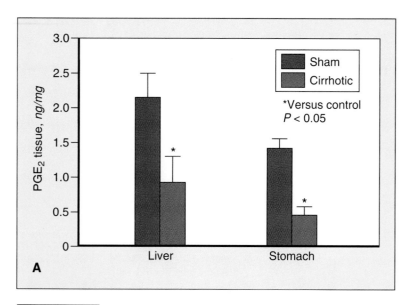

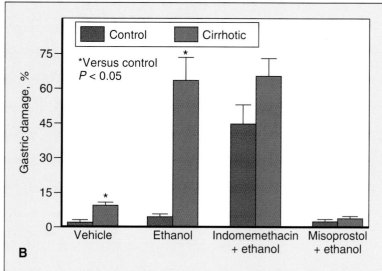

FIGURE 4-32.

Cirrhosis was induced by ligation of the common bile duct in rats (*n*=4–5 per group). **A**, Tissue prostaglandin level was significantly reduced in the liver and stomach in these cirrhotic rats (analysis of variance with contrasts; Mean±SEM). **B**, The gastric mucosa was exposed to 20% ethanol. The gastric mucosal damage induced by the 20% ethanol was significantly increased in the cirrhotic rats. The exacerbation was attenuated by misoprostol (analysis of variance with contrasts; Mean ± SEM). Data indicate that cirrhosis compromises mucosal defense by a mechanism associated with reduction of tissue prostaglandin. (*From* Beck *et al.* [28]; with permission.)

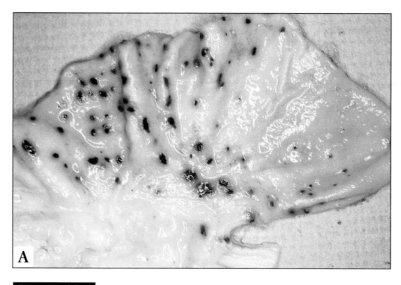

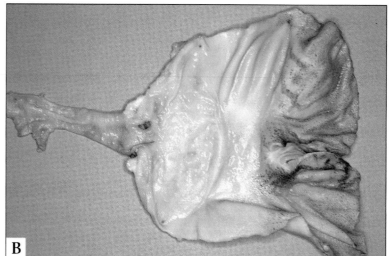

FIGURE 4-33.

Rabbits were immunized with thyroglobulin conjugates of prostaglandin E_2 and 6-keto-prostaglandin $F_{1\alpha}$. Gastroduodenal ulcers developed in these rabbits. Passive immunization of unimmunized rabbits with prostaglandin E_2-hyperimmune plasma also led to acute gastric ulcer formation. Examples of these ulcerations in the gastric body (**A**) and pyloroduodenal region (**B**) are shown. These observations confirm the essential role prostaglandins play in the mechanism of gastroduodenal mucosal defense. (*From* Redfern *et al.* [29]; with permission.)

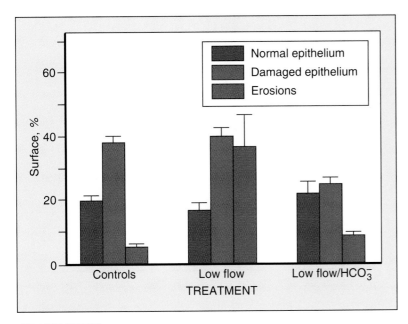

FIGURE 4-34.

Anesthetized cats were prepared for gastric blood flow measurement by microspheres and the gastric lumen was exposed to 2 mol/L NaCl, which induced a significant increase in gastric mucosal blood flow. Celiac artery occlusion to inhibit increase in blood flow (low flow) was associated with significant increased mucosal erosions. Intravenous bicarbonate dramatically reversed the exacerbation of gastric mucosal erosions in the corpus and fundus. Data suggest that the bicarbonate in blood is the basis of the protection afforded by the increased blood flow. (*From* Guttu *et al.* [30]; with permission.)

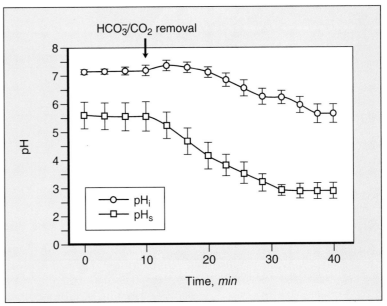

FIGURE 4-35.

Isolated Necturus salamander gastric antral mucosa was exposed to luminal acid. Intracellular pH (pH_i) and surface epithelial pH (pH_s) were monitored with microelectrodes. Removal of serosal bicarbonate (*arrow*) led to a reduction in pH_s and pH_i. The data suggest that a preepithelial buffer layer with pH gradient plays an important role in defense against luminal acid. (*From* Kiviluoto *et al.* [31]; with permission.)

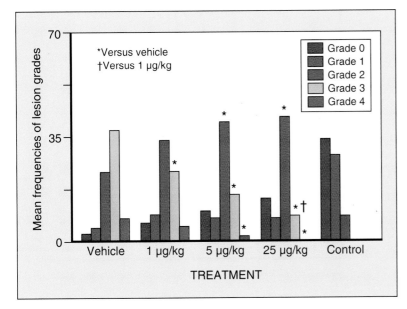

FIGURE 4-36.

Duodenal blood flow in anesthetized rats was measured by hydrogen gas clearance. Duodenal villous lesions were assessed after perfusion of the duodenum with 0.1 N HCl. Villous lesion grade was defined as 0 = normal, 1 = tip damage, 2 = tip to 25% length damage, 3 = 25% to 50% length damage, 4 = > 50% length damage. Rats were given vehicle or 16,16-dimethyl prostaglandin E_2 ($dmPGE_2$) subcutaneously in doses represented on the x axis. The significant reduction in deep (grade 3 and 4) damage by $dmPGE_2$ was associated with a significant increase in duodenal blood flow and alkaline secretion. (*From* Leung [23]; with permission.)

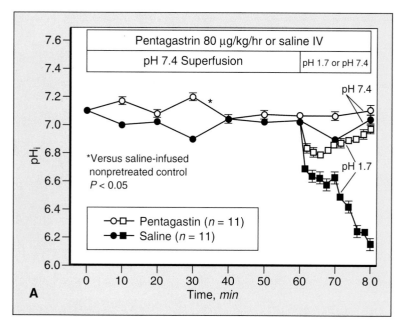

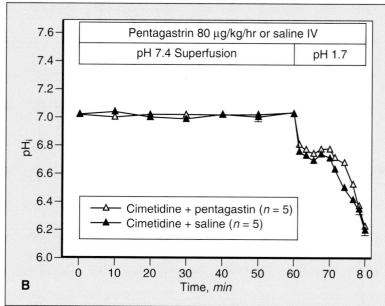

Gastric mucus gel thickness, intracellular pH (pH_i), gastric mucosal blood flow, and acid secretion were measured simultaneously in vivo, using a microfluorometric technique. Pentagastrin increased the pH_i of surface cells during superfusion with pH 7.4 buffer (**A**). During superfusion with pH 1.7 buffer, pentagastrin enhanced the rate of recovery of pH_i. **B**, Cimetidine eliminated the initial rise in pH_i and the enhanced recovery of pH_i towards baseline. Data not shown revealed that cimetidine abolished the increased blood flow associated with pentagastrin and increased mucus gel thickness in the absence of pentagastrin. These observations are consistent with the hypothesis that in the enhancement of defense during acid secretion, increase in blood flow is more important than increase in mucus. (*From* Nishizaki *et al.* [32]; with permission.)

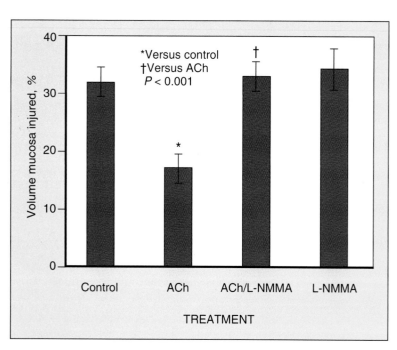

Rats were subjected to 30 minutes of gastric ischemia by celiac artery occlusion, followed by 15 minutes of reperfusion. Acidity in the gastric lumen was maintained by 100 mmol/L HCl during ischemia. The stimulator of endogenous nitric oxide synthesis acetylcholine (Ach) significantly reduced the gastric mucosal damage. The inhibitor of nitric oxide synthesis N_G-methyl-L-arginine (L-NMMA) reversed the effect of acetylcholine (analysis of variance with contrasts; Mean ± SEM). These data confirm reports that endogenous nitric oxide contributes to gastric mucosal defense. (*From* Andrews *et al.* [33]; with permission.)

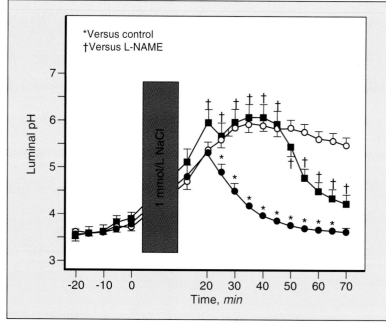

The output of bicarbonate (reflected by increase in luminal pH) from rat stomach mounted in an ex vivo chamber was measured. In control rats (*open circles*), topical 1 mol/L NaCl significantly increased luminal pH. The pH response was significantly attenuated by the nitric oxide synthesis inhibitor N^G-nitro-L-arginine (L-NAME), as shown by *closed circles*. The attenuation by L-NAME was reversed by L-arginine (*closed squares*) ($P < 0.05$. Mean ± SEM). Data suggest that nitric oxide is involved in the mechanism of the gastric alkaline response after damage with 1 mol/L NaCl. (*From* Takeuchi *et al.* [34]; with permission.)

ACKNOWLEDGEMENT

Supported by Veterans' Administration Medical Research Funds and in part by funds provided by the Cigarette and Tobacco Surtax Fund of the State of California through the Tobacco Related Disease Research Program of the University of California (1 RT 80). I would like to thank A. Bruce Ivie for his assistance in the preparation of the manuscript.

REFERENCES AND RECOMMENDED READING

1. Spychal RT, Goggin PM, Marrero JM, et al.: Surface hydrophobicity of gastric mucosa in peptic ulcer disease: Relationship to gastritis and *Campylobacter pylori* infection. *Gastroenterology* 1990, 98:1250–1254.

2. Nardone G, D'Armiento F, Corso G, et al.:Lipids of human gastric mucosa: Effect of *Helicobacter pylori* infection and nonalcoholic cirrhosis. *Gastroenterology* 1994, 107:362–368.

3. Mauch F, Bode G, Ditschuneit H, Malfertheiner P: Demonstration of a phospholipid-rich zone in the human gastric epithelium damaged by *Helicobacter pylori*. *Gastroenterology* 1993, 105:1698–1704.

4. Hills BA: Gastric mucosal barrier: Evidence for *Helicobacter pylori* ingesting gastric surfactant and deriving protection from it. *Gut* 1993, 34:588–593.

5. Lugea A, Mourelle M, Guarner F, et al.: Phosphatidylcholines as mediators of adaptive cytoprotection of the rat duodenum. *Gastroenterology* 1994, 107:720–727.

6. Bhaskar KR, Garik P, Turner BS, et al.: Viscous fingering of HCl through gastric mucin. *Nature* 1992, 360:458–461.

7. Holm L, Flemstrom G: Microscopy of acid transport at the gastric surface in vivo. *J Intern Med* 1990, 228(Suppl 1):91–95.

8. Endoh K, Kao J, Baker M, Leung FW: Involvement of α_2-adrenoceptors in mechanism of intragastric nicotine protection against ethanol injury in rat stomach. *Dig Dis Sci* 1993, 38:713–721.

9. Brown JF, Keates AC, Hanson PJ, Whittle BJR: Nitric oxide generators and cGMP stimulate mucus secretion by rat gastric mucosal cells. *Am J Physiol* 1993; 265:G418–G422.

10. Isenberg JI, Selling JA, Hogan DL, Koss MA: Impaired proximal duodenal mucosal bicarbonate secretion in patients with duodenal ulcer. *N Engl J Med* 1987, 316:374–379.

11. Knutson TW, Koss MA, Hogan DL, et al.: Acetazolamide inhibits basal and stimulated HCO_3^--secretion in human proximal duodenum. *Gastroenterology* 1995, 108:102–107.

12. Kaneko K, Guth PH, Kaunitz JD: In vivo measurement of rat gastric surface cell intracellular pH. *Am J Physiol* 1991, 261:G548–G552.

13. Nakamura K, Rokutan K, Marui N, et al.: Induction of heat shock proteins and their implication in protection against ethanol-induced damage in cultured guinea pig gastric mucosal cells. *Gastroenterology* 1991, 101:161–166.

14. Wong HM, Tepperman BL: Reduced glutathione modulates Ca^{2+}-mediated damage to rabbit isolated gastric mucosal cells. *Am J Physiol* 1994; 267:G1–G9.

15. Loguercio C, Taranto D, Beneduce F, et al.: Glutathione prevents ethanol induced gastric mucosal damage and depletion of sulfhydryl compounds in humans. *Gut* 1993, 34:161–165.

16. Gannon B, Browning J, O'Brien P, Rogers P: Mucosal microvascular architecture of the fundus and body of human stomach. *Gastroenterology* 1984, 86:866–875.

17. Holm L, Jagare A: Influence of tactile stimulation of the rat gastric mucosa on blood flow and acid output. *Am J Physiol* 1993; 265:G303–G309.

18. Masuda E, Kawano S, Nagano K, et al.: Endogenous nitric oxide modulates ethanol-induced gastric mucosal injury in rats. *Gastroenterology* 1995, 108:58–64.

19. Marroni N, Casadevall M, Panes J, et al.: Effects of chronic normovolemic anemia on gastric microcirculation and ethanol-induced gastric damage in rats. *Dig Dis Sci* 1994, 39:751–757.

20. Holzer P: Peptidergic sensory neurons in the control of vascular functions: Mechanisms and significance in the cutaneous and splanchnic vascular beds. *Rev Physiol Biochem Pharmacol* 1992, 121:49–146.

21. Iwata F, Leung FW: Misoprostol reverses the inhibition of gastric hyperemia and aggravation of gastric damage by tobacco cigarette smoke in the rat. *Scand J Gastroenterol* 1995, 30; 315–321.

22. Leung FW, Reedy TJ, Van Deventer GM, Guth PH: Reduction in index of oxygen saturation at margin of active duodenal ulcers may lead to slow healing. *Dig Dis Sci* 1989, 34:417–423.

23. Leung FW: Role of blood flow and alkaline secretion in acid-induced deep duodenal villous injury in rats. *Am J Physiol* 1991, 260:G339–G404.

24. Leung FW: Primary sensory nerves mediate in part the protective mesenteric hyperemia after intraduodenal acidification in rats. *Gastroenterology* 1993, 105:1737–1745.

25. Barreto JC, Smith GS, Tornwall MS, Miller TA: Protective action of oral N-acetylcysteine against gastric injury: Role of hypertonic sodium. *Am J Physiol* 1993, 264:G422–G426.

26. Endoh K, Kao J, Domek MJ, Leung FW: Mechanism of gastric hyperemia induced by intragastric hypertonic saline in rats. *Gastroenterology* 1993, 104:114–121.

27. Kao YCJ, Lichtenberger LM: Effect of 16,16-dimethyl prostaglandin E_2 on lipidic organelles of rat gastric surface mucous cells. *Gastroenterology* 1993, 104:103–113.

28. Beck PL, McKnight W, Lee SS, Wallace JL: Prostaglandin modulation of the gastric vasculature and mucosal integrity in cirrhotic rats. *Am J Physiol* 1993; 265:G453–G458.

29. Redfern JS, Blair AJ, Lee E, Feldman M: Gastrointestinal ulcer formation in rabbits immunized with prostaglandin E_2. *Gastroenterology* 1987, 93:744–752.

30. Guttu K, Sorbye H, Gislasow H, et al.: Role of bicarbonate in blood flow-mediated protection and repair of damaged gastric mucosa in the cat. *Gastroenterology* 1994, 107:149–159.

31. Kiviluoto T, Ahonen M, Back N, et al.: Preepithelial mucus-HCO_3^--layer protects against intracellular acidosis in acid-exposed gastric mucosa. *Am J Physiol* 1993; 264:G57–G63.

32. Nishizaki Y, Guth PH, Kim G, et al.: Pentagastrin enhances gastric mucosal defenses in vivo: Luminal acid-dependent and independent effects. *Am J Physiol* 1994; 267:G94–G104.

33. Andrews FJ, Malcontenti-Wilson C, O'Brien PE: Protection against gastric ischemia-reperfusion injury by nitric oxide generators. *Dig Dis Sci* 1994, 39:366–373.

34. Takeuchi K, Ohuchi T, Okabe S: Endogenous nitric oxide in gastric alkaline response in the rat stomach after damage. *Gastroenterology* 1994, 106:367–374.

35. Hills BA, Butler BD, Lichtenberger LM: Gastric mucosal barrier: Hydrophobic lining to the lumen of the stomach. *Am J Physiol* 1983, 244:G561–G568.

36. Schade C, Flemstrom G, Holm L: Hydrogen ion concentration in the mucus layer on top of acid-stimulated and -inhibited rat gastric mucosa. *Gastroenterology* 1994, 107:180–188.

37. Iwata F, Leung FW: Tobacco cigarette smoke aggravates gastric ulcer in rats by attenuation of ulcer margin hyperemia. *Am J Physiol* 1995, 268: G 153–G 160.

Chapter 5

Stomach and Duodenum: Injuries, Infections, and Inflammation

EDWARD LEE
BYRON CRYER

There are many agents that may result in injury or inflammation in the stomach and duodenum. For example, noxious agents such as nonsteroidal anti-inflammatory drugs or alcohol may result in gross gastroduodenal injury. Infectious agents such as *Helicobacter pylori* or *Treponema pallidum* may result in inflammation of the stomach or duodenum. As evidenced by the examples given, the etiologies that cause gastroduodenal injury are vastly different in that they share no apparent similarities. Despite the diverse nature of these insults, however, the potential gross and histologic gastroduodenal responses are relatively limited.

Strictly speaking, the term *gastritis* histologically describes an increase in the number of inflammatory cells in the gastric mucosa. Gastritis, however, is frequently used indiscriminately for gastric mucosal conditions with and without histologic inflammation. There may be agents such as nonsteroidal anti-inflammatory drugs that cause endoscopically assessed mucosal injury without an attendant increase in histologic inflammation. On the other hand, *H. pylori* infection commonly results in histologic inflammation without much endoscopically detectable injury. Such discrepancies have led to considerable confusion in establishing the definition and classification of gastritis.

This chapter presents a framework for the classification of the variety of insults that may result in the stomach or duodenum. Endoscopic injury, *ie, gastropathy*, will be differentiated from histologic injury (*ie, gastritis*). This chapter also provides descriptions of endoscopic, radiologic, or histologic characteristics observed in response to number of specific injurious or infectious agents.

GASTRITIS

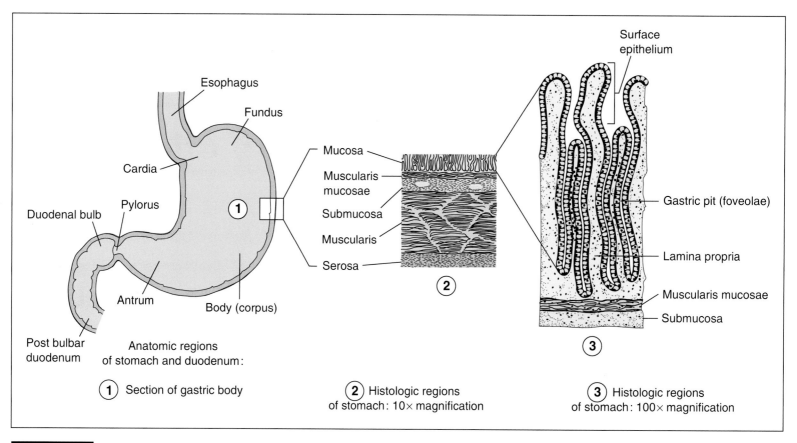

Esophagus

Fundus

Cardia

Pylorus

Duodenal bulb

Antrum

Body (corpus)

Post bulbar
duodenum

Anatomic regions
of stomach and duodenum:

Mucosa
Muscularis
mucosae
Submucosa
Muscularis
Serosa

Surface
epithelium

Gastric pit (foveolae)

Lamina propria

Muscularis mucosae
Submucosa

(1) Section of gastric body

(2) Histologic regions
of stomach: 10× magnification

(3) Histologic regions
of stomach: 100× magnification

FIGURE 5-1.

Gastritis: overview of anatomy and histology. Gastritis encompasses a heterogeneous group of gastric mucosal disorders, characterized by widespread injury at the gross and microscopic levels, which is usually associated with an acute, chronic, or mixed mucosal inflammatory cell component. Depending on etiology, gastritis may affect various mucosal regions of the stomach differentially. The cardia gland mucosa occupies an area 2 cm below the gastroesophageal junction. It is composed primarily of mucous glands.

The fundic gland mucosa covers both the gastric fundus and gastric body and is composed primarily of parietal and chief cells. The antral gland mucosa covers the anatomic antrum and is composed primarily of mucus cells and gastrin-producing cells. On microscopic evaluation of gastric biopsies, the increased inflammatory cell infiltrate in gastritis will primarily involve the mucosal layer. With different types of gastritis, various parts of the gastric mucosa may be variably involved (surface epithelium versus gastric pits) and the predominant type of inflammatory cells may vary (*eg*, lymphocyte, neutrophil, eosinophil, or granuloma formation).

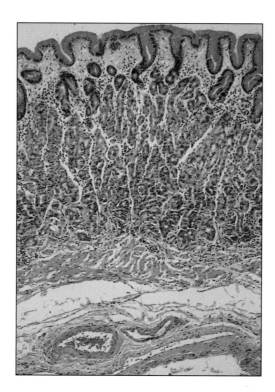

FIGURE 5-2.

Normal fundic mucosa. The figures in this chapter review various types of gastritis and associated features. Before reviewing abnormal gastric mucosal histology, however, a histologic orientation of normal fundic mucosa is presented. In biopsies of normal fundic mucosa, small numbers of lymphocytes and plasma cells are normally found within the lamina propria, the space between the glands and epithelial cells that is comprised of connective tissue. In noninflamed gastric biopsies, neutrophils are not normally present.

TABLE 5-1. GENERAL CLASSIFICATION OF GASTRITIS

Category	Nomenclature	Diagnostic modality	Etiology
Endoscopic	Gastropathy	Endoscopy	NSAIDs, physiologic stress, alchohol, chemical agents, and idiopathic
Histologic			
Acute	Acute erosive hemorrhagic gastritis	Endoscopic biopsy and histologic evaluation	NSAIDs, physiologic stress, alchohol, chemical agents, and idiopathic
Chronic			
Nonspecific	Chronic active superficial gastritis Chronic superficial gastritis Chronic atrophic gastritis	Endoscopic biopsy and histologic evaluation	Helicobacter pylori, autoimmune, and bile reflux
Specific	Depends on etiology	Endoscopic biopsy and histologic evaluation	Bacterial, viral, fungal parasitic, granulomatous, eosinophilic, and hypertrophic

TABLE 5-1.

General classification of gastritis. Gastritis may be determined endoscopically or histologically. Endoscopic gastritis is defined by gross findings of mucosal erosions or focal hemorrhagic lesions. On mucosal biopsy of these endoscopic abnormalities, epithelial and vascular changes predominate and, about half the time, no increased inflammatory cell infiltrate is present.

Classifications of histologic gastritis vary because there is no general agreement on its classification. Histologic gastritis, by definition, is associated with increased mucosal inflammation on microscopic examination and, in our classification, is separated into acute and chronic forms. Acute erosive hemorrhagic gastritis is the histologic correlate of acute mucosal injury detected endoscopically. Chronic gastritis is divided into nonspecific and specific categories.

Before the discovery of the involvement of *Helicobacter pylori*, few of the nonspecific forms of gastritis could be linked to a single etiologic agent or disease process. Most of the nonspecific forms now, however, appear to be related to the effects of *H. pylori*. Morphologically, nonspecific gastritis is characterized by variable microscopic patterns, and, depending on the pattern, can be further classified as chronic active superficial gastritis, chronic superficial gastritis, or chronic atrophic gastritis. Specific histologic gastritis is associated with a specific etiologic agent or disease process and most forms have a distinctive morphology. NSAIDs—nonsteroidal anti-inflammatory drugs.

EROSIVE GASTRITIS: VIEWED BY ENDOSCOPY

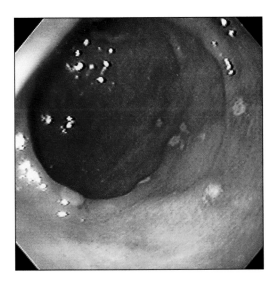

FIGURE 5-3.

Endoscopic erosive gastritis. The observations of multiple erosive and hemorrhagic lesions may be defined endoscopically as gastritis. This figure is an example of endoscopic erosive gastritis. Common settings that may lead to endoscopic gastritis include use of nonsteroidal anti-inflammatory drugs, alcohol abuse, and the physiologic stress associated with serious illnesses (stress gastritis). Other less common causes include ingestion of corrosives, chemotherapeutic agents, or irradiation. There may also be no known demonstrable associated factor present (idiopathic). (*Courtesy of* W. Harford, Dallas, TX)

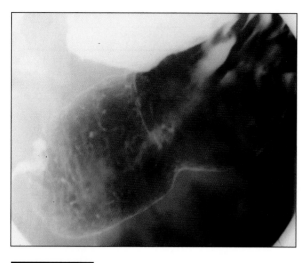

FIGURE 5-4.

Erosive gastritis on upper gastrointestinal barium examination. Superficial gastric erosions appear radiographically as multiple tiny flecks of barium, which represent the erosions, surrounded by radiolucent halos, which represent surrounding mounds of edematous mucosa. Superficial gastric erosions can also appear as flat defects that coat with barium without surrounding reaction and are represented by reproducible linear streaks or dots of contrast. This barium study is an example of the radiographic appearance of erosive gastritis showing multiple tiny flecks, some surrounded by halos. It also shows areas of coalescence of lesions into linear streaks. (*Courtesy of* W. L. Peterson, Dallas TX)

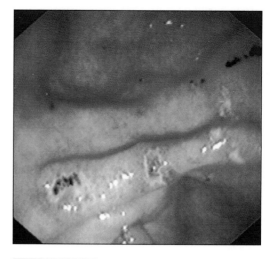

FIGURE 5-5.

Gastritis. Aspirin and other nonsteroidal anti-inflammatory drugs (NSAIDs). As shown in this figure, ingestion of aspirin and other NSAIDs can produce acute gastric mucosal erosions and subepithelial hemorrhages. Although found in all gastric locations, these NSAID–associated lesions have a predilection for the fundus and body. The constellation of multiple small erosions and multiple small submucosal hemorrhages throughout the stomach is very suggestive of NSAID use. On microscopic evaluation, the occurrence of a mucosal inflammatory infiltrate is not greater than that expected for age-matched controls who are not taking NSAIDs. Thus, NSAIDs do not actually cause a histologic gastritis. A more appropriate term for this condition is *NSAID gastropathy.*

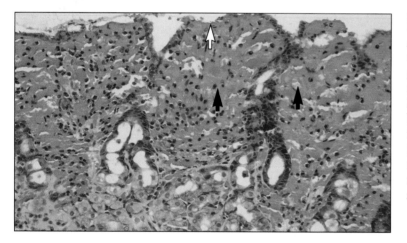

FIGURE 5-6.

Acute erosive hemorrhagic gastritis. As already mentioned, acute erosive hemorrhagic gastritis is the histologic correlate for the gross mucosal injury (erosions and hemorrhage) associated with agents such as nonsteroidal anti-inflammatory drugs. As shown here, the histologic features are erosions (*open arrow*) as evidenced by denuding of surface epithelium with necrosis of the glands involving the superficial third of the mucosa and hemorrhage (*closed arrow*) also involving the superficial portion of the gastric mucosa. It is this lack of penetration of the necrosis down to the muscularis layer that differentiates acute erosive gastritis from acute ulceration.

CONDITIONS RELATED TO ALCOHOL CONSUMPTION

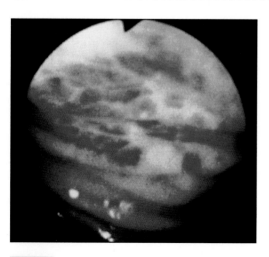

FIGURE 5-7.

Endoscopic gastritis: alcohol. Alcohol consumption can result in endoscopic mucosal abnormalities termed *alcoholic hemorrhagic gastritis*. As shown in this figure, endoscopically such patients will have multiple subepithelial hemorrhages without any visible breaks in the mucosa. The appearance has been described as that of "blood under plastic wrap". These lesions are mainly confined to the body and fundus of the stomach and are infrequently seen in the antrum. The histology of hemorrhagic alcoholic gastritis is shown in Figure 5-8. (*From* Laine and Weinstein [1]; with permission.)

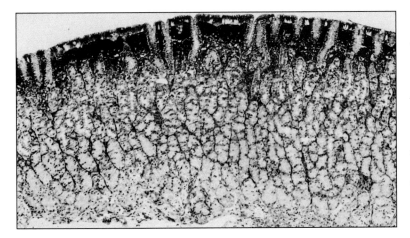

FIGURE 5-8.

Alcoholic hemorrhagic gastritis: histologic features. As seen in this figure, alcoholic hemorrhagic gastritis is depicted microscopically as superficial hemorrhage, occurring primarily in the foveolar regions, and has a band-like distribution in the interpit regions. The overlying epithelium is intact. In the adjacent, nonhemorrhagic mucosa (not shown), edema, which may extend into the deeper glandular zones, may be a prominent feature. Inflammatory infiltrate, if present, is usually mild at best. Thus the term *gastritis*, which suggests a mucosal inflammatory infiltrate, is an inaccurate description of this lesion. *Alcoholic subepithelial hemorrhages* or *alcoholic gastropathy* may be more appropriate terms to describe what has usually been referred to as *alcoholic hemorrhagic gastritis*. Because the gastric surface epithelium remains intact, gastric erosions are not usually seen with this condition. (*From* Laine and Weinstein [1]; with permission.)

CHRONIC GASTRITIS

TABLE 5-2. CHRONIC GASTRITIS: NONSPECIFIC GASTRITIS-*HELICOBACTER PYLORI*

CLASSIFICATIONS OF CHRONIC GASTRITIS

CATEGORY	NOMENCLATURE	ETIOLOGY
Nonspecific	Chronic active superficial gastritis or Chronic superficial gastritis or Chronic atrophic gastritis	*H. pylori*, autoimmune and bile reflux
Specific	Depends on etiology	Bacterial, viral, fungal, parasitic, granulomatous, eosinophilic, and hypertrophic

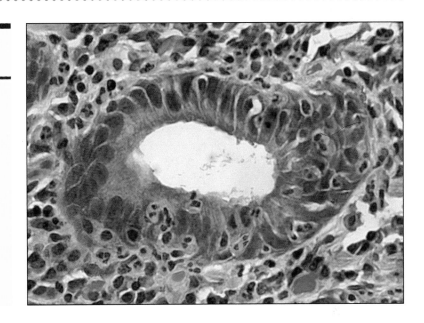

TABLE 5-2 AND FIGURE 5-9.

Chronic gastritis: nonspecific gastritis, *Helicobacter pylori*. As we move into the chronic gastritides, the classification of chronic gastritis is presented again for review. Nonspecific histologic gastritis is characterized by various patterns of gastric mucosal inflammation (as compared with the specific forms of gastritis that usually have a predictable pattern of mucosal inflammation). Nonspecific histologic gastritis is more precisely called *nonerosive nonspecific gastritis*, and since the discovery of *H. pylori*, it is almost always noted in association with this organism. Therefore, most cases of nonerosive nonspecific gastritis are said to be caused by *H. pylori*. *H. pylori* appear as small rods with a central bend or curve that are found beneath the mucus coat overlying surface epithelial cells. Although there are special stains to detect *H. pylori*, the organism can usually be easily seen on high-power microscopic examination of a hematoxylin and eosin–stained section as shown in this figure of a fundic mucosal biopsy with chronic active superficial gastritis; *H. pylori* is visible overlying the surface epithelium of the pits.

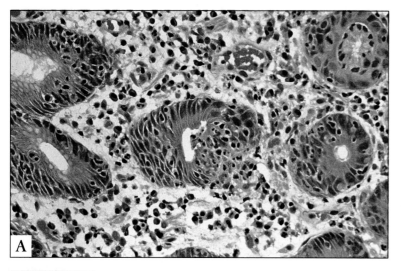

FIGURE 5-10.

Nonerosive nonspecific gastritis: activity. The type of mucosal inflammatory infiltrate will determine the activity of the biopsy. **A,** Chronic active superficial gastritis is defined by an increase in both acute (neutrophils) and chronic (lymphocytes and plasma cells) inflammatory cells in the lamina propria. **B,** Chronic superficial gastritis is defined by an increase in only chronic inflammatory cells (lymphocytes and plasma cells) in the lamina propria. In this example of chronic superficial gastritis, note the markedly diminished number of neutrophils, the lack of neutrophil infiltration of the glands, and the numerous *Helicobacter pylori* present in the pits.

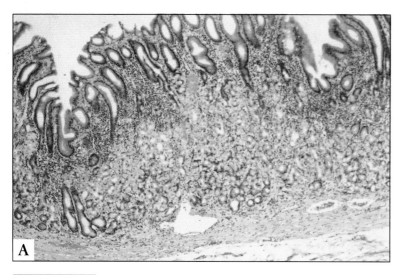
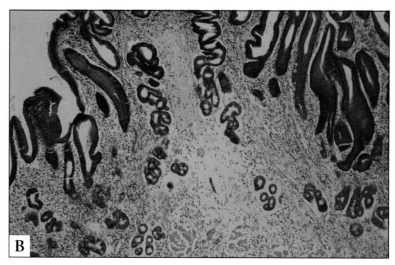

FIGURE 5-11.

Nonerosive nonspecific gastritis: depth of inflammation. Nonerosive nonspecific gastritis is also defined by depth (severity) of mucosal inflammation. **A,** The least severe grade is chronic superficial gastritis in which the inflammation is confined to the gastric pit (foveolar) region. The glandular compartment is usually unaffected. **B,** In the higher grade, chronic atrophic gastritis, inflammation extends down into the mucosa to involve the glandular compartment and variable degrees of glandular atrophy may be present. Note in this example of chronic atrophic gastritis that a number of glands have been lost through destruction by inflammatory cells.

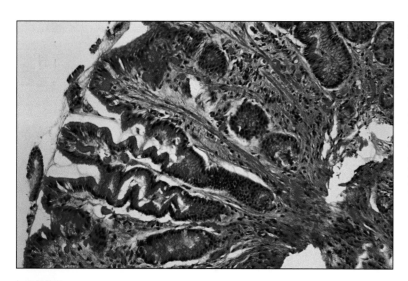

FIGURE 5-12.

Foveolar hyperplasia. Chronic inflammation of the gastric pits may lead to an increase in pit (foveolar) mitotic activity, ultimately resulting in pit elongation or foveolar hyperplasia. As shown, in addition to having become elongated, the gastric pits become more tortuous and develop a corkscrew appearance. Foveolar hyperplasia is the product of chronic inflammation associated with a number of conditions including gastropathy resulting from use of nonsteroidal anti-inflammatory drugs, Ménétrier's disease, hyperplastic polyps, and alkaline reflux gastritis in patients who have undergone partial gastric resections or gastrojejunostomies.

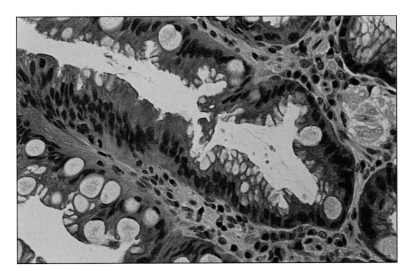

FIGURE 5-13.

Intestinal metaplasia. The presence of intestinal metaplasia is characterized by a change of mucosal pattern from gastric type of epithelium to either a small intestinal type (paneth cells), colonic type (goblet cells), or both. In the stomach, intestinal metaplasia can occur in any gastric region and may arise in response to chronic injury such as in gastritis, especially chronic atrophic gastritis. Intestinal metaplasia is usually found in the pit region of the surface epithelium. This example demonstrates goblet cells lining many of the gastric pits.

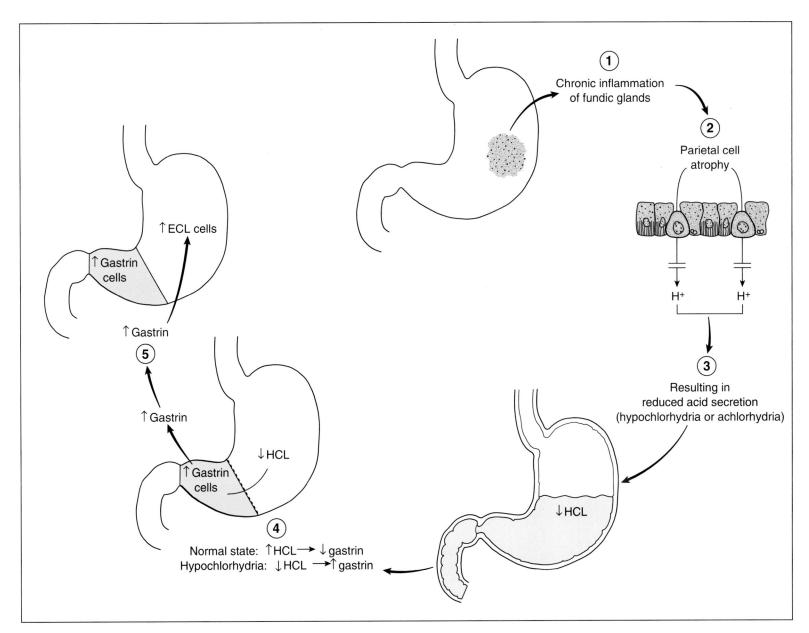

FIGURE 5-14.

Endocrine consequences of chronic atrophic gastritis. Chronic severe fundic gastritis may affect gastric endocrine cells through the following sequence of events:
1) Chronic glandular inflammation
2) Atrophy of parietal cells
3) Parietal cell atrophy will result in reduced acid secretion (hypochlorhydria or achlorhydria)

4) In the normal stomach, gastric acid produced by parietal cells in the gastric body will reduce production of gastrin by gastrin cells in the antrum; in states of reduced gastric acid secretion, the normal feedback inhibition of gastrin is diminished, thus resulting in increased numbers of gastrin cells in the antrum and increased gastrin production
5) Elevated gastrin levels will stimulate proliferation of enterochromaffin-like (ECL) cells in the gastric body

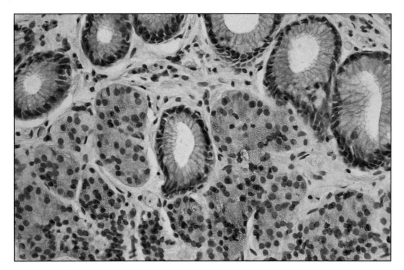

FIGURE 5-15.

Enterochromaffin-like cell (ECL) hyperplasia. ECL cells are endocrine cells normally present and scattered among other cells in the fundic mucosa. The cytoplasm of ECL cells is filled with core granules that stain with the immunostain chromogranin. As shown in Figure 5-14, hypergastrinemia associated with severe atrophic fundic gastritis may lead to ECL cell hyperplasia. Shown here is an example of ECL cell hyperplasia. Note the cells with bland nuclei and a generous amount of clear cytoplasm lining the gastric glands. The immunostaining (brown pigment) highlights the increased number of ECL cells.

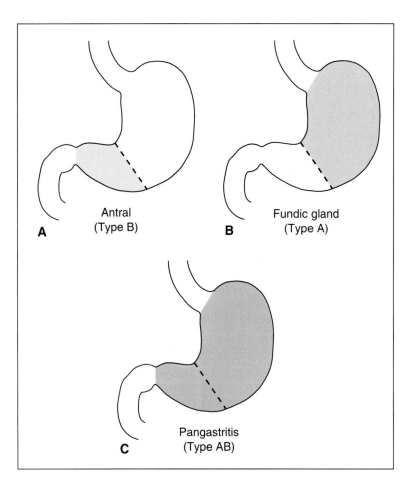

FIGURE 5-16.

Topographic distributions of nonerosive, nonspecific gastritis. The three panels of this figure demonstrate the three major gastric topographic distributions for non-specific gastritis.

A, Antral gastritis, also referred to as *type B*, is almost always associated with *Helicobacter pylori*. In duodenal ulcer patients, more than 90% have antral gastritis, and 50% to 80% of gastric ulcer patients have this type of gastritis. Type B gastritis is most intense in the antrum. It commonly coexists, however, with a less severe inflammation in the fundic mucosa.

B, Fundic gastritis, also referred to as *type A*, is most intense in the body of the stomach. This pattern of gastritis is seen in pernicious anemia. Although type A gastritis is most intense in body of the stomach and has been described to "spare the antrum", it is frequently associated with a less severe antral gastritis. Thus, type B and A gastritis are actually pangastritides with the predominance of inflammation confined to either the gastric antrum or body.

C, A third type of gastritis, a pangastritis (*Type AB*), has been described and is represented by gastritis in the antrum and body. Type AB gastritis most likely represents proximal extension of Type B gastritis and is also highly associated with *H. pylori* colonization.

There is a fourth topographic pattern of gastritis (not shown) called *multifocal atrophic gastritis*, which begins in the region of the incisura and extends out both proximally and distally and is commonly associated with intestinal metaplasia. (*Adapted from* Weinstein [2]; with permission).

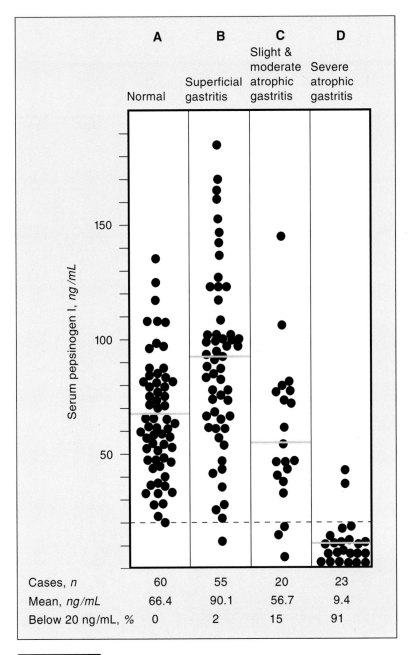

	A	B	C	D
	Normal	Superficial gastritis	Slight & moderate atrophic gastritis	Severe atrophic gastritis
Cases, *n*	60	55	20	23
Mean, *ng/mL*	66.4	90.1	56.7	9.4
Below 20 ng/mL, %	0	2	15	91

FIGURE 5-17.

Serum pepsinogens and chronic gastritis. Pepsinogens, which are gastric proteolytic enzymes, are synthesized by chief and mucus cells and are released into gastric juice and into serum. Two classes of serum pepsinogens can be immunologically detected: pepsinogen I and pepsinogen II.

As shown in this figure, serum pepsinogen levels may vary according to the stage of gastritis. In response to *Helicobacter pylori* infection (chronic active superficial gastritis), serum pepsinogen levels will rise (**A** and perhaps **B**). Eradication of *H. pylori* will decrease serum pepsinogen back towards normal. With continuing chronic gastritis (**C** and **D**), there is progressive loss of fundic gland mucosa (atrophy) with parallel decreases in serum pepsinogens. In severe chronic atrophic gastritis (*D*), where there has been profound loss of fundic mucosa, serum pepsinogen levels are very low.

Pepsinogen I is synthesized primarily in the gastric body, whereas pepsinogen II is made in the gastric body and antrum. In chronic atrophic (Type A) gastritis, primarily the fundic gland mucosa is involved and the antrum is spared, resulting in very low pepsinogen I concentrations, whereas pepsinogen II concentrations are maintained or slightly reduced. Because of the disproportionate reduction in pepsinogen I compared with pepsinogen II, the serum pepsinogen I:II ratio in atrophic gastritis is very low and can be used to screen patients for this disorder. (*From* Varis and Isokoski [3]; with permission.).

TABLE 5-3. CHRONIC GASTRITIS: SPECIFIC (DISTINCTIVE) GASTRITIS

INFECTIONS

Bacterial
   Tuberculosis
   Syphilis
   Phlegmonous and emphysematous gastritis
Viral
   Cytomegalovirus
   Herpesviruses
Fungal
   Candidiasis
   Histoplasmosis
   Mucormycosis
   Cryptococcosis
   Aspergillosis
Parasites and Nematodes
   Cryptosporidiosis
   Strongyloidiasis
   Amebiasis
   Toxoplasmosis
   Pneumocystis carinii infection

GASTROINTESTINAL TRACT DISEASE

Crohn's disease
Eosinophilic gastroenteritis
Systemic disease
   Sarcoid
   Graft-vs-host disease
   Chronic granulomatous disease
Miscellaneous (unknown association)
   Ménétrier's disease
   Focal lymphoid hyperplasia
   Granulomatous gastritis

TABLE 5-3.

Chronic gastritis: specific or distinctive gastritis. The designation specific or distinctive gastritis refers to histologic features that are suggestive of a specific diagnosis. Viewed endoscopically, these disorders may or may not have mucosal abnormalities. Listed in this table are some of the various etiologies that have been associated with a specific form of gastritis. Compared with the nonspecific forms of gastritis, the specific forms are rarer. A few examples of cases of specific gastritis follow in Figures 5-18 to 5-35. (*Adapted from* Weinstein [2]; with permission.)

GASTRIC GRANULOMA

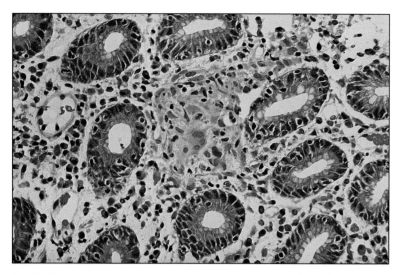

TABLE 5-4. CONDITIONS ASSOCIATED WITH GASTRIC GRANULOMAS

Infectious
   Tuberculosis
   Syphilis
   Histoplasmosis and other fungal infections
   Parasites
Noninfectious systemic disease
   Crohn's disease
   Sarcoidosis
   Chronic granulomatous disease
   Allergic granulomatosis
Miscellaneous
   Foreign body
   Idiopathic

FIGURE 5-18.

Gastric granuloma. Granulomas in the gastric mucosa may be associated with a variety of systemic and infectious diseases such as Crohn's disease, tuberculosis, sarcoidosis, syphilis, and fungal infections. Granulomas may also form in response to a foreign body such as talc or silica that has become embedded in the gastric mucosa. In some instances, no etiology can be found, and this histologic observation is defined *idiopathic granulomatous gastritis*. Gastric granulomas are most commonly located in the antrum.

TABLE 5-4.

Conditions associated with gastric granulomas. (*Adapted from* Weinstein [2]; with permission.).

GASTRIC SYPHILIS

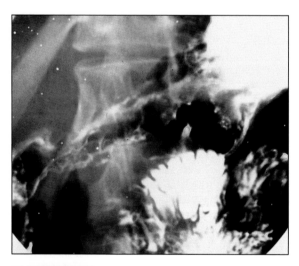

FIGURE 5-19.

Gastric syphilis: upper gastrointestinal barium examination. Gastric syphilis is caused by infection with the organism *Treponema pallidum*. Gastric involvement usually presents in the secondary stage of the disease. On upper gastrointestinal system barium studies, gastric syphilis may be manifested as discrete, nodular gummalike lesions. Diffuse involvement of the stomach with a predominance of antral involvement is, however, more common. Swelling and thickening of the gastric wall can result in mural rigidity and narrowing of the lumen. As seen in this upper gastrointestinal barium study, diffuse thickening of the gastric wall resulted in narrowing of the antrum and scattered gummatous polyps. Luminal narrowing produces a tubular deformity or a funnel-shaped defect in which the apex of the funnel is at or near the pylorus. (*Courtesy of* Mark Feldman, Dallas, TX)

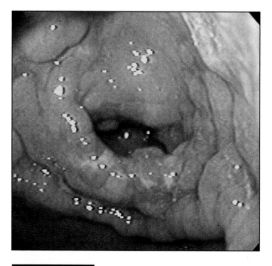

FIGURE 5-20.

Gastric syphilis: endoscopic manifestations. Endoscopically gastric syphilis usually presents as thick gastric folds with submucosal infiltration and multiple erosions. The endoscopic picture is suggestive of gastric carcinoma. Shown in this figure is the gastric antrum of a patient with syphilis that endoscopically demonstrates massive submucosal infiltration and erosions. (*Courtesy of* Mark Feldman, Dallas, TX)

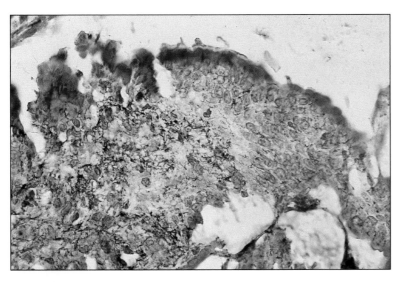

FIGURE 5-21.

Gastric syphilis: histology. Histologically, *Treponema pallidum* is demonstrated in gastric biopsies either by silver staining or by fluorescent antibody staining. Histologic demonstration of the corkscrew appearance of the organisms in gastric biopsies is required for diagnosis. This figure shows a gastric body biopsy from the patient shown in Figure 5-20. It has been silver stained and demonstrates the organisms present. Granulomas would be another suggestive feature but not diagnostic for gastric syphilis. Other than the findings mentioned, the histology of gastric syphilis demonstrates a nonspecific inflammatory response.

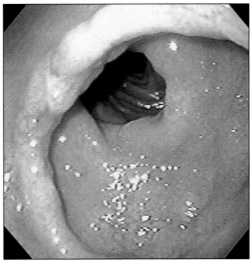

FIGURE 5-22.

Gastric syphilis: posttherapy. Following appropriate antibiotic therapy for syphilis, the radiographic, endoscopic, and histologic abnormalities of gastric syphilis can be expected to resolve. This figure is an endoscopic photograph of the antrum of the gastric syphilis patient shown in Figure 5-20, 1 month after treatment with benzathine penicillin. As noted previously, the massive submucosal infiltration seen earlier has almost completely abated. (*Courtesy of* M. Feldman, Dallas, TX)

GASTRIC HISTOPLASMOSIS

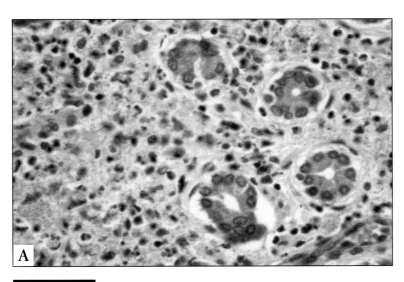

A **B**

FIGURE 5-23.

Gastric histoplasmosis. Gastric histoplasmosis usually occurs in the setting of disseminated histoplasmosis and is caused by the organism *Histoplasma capsulatum*. Although it may be found worldwide, it is concentrated in the Ohio, Missouri, and Mississippi river valleys and is transmitted by bats, chickens, and other birds through their droppings. Endoscopically it may appear as an ulceration, mass lesions, or thickened folds. On biopsy, organisms can be identified with silver staining. Diagnosis is confirmed by a positive culture, presence of typical organisms in granulomas on gastric biopsy, or by high-complement fixation titers. These figures show gastric biopsies from a patient with disseminated histoplasmosis. **A,** Low-power view of a hematoxylin and eosin stained section in which macrophage and histoplasma infiltration widely separating the glands can be appreciated. **B,** High-power view of a periodic acid–Schiff stained section wherein the macrophages and isolated organisms are better appreciated. (*Courtesy of* E. Bigio, Dallas, TX)

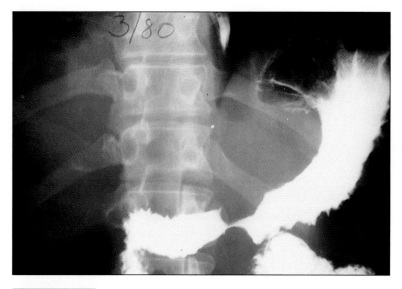

FIGURE 5-24.

Crohn's disease: upper gastrointestinal barium examination. Although Crohn's disease can involve any portion of the gastrointestinal tract, clinically apparent isolated gastric Crohn's disease is a rare entity. Gastric Crohn's disease usually involves the antrum and pylorus. When gastric Crohn's disease is present, usually the proximal duodenum or other parts of the small and large intestines are involved as well. As in this figure, barium studies of the upper gastrointestinal tract may reveal gastric deformity with enlarged nodular folds, poor distensibility, and deformed pylorus. (*Courtesy of* M. Feldman, Dallas, TX)

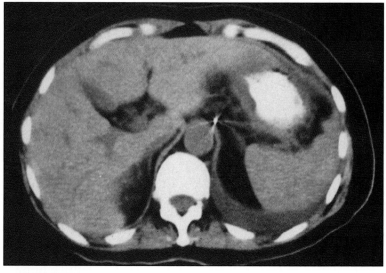

FIGURE 5-25.

Crohn's disease seen using computed tomographic scan. Because transmural inflammation is seen in Crohn's disease, gastric wall thickening is a characteristic finding. In this computed tomographic scan of the abdomen with contrast, diffuse thickening of the wall of the stomach is seen. Endoscopy in such patients reveals aphthoid and serpiginous erosions, ulcerations, and mucosal irregularities. (*From* Cary *et al.* [4]; with permission.)

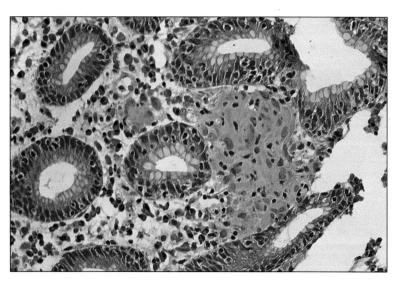

FIGURE 5-26.

Crohn's disease: histology. Histologically, gastric Crohn's disease appears as an idiopathic granulomatous gastritis. Thus, in the absence of other clinical manifestations to suggest Crohn's disease, the diagnosis is difficult to make solely on the basis of histologic evidence. This figure shows two (one large and one small) granulomas (nodular collections of histiocytes) within the lamina propria. Acute and chronic inflammatory infiltrates involving the lamina propria are also present.

■ EOSINOPHILIC GASTRITIS

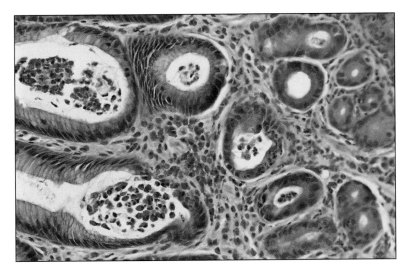

FIGURE 5-27.

Eosinophilic gastritis. The view of this condition represents the gastric component of the more generalized eosinophilic gastroenteritis. Endoscopically, usually no gross abnormality is present. Although all parts of the stomach may be involved, the eosinophilic infiltrate has a predilection for the antrum. This figure above demonstrates a gastric biopsy with numerous eosinophils most abundant in the superficial lamina propria and the lumen of the pits. On deeper sections the infiltrate may extend down into the muscularis mucosa. No ulceration, granulomas, or parasites were present. Such findings are consistent with a diagnosis of eosinophilic gastritis, a nonspecific diagnosis with a large differential that includes allergy, collagen vascular disorders such as Churg-strauss syndrome or polyarteritis nodosa, parasitic infections such as schistosomiasis and strongyloidiasis, and lymphoma.

■ MÉNÉTRIER'S DISEASE

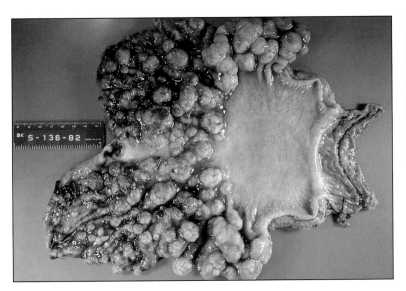

FIGURE 5-28.

Ménétrier's disease. The clinical features diagnostic of Ménétrier's disease are giant folds, especially in the fundus and body of the stomach, protein-losing enteropathy with hypoalbuminemia, hypochlorhydria in advanced stages, and a marked increase in mucosal thickness overall. As shown in this figure, its gross pathological characteristics are enlarged gastric folds in the gastric body that typically spare the antrum. These folds have a nodular or polypoid configuration and may have associated erosions or ulcerations.

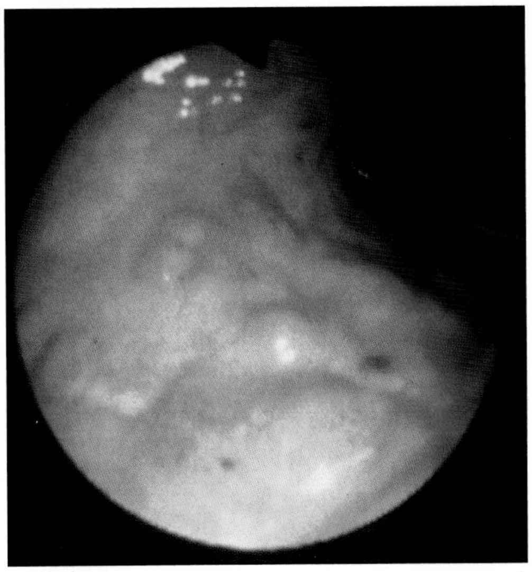

FIGURE 5-29.

Ménétrier's disease: endoscopic characteristics. In common with the view shown in Figure 5-28, on endoscopy in Ménétrier's disease, large nodular gastric folds may also be appreciated. Shown is an endoscopic image of the gastric body taken from the retroflexed endoscopic angle of nodular- and polypoid-appearing gastric folds in a patient with Ménétrier's disease. (*Courtesy of* M. Feldman, Dallas, TX)

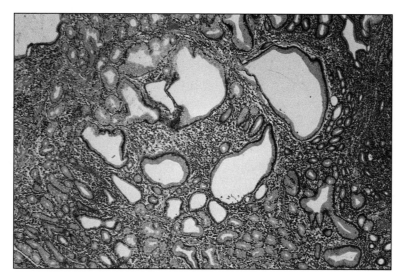

FIGURE 5-30.

Ménétrier's disease: histologic characteristics. Histologically, Ménétrier's disease is characterized by marked elongation and cystic dilation of glands lined by foveolar epithelium and glandular atrophy. The lamina propria has a dense chronic (lymphocytic) inflammatory infiltrate.

■ OTHER CAUSES

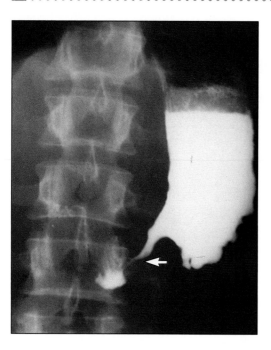

FIGURE 5-31.

Ingestion of caustic substances. Ingestion of caustic agents (typically, they are strongly acidic, but similar effects with strong alkaline substances may also be seen) can cause gastric injury, especially in the antrum. Pathologically, caustic injuries to the gastric mucosa are classified as a continuum starting with superficial injury associated with inflammation, edema, and erythema which generally does not result in scar or stricture formation (first degree).

The next levels of injury are characterized by inflammation, granulation tissue, and ulceration extending down to the muscularis (second degree) or penetration which extends through the gastric wall (third degree). From 2 to 3 weeks following second- and third-degree gastric injuries, a fibroblastic reaction develops most prominently in the antrum, which can result in antral stricturing.

The upper gastrointestinal system barium study shown here is from a patient who had ingested a caustic agent. Note the long tapering antral stricture (*open arrow*) resulting from luminal compression from extensive mucosal scarring noted radiographically as a nodular mass effect. The same nodularity resulting from scarring is also noted in the gastric body along the greater curvature. (*Courtesy of* M. Feldman, Dallas, TX)

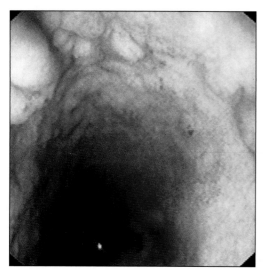

FIGURE 5-32.

Nodular duodenitis. When inflammation involves the duodenum, endoscopically it may be manifested in various ways including hyperemia, edema, large folds, nodularity (psuedopolyps), friability, erosions, or hemorrhage. This patient has one variant of duodenal inflammation, nodular duodenitis. Based on this endoscopic appearance, differential diagnoses include Brunner's gland hyperplasia, adenomatous and villous polyps, lymphoid aggregates, lymphoma, Crohn's disease, parasitic infection, and pancreatic rests. Accordingly, confirmation of diagnosis requires biopsy and histologic inspection.

TABLE 5-5. GASTRIC AND DUODENAL INFECTIONS IN AIDS

INFECTIOUS AGENTS ASSOCIATED WITH GASTRITIS AND DUODENITIS IN AIDS

Bacteria
  Salmonella
    Mycobacterium avium-intracellulare
    Mycobacterium tuberculosis

Viruses
  Cytomegalovirus
    Herpes simplex virus

Protozoa
  Cryptosporidium
  Isospora belli
    Microsporidia
    Giardia lamblia

Fungal
  Histoplasmosis
    Coccidiomycosis

TABLE 5-5.

Gastric and duodenal infections in AIDS. A wide range of bacterial, viral, protozoal, and fungal organisms may cause gastritis and duodenitis in patients with AIDS.

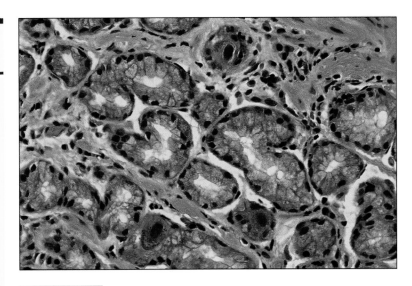

FIGURE 5-33.

Cytomegalovirus. Although cytomegalovirus infection may be found in the stomach or duodenum, it may also be found anywhere in the gastrointestinal tract. It may also be found in normal hosts. However, cytomegalovirus gastritis occurs more frequently in patients who are in immunocompromised states such as those with AIDS or transplant recipients. Endoscopically, the gastroduodenal mucosa may have a variety of appearances ranging from normal to ulceration. As shown in this figure from a gastric biopsy, the characteristic feature on histology is enlarged cells with enlarged nuclei that contain eosinophilic inclusion bodies.

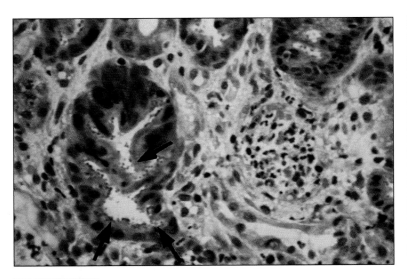

FIGURE 5-34.

Cryptosporidium. This pathogen is a common cause of self-limited diarrhea in healthy hosts, particularly in travelers or in those who work with animals. In AIDS patients, however, infection with this organism produces a chronic voluminous diarrhea and is probably the most common cause of diarrhea in AIDS. However, all of the other organisms listed in Table 5-4 may produce diarrhea in AIDS. The small bowel is the most common site for *Cryptosporidium*, although the organism can be found in all gastrointestinal regions. As shown above, small bowel biopsy will demonstrate *Cryptosporidium* on the apical surface of intestinal epithelial cells, villous atrophy, and crypt hypertrophy. (*From* Cello [5]; with permission.)

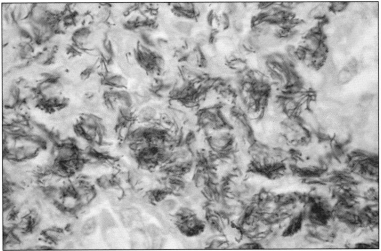

FIGURE 5-35.

Mycobacterium avium-intracellulare. Small intestinal involvement by mycobacterium may be with either *Mycobacterium avium-intracellulare* or *Mycobacterium tuberculosis*, although in the duodenum, infections with *M. avium-intracellulare* are more common. Either may present clinically with diarrhea, obstruction, or abdominal pain. Endoscopically, duodenal *M. avium-intracellulare* may appear as fine, white mucosal nodules. Histologic features on hematoxylin and eosin stain are "foamy macrophages" (macrophages distended with organisms) and blunted and widened villae associated with an enteritis producing a histologic appearance similar to Whipple's disease. On acid-fast stain, as shown in this figure, the lamina propria is infiltrated with foamy macrophages and acid-fast bacilli. (*Courtesy of* M. Feldman, Dallas, TX)

REFERENCES AND RECOMMENDED READING

1. Laine L, Weinstein WM:Histology of hemorrhagic "gastritis": A prospective evaluation. *Gastroenterology* 1988, 94:1254–1262.

2. Weinstein WM: Gastritis and gastropathies. In *Gastrointestinal Disease, edn. 5*. Edited by Sleisenger MH, Fordtran JS. Philadelphia: WB Saunders; 1993:549.

3. Varis K, Isokoski M: Screening of type A gastritis. *Ann Clin Res* 1981, 13:133-138.

4. Cary ER, Tremaine WJ, Banks PM, Nagorney DM: Case Report: Isolated Crohn's disease of the stomach. *Mayo Clin Proc* 1989, 64:776–779.

5. Cello JP: *AIDS-Related Diarrhea*. East Hanover, NJ: Sandoz;1992.

Chapter 6

Helicobacter Pylori

Byron Cryer
Edward Lee

Helicobacter pylori is the most common bacterial infection in humans. This organism was first discovered in 1982 when Warren [1] and Marshall [2], two Australian investigators, reported spiral organisms in gastric mucosal biopsies of patients with chronic active gastritis. Since its discovery, *H. pylori* gastritis has been associated with peptic ulcer disease, gastric adenocarcinoma, and gastric lymphoma. Among these diseases, the strongest association is with *H. pylori* and peptic ulcers. Eradication of *H. pylori* infection with antibiotics results in a dramatic reduction in ulcer recurrence.

Epidemiologic studies have shown that greater than 1 billion people worldwide are infected with *H. pylori*. However, only a small number of infected subjects ever develop one of the diseases associated with *H. pylori*. Thus, there are other, as of yet, unidentified factors that determine which asymptomatically infected individuals will ultimately develop an *H. pylori*–related disease.

This chapter will review a number of areas pertaining to *H. pylori* and its associated diseases. First, structural and biochemical characteristics of the organism will be discussed. Also reviewed are *H. pylori* epidemiology, diagnostic tests available to identify the infection, disease associations, and treatment options.

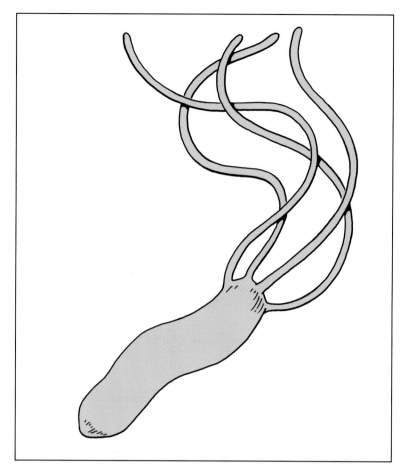

FIGURE 6-1.

Morphology and taxonomy. *Helicobacter pylori* is a spiral-shaped, gram-negative bacterium with four to six unipolar sheathed flagella. It is found within the stomach and duodenum of humans. The organism was first named *Campylobacter*-like ("curved rod") organism, then *Campylobacter pylori*. Its name was later changed to *H. pylori*, however, when biochemical and genetic characterization showed that it was not a member of the *Campylobacter* genus. *H. pylori* infections can be observed in healthy patients and in patients with a variety of gastrointestinal disease. *H. pylori*'s unique features, its helical shape and flagella, assist its movement through the gastric mucus layer.

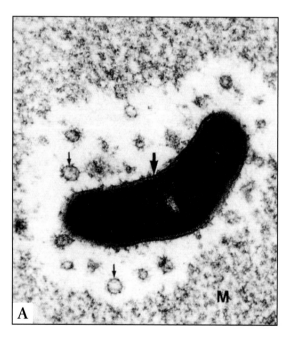

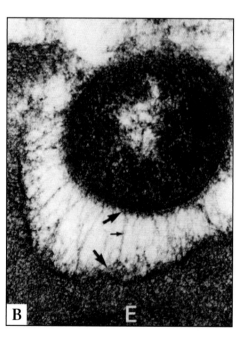

FIGURE 6-2.

Two electron micrographs from the gastric antrum of a *Helicobacter pylori*–infected patient. **A**, *H. pylori* is lying in finely granular mucus (M), yet slightly separated from the mucus by an electron-lucent, less granular zone containing membrane-bound glycocaliceal bodies (*small arrows*). *H. pylori* also has a glycocalyx, which is a flocculent layer coating its limiting membrane (*large arrow*). Special adhesions aid in *H. pylori*'s adherence to gastric epithelium. **B**, A cross-section of the organism linked to a gastric epithelial cell (E). Fine filamentous strands of glycocalyx-like material (*small arrow*) extend between *H. pylori* and gastric epithelial cell membranes. These strands link the glycocalyx of *H. pylori* to the glycocalyx of gastric epithelial cells (*large arrows*). (*From* Thomsen *et al.* [3]; with permission)

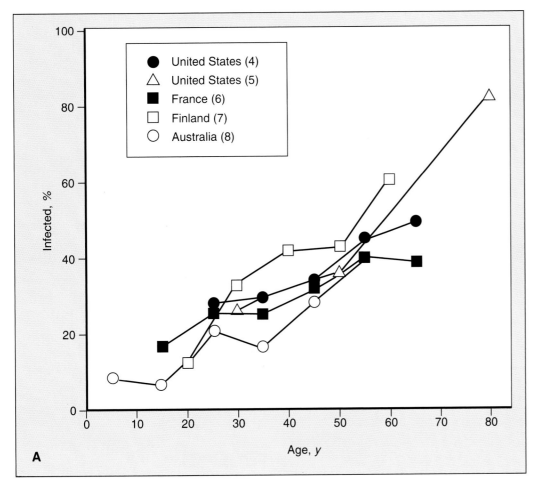

A

FIGURE 6-3.

Prevalence by age and country of origin. The prevalence of *Helicobacter pylori* colonization in healthy individuals varies greatly with age and country of origin. **A,** In developed countries, it is uncommon for children to be infected with *H. pylori*, whereas up to 50% of adults older than 60 years of age are infected. **B,** These rates of infection compare with underdeveloped countries where approximately 40% of children younger than 10 are infected with *H. pylori* and, depending on the country, this percentage may increase to greater than 80% by 50 years of age. The mode of transmission of *H. pylori* is thought to be person-to-person through fecal-oral or oral-oral routes. In underdeveloped countries, where many people live in close quarters or where sanitation systems are less advanced or nonexistent, greater opportunities for transmission of *H. pylori* may exist. (*Adapted from* Taylor and Blaser [10]; with permission.)

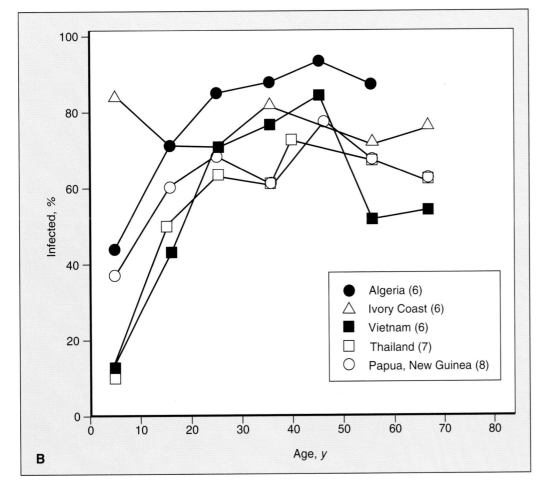

B

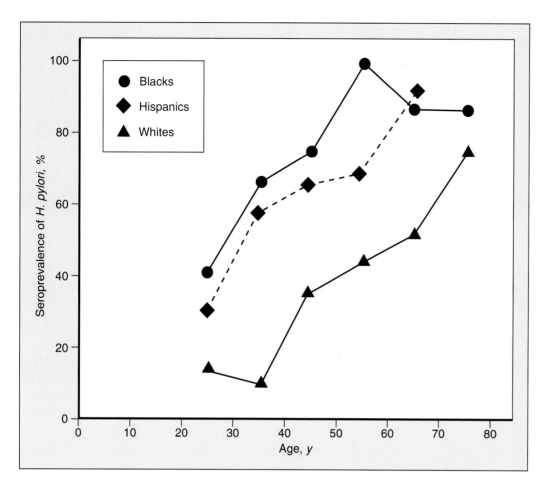

FIGURE 6-4.

Prevalence by ethnic group. In developed countries such as the United States, prevalence of *Helicobacter pylori* varies among different ethnic groups matched for socioeconomic status. (*Data from* Malaty *et al.* [11].)

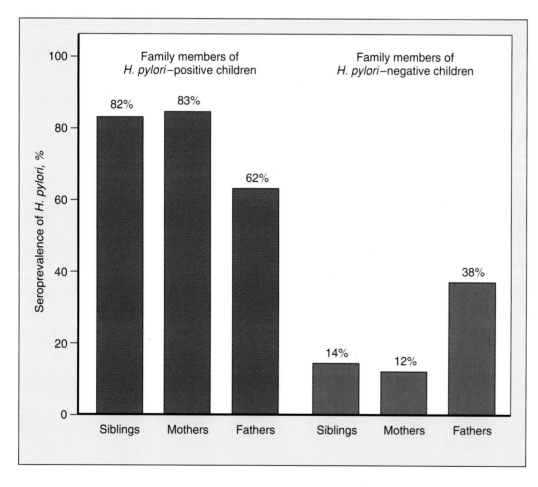

FIGURE 6-5.

Clustering of organism within families. Support for person-to-person transmission of *Helicobacter pylori* comes from studies of children in institutions of custodial care and from studies of families in which there is at least one infected child. As seen in the results of the study above, family members of a child infected with *H. pylori* are more likely to be infected than family members of an uninfected child. (*Data from* Drumm *et al.* [12].)

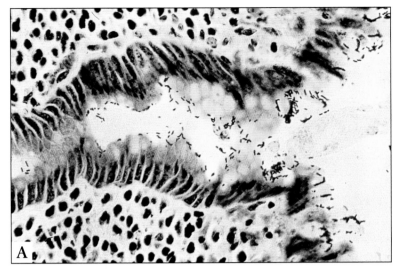

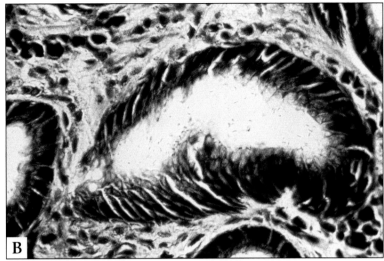

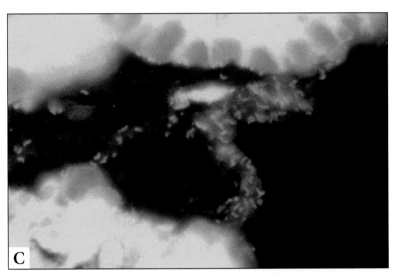

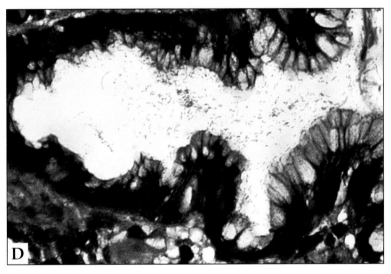

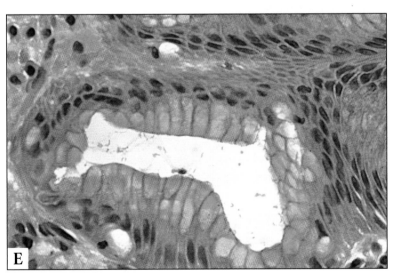

FIGURE 6-6.

Histologic stains. *Helicobacter pylori* infection can be identified in a number of ways. Histologic identification of the organisms in gastric mucosal biopsies is one method of directly assessing *H. pylori* infection. As shown, at high-power magnification, *H. pylori* can be easily identified. There are a number of special histologic stains that can be used to identify *H. pylori*. These include the Warthin-Starry silver stain (**A**), Giemsa stain (**B**), acridine orange stain (**C**), and Gimenez stain (**D**). However, *H. pylori* can be almost as easily identified using the routine hematoxylin and eosin stain (**E**) as with the other special stains. (From Peterson *et al* [13] with permission.)

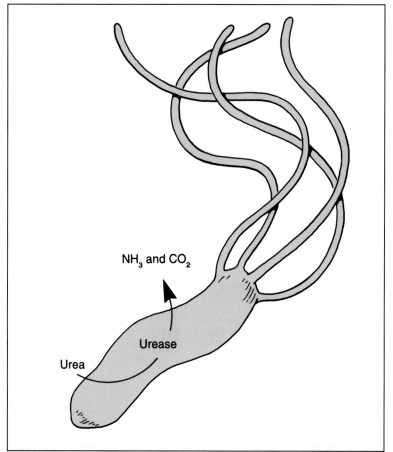

FIGURE 6-7.

Urease. *Helicobacter pylori* produces several different enzymes, one of which is urease, which helps it adapt to the hostile gastric environment. Urease will metabolize urea to NH_3 and CO_2. Urease is not normally present in mammalian cells, but is found in *H. pylori*. Thus, the presence of urease activity within the stomach is sensitive and specific for the presence of *H. pylori*. Two tests for *H. pylori*, the urea breath test and the rapid urease assay, both indirectly test for presence of *H. pylori* through assessment of urease activity.

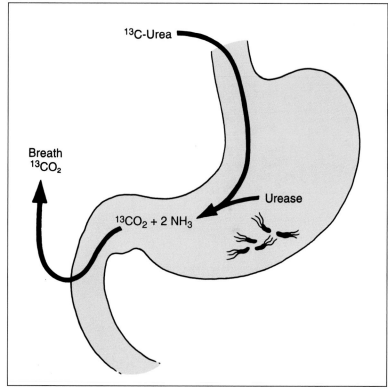

FIGURE 6-8.

Urea breath tests (C^{13} and C^{14}). Diagnosis of *Helicobacter pylori* by the urea breath test is based on urease metabolism of ingested urea. Either C^{14}– or C^{13}–labeled urea is ingested. (The C^{13}–labeled urea is a nonradioactive carbon isotope). If *H. pylori* is present, urea is metabolized to ammonia and carbon-labeled carbon dioxide. The labeled carbon dioxide is then excreted in breath as labeled carbon dioxide, which is then collected and quantified. Although this illustration demonstrates the breath test using C^{13}, the urea breath test can be similarly performed using C^{14}.

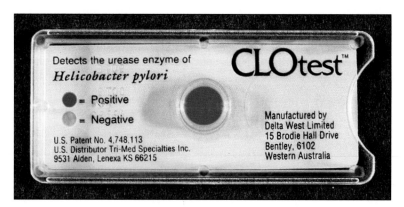

FIGURE 6-9.

Rapid urease tests. Another indirect test for *Helicobacter pylori*, the rapid urease test, is based on metabolism of urea by urease. In this test, a mucosal biopsy is inoculated into a well that contains urea and a pH-sensitive dye (phenol red). If urease is present in the biopsy, urea in the medium is converted to NH_4^+, which will raise the pH. In response to an elevation in pH, the pH sensitive dye causes the well to change colors. This figure is an example of a rapid urease test, the CLOtest^{TM} (Delta West Limited, Bentley, Western Australia). In this test, presence of *H. pylori* in a mucosal biopsy will be evidenced by a color change from yellow to red.

TABLE 6-1. TESTS FOR *HELICOBACTER PYLORI* INFECTION

NONINVASIVE			
TEST	SENSITIVITY, %	SPECIFICITY, %	COMMENTS
Serology	88–96	86–95	Antibody titers do not return to negative after eradication of *H. pylori*; thus, serology is not a suitable test to document effectiveness of eradication
Urea breath tests	90–100	89–100	Because this test has high sensitivity and specificity and is noninvasive, when commercially available, it will be useful for documentation of *H. Pylori* eradiction

INVASIVE			
TEST	SENSITIVITY, %	SPECIFICITY, %	COMMENTS
Histology	93–99	95–99	Requires histologic evaluation of mucosal biopsy; thus, it is expensive
Rapid urease test (CLOtest™, Delta West Limited, Bentley, Western Australia)	89–98	93–98	Inexpensive, it can provide relatively rapid diagnosis
Culture	77–92	100	Technically difficult and accuracy varies with laboratory; also expensive

TABLE 6-1.

The tests for diagnosis of *Helicobacter pylori* can be categorized noninvasive (*ie*, do not require endoscopy) or invasive (*ie*, require endoscopy). The advantages and disadvantages of each diagnostic method are listed. When the urea breath test is commercially available, it will be a good test for *H. pylori* screening and for follow-up of efficacy of *H. pylori* eradication because it is noninvasive and has good sensitivity and acceptable specificity.

TABLE 6-2. ASSOCIATION OF *HELICOBACTER PYLORI* WITH GASTROINTESTINAL DISEASE

GROUP	SEROPREVALENCE OF *H. PYLORI* INFECTION, %
Healthy subjects	20*
Chronic active gastritis	100
Duodenal ulcer	>90
Gastric ulcer	50–80
Gastric adenocarcinoma	90
Gastric lymphoma	85

*Will vary with age and ethnic group

TABLE 6-2.

Association of *Helicobacter pylori* with gastrointestinal disease. As shown in the previous figures (Figs. 6-3, 6-4, 6-5), *H. pylori* may be found in healthy asymptomatic individuals, and rates of infection vary depending on age, country of origin, and ethnic group. In this table however, individuals with certain gastrointestinal diseases have higher rates of *H. pylori* infection than nondiseased, healthy subjects.

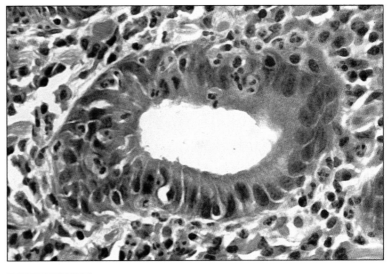

FIGURE 6-10.

Helicobacter pylori and chronic active gastritis. *H. pylori* infection causes a chronic nonerosive, nonspecific gastritis in the antrum and fundus. The preferred terminology for the above type of *H. pylori*–related gastritis is *chronic active superficial gastritis*. As shown in this figure, inflammation in chronic active superficial gastritis is superficial, *ie*, confined to the region around the gastric pits (foveolae). The infiltrate is characterized by an increase in both acute (neutrophils) and chronic (lymphocytes and plasma cells) inflammatory cells in the lamina propria. Neutrophils are seen invading the glandular epithelial cells and *H. pylori* is visualized within the glandular lumen. The deeper glandular region (not shown) is usually unaffected in this type of gastritis.

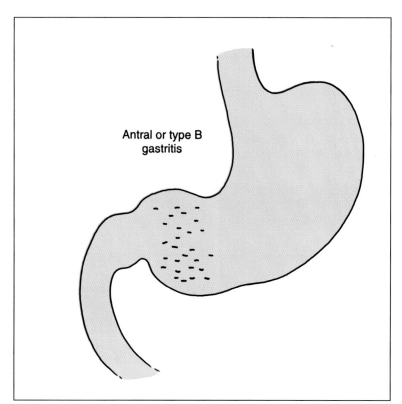

FIGURE 6-11.

Antral (type B) gastritis. Gastric infection with *Helicobacter pylori* causes mucosal inflammation that is concentrated in the gastric antrum. This pattern of inflammation is referred to as *type B gastritis*. Although type B gastritis is most intense in the antrum, it commonly coexists with a less severe inflammation in the fundus. Almost all (95%) patients who have this pattern of gastritis will concurrently be infected with *H. pylori*. As discussed in Chapter 5, this gastritis is characterized histologically and is usually not associated with gross endoscopic abnormalities.

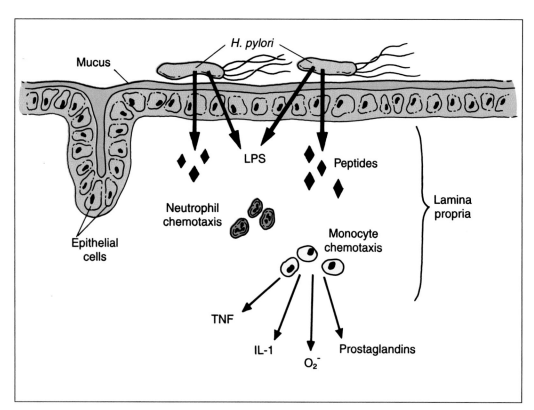

FIGURE 6-12.

Helicobacter pylori's initiation of mucosal inflammation. *H. pylori* resides in the mucus layer overlying the gastric epithelium. In the lamina propria, there is almost always an associated inflammatory infiltrate. Because the epithelial layer (which falls between *H. pylori* and the inflammatory cells) is intact, secondary mediators (and not *H. pylori*) evoke mucosal inflammatory cells. *H. pylori* secretes factors, a peptide, and lipopolysaccharides (LPS), which are chemotactic for neutrophils and monocytes. Characterization of the peptide reveals that it is heat, acid, and alkali stable. It has a molecular weight of approximately 3000. The inflammatory cells, once recruited, will then release oxygen radicals, prostaglandins, interleukin 1 (IL-1), and tumor necrosis factor (TNF) that will further promote additional inflammation.

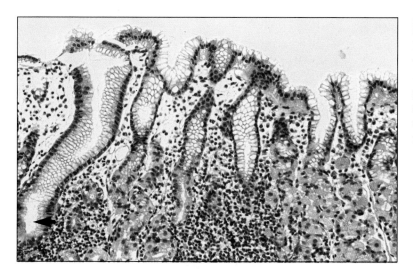

FIGURE 6-13.

Lymphoid follicle. *Helicobacter pylori* infection can be associated with mucosal lymphoid follicles as shown. Also seen are *H. pylori* (*arrow*) within the base of gastric pits. Histologic identification of gastric lymphoid follicles, not normally observed in an uninfected stomach, strongly suggests a coexisting *H. pylori* infection, even if the organisms are not visualized in the same section as the lymphoid follicle.

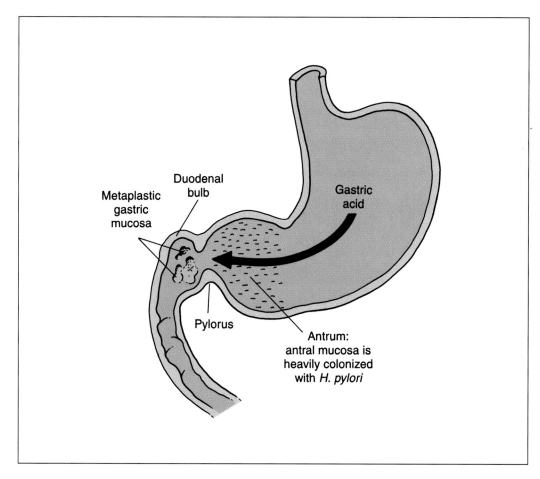

FIGURE 6-14.

Gastric metaplasia in the duodenal bulb and duodenal ulcer pathogenesis. The current hypothesis regarding formation of duodenal gastric metaplasia is that it develops in response to duodenal acid exposure, thus leading to direct epithelial damage or secondary inflammation. These injured duodenal areas may heal by acquiring gastric epithelium, which might be better adapted than duodenal epithelium for acid exposure. After gastric metaplasia has occurred, these areas provide a site for *Helicobacter pylori* adherence. This may contribute to the pathogenesis of duodenal ulceration.

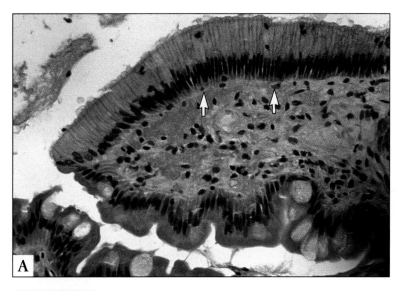

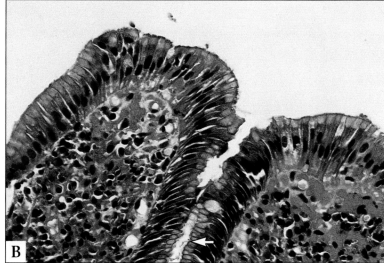

FIGURE 6-15.

Histology of gastric metaplasia. As reviewed in Figure 6-14, metaplasia gastric tissue first forms in the duodenum, and later *Helicobacter pylori* may attach to these duodenal sites. Thus, gastric metaplasia may occur in some subjects who have not yet been infected with *H. pylori*. **A,** Gastric (foveolar) epithelial cells (*open arrows*) are adjacent to duodenal mucosal epithelial cells. *H. pylori* needs gastric epithelium as a pre-requisite for its attachment as there are specific adhesins for *H. pylori* on gastric epithelial cells. Thus, when *H. pylori* is found in the duodenum, it is always in association with metaplastic gastric tissue. **B,** Duodenal biopsy with metaplastic gastric epithelial cells (*open arrow*) adjacent to duodenal epithelium. *H. pylori* are visible overlying the surface of the metaplastic gastric mucosa.

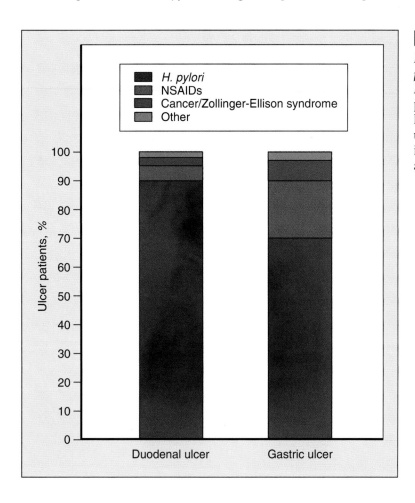

FIGURE 6-16.

Helicobacter pylori and peptic ulcer disease. The assumption that *H. pylori* causes peptic ulcer disease is based on two lines of evidence. *H. pylori* has a higher prevalence in gastric and duodenal ulcer patients than in noninfected, healthy controls. Although *H. pylori* has a stronger association with duodenal ulcers than with gastric ulcers, *H. pylori* is the most common cause of gastric ulcers. Depending on the series, *H. pylori* has been associated from 50% to 80% of all gastric ulcers. NSAIDs—nonsteroidal anti-inflammatory drugs.

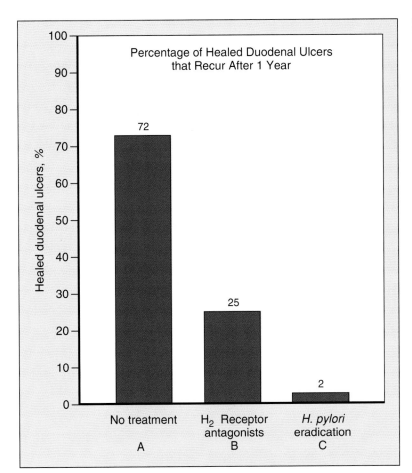

FIGURE 6-17.

Helicobacter pylori and peptic ulcer disease. The second major proof that *H. pylori* causes peptic ulcer disease is that when duodenal ulcers are healed by eradication of *H. pylori* (**C**), rates of recurrent ulcers are much lower than when ulcers are healed but *H. pylori* is not eradicated (**A** and **B**). (*Data from* Freston [14] and Tytgat and Rauws [15].)

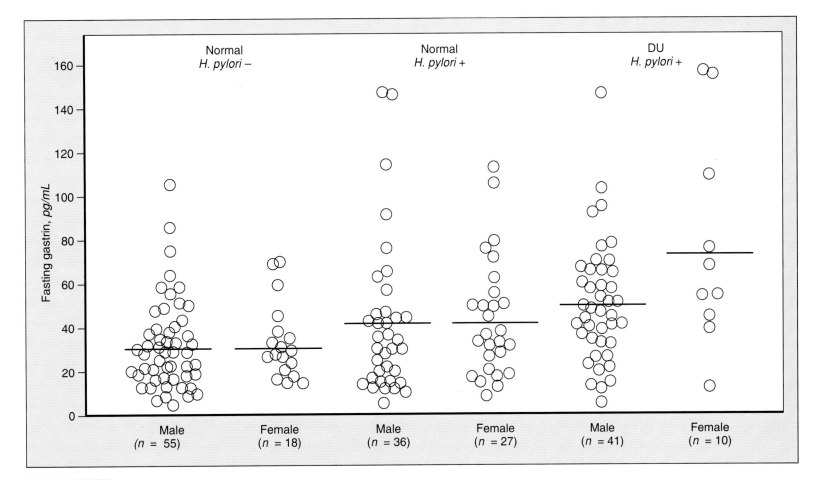

FIGURE 6-18.

Helicobacter pylori and serum gastrin concentrations. In both ulcer and nonulcer (normal) patients, *H. pylori* infection is associated with an increase in serum gastrin concentrations. Shown above are fasting serum gastrin (pg/mL) concentrations in normal subjects with and without *H. pylori* infections and duodenal ulcer (DU) patients as a function of gender. Mean values are represented by *horizontal bars*. (*From* Peterson *et al.* [16]; with permission.)

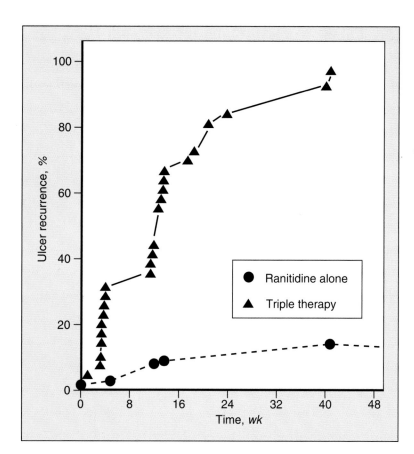

FIGURE 6-19.

Effect of *Helicobacter pylori* eradication on duodenal ulcer recurrence. In the results of the study, when triple therapy (bismuth, metronizadole, and either amoxicillin or tetracycline) is given for *H. pylori* eradication and is added to ranitidine for duodenal ulcer healing, duodenal ulcer recurrence rates at 1 year are much lower than when initial healing is accomplished with ranitidine alone. After the treatment period of ulcer healing, no ulcer maintenance therapy was given. (*From* Graham *et al.* [17]; with permission.)

TABLE 6-3. COMPARISON OF TREATMENT REGIMENS FOR ERADICATION OF *HELICOBACTER PYLORI*

REGIMEN	6-WEEK HEALING RATE, %	ERADICATION, %	RELAPSE RATE, %
Ranitidine, tetracycline, metronidazole, bismuth	80	90	12
Ranitidine, metronidazole, amoxicillin	92	89	8
Omeprazole, amoxicillin	100	60–80	9

TABLE 6-3.

Comparison of treatment regimens for eradication of *Helicobacter pylori*. Several different regimens are effective for *H. pylori* eradication. Three of the more commonly used regimens are listed above. Although there are small differences in rates of healing, eradication, and relapse, a common feature of all *H. pylori* eradication regimens is that if *H. pylori* is eradicated, then recurrence rates will be low for duodenal and gastric ulcers. For effective eradication of *H. pylori*, it is important that a combination of agents be used. There is no form of monotherapy that is effective for *H. pylori* eradication.

HELICOBACTER PYLORI AND GASTRIC CANCER

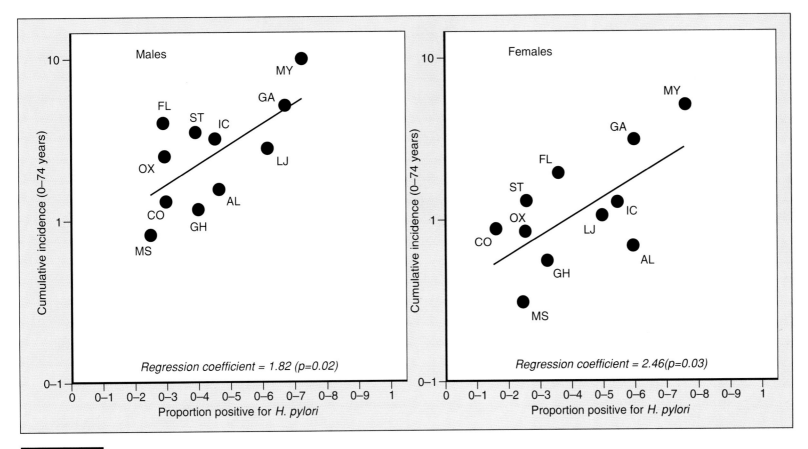

FIGURE 6-20.

Epidemiology and geographic data. Incidence and mortality rates from gastric cancer by *Helicobacter pylori* seropositivity. Epidemiologic data indicate that gastric cancer occurs more frequently in certain populations that also have higher rates of *H. pylori* infection. In this figure, in various populations, rates of *H. pylori* infection and rates of gastric adenocarcinoma are shown for both males (*left*) and females (*right*). Rates of *H. pylori* infection correlate with rates of gastric adenocarcinoma. Areas with low rates of *H. pylori* are associated with lower rates of gastric cancer and the reverse. AL—Algiers; CO—Copenhagen; FL—Florence; GA—Gaia; GH—Ghent; IC—Iceland; LJ—Ljubljana; MS—Minneapolis-St. Paul; MY—Miyagi; OX—Oxford; ST—Stoke. (*From* Eurogast Study Group [18]; with permission.)

TABLE 6-4. SEROPREVALENCE OF *HELICOBACTER PYLORI* 6 TO 14 YEARS BEFORE DIAGNOSIS OF GASTRIC CANCER IN NESTED CASE-CONTROL STUDIES

STUDY	CASES, *n*	CONTROLS, *n*	FOLLOW-UP, *y*	ODDS RATIO	95% CONFIDENCE INTERVAL
Forman [16]	29	116	6.0	2.8	1.0 to 8.0
Nomura [17]	109	109	13.0	6.0	2.1 to 17.3
Parsonnet [18]	108	108	14.2	3.6	1.8 to 7.3

TABLE 6-4.

In the results of three studies that are given, stored sera from patients with gastric adenocarcinoma and control subjects without cancer were analyzed for *Helicobacter pylori*. Sera were collected at time intervals ranging from 6 to 14 years before the diagnosis of cancer. Those who were infected with *H. pylori* at some point in the past ultimately had an incidence of gastric cancer that was three to six times higher than those who had not been infected with *H. pylori*. (*Data from* Forman *et al.* [19], Nomura *et al.* [20], and Parsonnet *et al.* [21].)

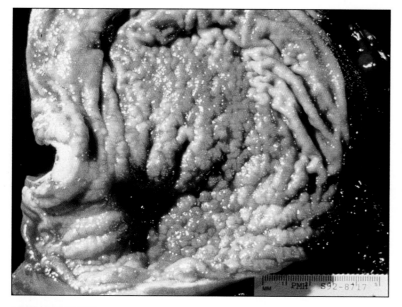

```
                    ┌──────────────┐
                    │   H. pylori  │
                    └──────┬───────┘
                           ▼
        ┌──────────────────────────────────┐
        │ Chronic active superficial gastritis │
        └──────────────────┬───────────────┘
                           ▼
        ┌──────────────────────────────────┐
        │    Chronic atrophic gastritis    │
        └──────────────────┬───────────────┘
                           ▼
        ┌──────────────────────────────────┐
        │     Chronic atrophic gastritis   │
        │     with intestinal metaplasia   │
        └──────────────────┬───────────────┘
                           ▼
        ┌──────────────────────────────────┐
        │            Dysplasia             │
        └──────────────────┬───────────────┘
                           ▼
        ┌──────────────────────────────────┐
        │      Gastric adenocarcinoma      │
        └──────────────────────────────────┘
```

FIGURE 6-21.

Characteristics of gross pathology. As shown in earlier figures, *Helicobacter pylori* is epidemiologically associated with adeno-carcinoma of the gastric body and antrum. This association of *H. pylori* is not, however, seen with adenocarcinomas of the gastric cardia. Shown is a resected stomach with diffuse gastric adenocarcinoma of the "linitis plastica" type. A very large, deep ulcer is seen at the junction of the gastric body and antrum. Diffuse thickening of the entire stomach is seen as producing multiple, nodular folds. On microscopic sections, *H. pylori* and adenocarcinoma were both visualized. (*Courtesy of* C. Vardaman, Dallas, TX)

FIGURE 6-22.

Relationship of *Helicobacter pylori* to gastric cancer. Sequence of gastric mucosal histologic events through which chronic gastric inflammation may predispose to gastric adenocarcinoma is shown. *H. pylori* is the major cause of chronic active superficial gastritis which, in some patients, may progress to chronic atrophic gastritis. As important as *H. pylori* appears to be in gastric cancer, however, other cofactors must also play a role. Only a small proportion of patients progress to atrophic gastritis, much less dysplasia and adenocarcinoma. At this time it is uncertain whether eradication of *H. pylori* in infected, but otherwise healthy, subjects will prevent gastric cancer or reduce its incidence.

TABLE 6-5. *HELICOBACTER PYLORI* AND GASTRIC NON-HODGKIN'S LYMPHOMAS

	CASES, *n*	INFECTED, %	MATCHED CONTROLS INFECTED, %	ODDS RATIO	95% CONFIDENCE INTERVAL
Gastric non-Hodgkin's lymphoma	33	85	55	6.3*	2.0 to 19.9
Nongastric non-Hodgkin's lymphoma	31	65	59	1.2	0.5 to 3.0

*P=0.02

TABLE 6-5.

Non-Hodgkin's lymphoma of the stomach is a rare disorder that accounts for only 3% of gastric malignancies, but is the most common type of extranodal lymphoma. Epidemiologic data have suggested an association between *H. pylori* infection and gastric lymphomas. Similar to the nested case control studies previously described, in this study, stored sera from patients with non-Hodgkin's gastric lymphomas and control subjects without cancer were analyzed for *H. pylori*. The sera were collected years before the diagnosis of gastric lymphoma. Patients with non-Hodgkin's gastric lymphoma were six times more likely to have been previously infected with *H. pylori* than were control subjects without lymphoma.

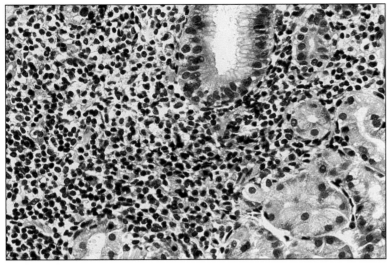

FIGURE 6-23.

Dense lymphoid infiltrate. Mucosa-associated lymphoid tissue lymph-omas (MALT), which constitute a subset of non-Hodgkin's lymphoma, are low-grade clonal neoplasms of B-cell lymphocytes that are thought to arise from lymphoid aggregates in the lamina propria. Epidemiologic data suggest that *H. pylori* infection is also associated with MALT lymphomas of the stomach. Shown is a gastric biopsy demonstrating a dense lymphoid infiltrate, possibly a precursor phenomenon to gastric MALT lymphoma. Note the numerous monotonous appearing lymphoid cells. This lymphoid aggregate is not yet felt to represent a MALT lymphoma.

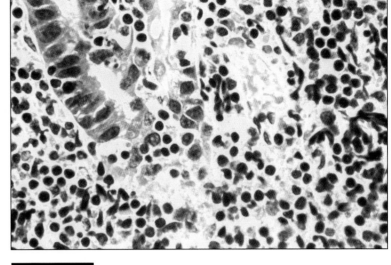

FIGURE 6-24.

Lymphoepithelial lesion. The transition from a *Helicobacter pylori*–related dense lymphoid infiltrate to a true mucosa-associated lymphoid tissue (MALT) lymphoma is felt to be represented histologically by the appearance of numerous lymphoepithelial lesions (LEL). Although LELs on histology are strongly suggestive of a MALT lymphoma, the diagnosis is confirmed through demonstration of monoclonality using gene rearrangement studies. As shown, a dense lymphoid infiltrate and glandular dropout are both present. The LEL is characterized by gland infiltration and destruction by lymphocytes.

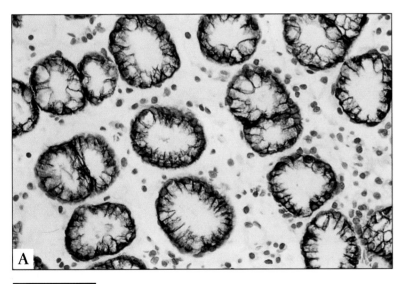

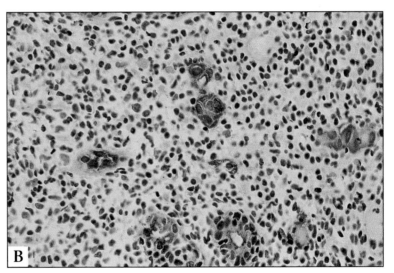

FIGURE 6-25.

Cytokeratin stains. As shown earlier in Figure 6-23, loss of gastric glands through destruction by invading lymphocytes is a characteristic feature of mucosa-associated lymphoid tissue (MALT) lymphomas. The loss of gastric glands is best appreciated on a cytokeratin stain, a stain which will highlight the gastric glands. A, A cytokeratin stain of normal gastric mucosa. Characteristic features are a normal number of gastric glands that are outlined graphically by the cytokeratin stain and the sparse population of plasma cells and lymphocytes in the lamina propria which do not invade the gastric glands. B, A cytokeratin-stained section of a biopsy of a MALT lymphoma. Compared with A (normal mucosa), note the significant "glandular dropout," lymphoepithelial lesions, and dense lymphoid infiltrate.

TABLE 6-6. REGRESSION OF GASTRIC MUCOSA-ASSOCIATED LYMPHOID TISSUE (MALT) LYMPHOMA WITH *HELICOBACTER PYLORI* ERADICATION

RESPONSE TO *H. PYLORI* ERADICATION	PATIENTS, *n**
Regression of MALT lymphoma	6
Reduction of MALT lymphoma	19
Persistence of MALT lymphoma	4
Status uncertain	3

*Total equals 32

TABLE 6-6.

Regression of gastric mucosa-associated lymphoid tissue (MALT) lymphoma with *Helicobacter pylori* eradication. Further evidence for a etiologic role of *H. pylori* in gastric MALT lymphomas comes from studies in which MALT lymphomas have been observed to regress after *H. pylori* eradication. In results of this study, 32 patients with MALT lymphoma and *H. pylori* were treated with antibiotics to eradicate *H. pylori*. Six patients showed regression and 19 patients showed a reduction in their MALT lymphomas with *H. pylori* eradication.

TABLE 6-7. GUIDELINES FOR ANTIBIOTIC THERAPY OF *HELICOBACTER PYLORI* INFECTION

	TREATMENT INDICATED?	
PATIENT STATUS	*H. PYLORI* NEGATIVE	*H. PYLORI* POSITIVE
Asymptomatic (No ulcer)	No	No
Nonulcer dyspepsia	No	No
Gastric ulcer	No	Yes
Duodenal ulcer	No	Yes
Gastric adenocarcinoma	No	No
Gastric mucosa-associated lymphoid tissue lymphoma	No	Yes

TABLE 6-7.

Guidelines for antibiotic therapy of *Helicobacter pylori* infection. (*From* NIH Consensus Development Panel [22].)

■ REFERENCES AND RECOMMENDED READING

1. Warren JR: Unidentified curved bacilli on gastric epithelium in active chronic gastritis (letter). *Lancet* 1983, 2:1273.

2. Marshall BJ: Unidentified curved bacilli on gastric epithelium in active chronic gastritis (letter). *Lancet* 1983, 2:1273–1275.

3. Thomsen LL, Gavin JB, Tasman-Jones C: Relation of *Helicobacter pylori* to the human gastric mucosa in chronic gastritis of the antrum. *Gut* 1990, 31:1230–1236.

4. Dooley CP, Fitzgibbons PL, Cohen H, *et al.*: Prevalence of *Helicobacter pylori* infection and histologic gastritis in asymptomatic persons. *N Engl J Med* 1989, 321:1562–1566.

5. Graham DY, Klein PD, Opekun AR, Boutton TW: Effect of age on the frequency of active *Campylobacter pylori* infection diagnosed by the ^{13}C-urea breath test on normal subjects and patients with peptic ulcer disease. *J Infect Dis* 1988, 157:777–780.

6. Megraud F, Brassens-Rabbe M-P, Denis F, *et al.*: Seroepidemiology of *Campylobacter pylori* infection in various populations. *J Clin Microbiol* 1989, 27:1870–1873.

7. Kosunen TU, Hook J, Rautelin HI, Myllyla G: Age-dependent increase of *Campylobacter pylori* antibodies in blood donors. *Scand J Gastroenterol* 1989, 24:110–114.

8. Mitchell HM, Lee A, Berkowicz J, Borody T: The use of serology to diagnose active *Campylobacter pylori* infection. *Med J Aust* 1988, 149:604–609.

9. Perez-Perez GI, Bodhidatta L, Wongsrichanalai J, *et al.*: Seroprevalence of *Campylobacter pylori* infections in Thailand. *J Infect Dis* 1990, 161:1237–1241.

10. Taylor DH, Blaser MJ: The epidemiology of *Helicobacter pylori* infection. In *Helicobacter pylori in Peptic Ulceration and Gastritis*. Edited by Marshall BJ, McCallum RW, Guerrant RL. Boston: Blackwell Scientific; 1991:46–54.

11. Malaty HM, Evans DG, Evans DJ Jr, Graham DY: *Helicobacter pylori* in Hispanics: Comparison with blacks and whites of similar age and socioeconomic class. *Gastroenterology* 1992, 103:813–816.

12. Drumm B, Perez-Perez GI, Blaser MJ, Sherman PM: Intrafamilial clustering of *Helicobacter pylori* infection. *N Engl J Med* 1990, 322:359—363.

13. Peterson WL, Lee E, Feldman M: Relationship between *Campylobacter pylori* and gastritis in healthy humans after administration of placebo or indomethacin. *Gastroenterology* 1988, 95:1185–1197.

14. Freston JW: H$_2$-receptor antagonists and duodenal ulcer recurrence: Analysis of efficacy and commentary on safety, costs, and patients selection. *Am J Gastroenterol* 1987, 82:1242–1249.

15. Tytgat GNJ, Rauws EAJ: *Campylobacter pylori* and its role in peptic ulcer disease. *Gastroenterol Clin North Am* 1990, 19:183–196.

16. Peterson WL, Barnett CC, Evans DJ Jr, *et al.*: Acid secretion and serum gastrin in normal subjects and patients with duodenal ulcer: The role of *Helicobacter pylori*. *Am J Gastroenterol* 1993, 88:2038–2043.

17. Graham DY, Lew GM, Klein PD, *et al.*: Effect of treatment of *Helicobacter pylori* infection on the long-term recurrence of gastric or duodenal ulcer: A randomized, controlled study. *Ann Intern Med* 1992, 116:705–708.

18. The Eurogast Study Group: An international association between *Helicobacter pylori* infection and gastric cancer. *Lancet* 1993, 341:1359–1362.

19. Forman D, Newell D, Fullerton F, *et al.*: Association between infection with *Helicobacter pylori* and risk of cancer: Evidence from a prospective investigation. *BMJ* 1991, 302:1302–1305.

20. Nomura A, Stemmermann GN, Chyou P, *et al.*: *Helicobacter pylori* infection and gastric carcinoma among Japanese Americans in Hawaii. *N Engl J Med* 1991, 325:1132–1162.

21. Parsonnet J, Friedman GD, Vandersteen DP, *et al.*: *Helicobacter pylori* infection and the risk of gastric carcinoma. *N Engl J Med* 1991, 325:1127–1131.

22. NIH Consensus Development Panel: *Helicobacter pylori* in peptic ulcer disease. *JAMA* 1994, 272:65–69.

Chapter 7

Peptic Ulcer Disease

C. Mel Wilcox

Benign ulcerative lesions of the stomach and duodenum, collectively termed *peptic ulcer disease,* have been recognized for many years as an important cause of morbidity and potential mortality. These gastroduodenal lesions may be the end result of a variety of heterogenous processes. Superficial lesions caused by denudation of the surface epithelium, termed *erosions,* may sometimes be difficult to distinguish both radiographically and endoscopically from small ulcers. True ulceration represents a mucosal defect extending into the muscularis mucosa. Over the past decade, the etiologic association of *Helicobacter pylori* with peptic ulcer has been conclusively established. The epidemiology and pathophysiologic consequences of gastritis resulting from *H. pylori* reconcile several features associated with peptic ulcer disease. This association has profoundly changed our current approach to diagnosis and treatment of ulcer disease.

Peptic ulcer disease is a common condition. It has been estimated that 5% to 10% of the population of the United States may develop a peptic ulcer. Although the incidence of peptic ulcer disease appears to be decreasing, the use of both prescription and over-the-counter nonsteroidal anti-inflammatory drugs has increased the incidence of ulcerative disease of the stomach. Nevertheless, ulcer disease continues to be associated with significant morbidity, primarily from complications such as bleeding and perforation.

Peptic ulcer disease may usually be suspected when the patient presents with the typical complaint of epigastric abdominal pain. The pain usually occurs either between meals or at night. Eating often relieves the pain, although in some patients, eating may cause or exacerbate the pain or may result in nausea and vomiting. Ulcer disease may present acutely with bleeding or perforation in the absence of prior abdominal complaints. The barium upper gastrointestinal radiologic series remains a useful diagnostic tool, although sensitivity varies depending on the size and location of the ulcer. Endoscopic examination has the highest sensitivity and may be more appropriate for patients with a complication such as bleeding or when a gastric malignancy is clinically suspected. Given the association of *H. pylori* with peptic ulcer and that noninvasive tests are now available for diagnosis of this infection, diagnostic strategies for peptic ulcer may change in the future. Currently, however, endoscopy represents the standard criterion for diagnosis of peptic ulcer.

Current clinical therapeutic techniques effectively treat peptic ulcer. Over the past 3 decades, treatment regimens have advanced from high-dose antacids to H₂-receptor blockers and, more recently, to proton pump inhibitors such as omeprazole.

The latter agents effectively abolish gastric acid secretion. Nevertheless, despite the efficacy of these drugs, ulcer recurrence remains almost uniform. Effective antibiotic therapy to eradicate *H. pylori*, however, has dramatically changed the natural history of ulcer disease, so that, in many patients, ulcer disease may be cured. Surgery still represents an important therapeutic option, particularly in those patients with a complication such as perforation, pyloric obstruction, or significant hemorrhage.

EPIDEMIOLOGY

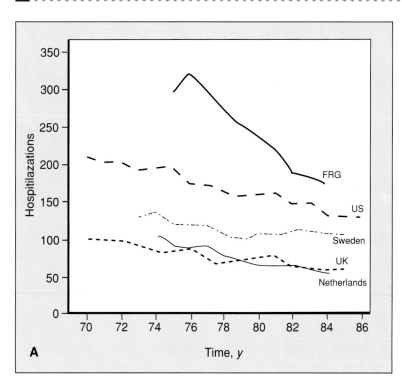

A

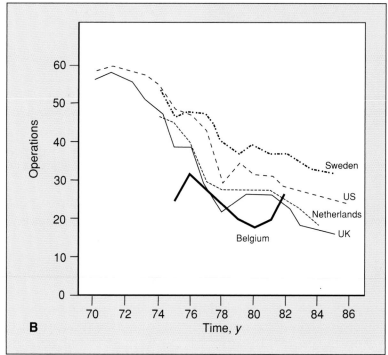

B

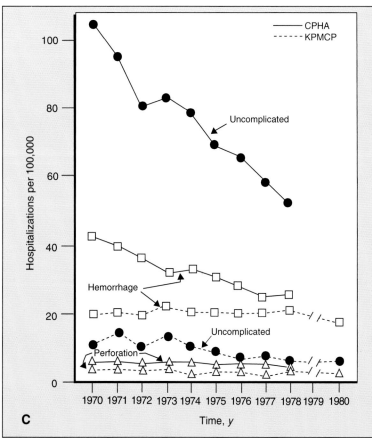

C

FIGURE 7-1.

Trends in the epidemiology of peptic ulcer. Studies undertaken in the United States, as well as in other developed countries, suggest that the incidence of peptic ulcer has been decreasing over the past several decades. **A,** This decreasing incidence has been manifested by significant reductions in hospitalizations for peptic ulcer. **B,** Other important trends include decreases in loss of work and elective surgery for peptic ulcer. **C,** However, incidence of bleeding peptic ulcer and perforation remains little changed. Interestingly, these changes in the incidence of peptic ulcer occurred before the introduction of the first H₂-receptor antagonist (cimetidine) in 1977.

(Continued on next page)

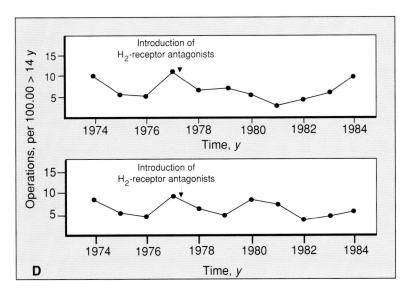

FIGURE 7-1. (CONTINUED)

D, In addition, use of these agents has not decreased the rate of surgery for complicated ulcers (*eg*, bleeding, perforation). Given that ulcers rarely result in death, changes in mortality have been much less significant. CPHA—Commission on Professional and Hospital Activities (National); FRG—Federal Republic of Germany (the former West Germany); KPMCP—Kaiser-Permanente Medical Care Program. (**A** and **B**, *From* Bloom [1]; with permission.) (**C**, *From* Kurata and Haile [2]; with permission.) (**D**, *From* Christensen *et al.* [3]; with permission.)

PATHOGENESIS

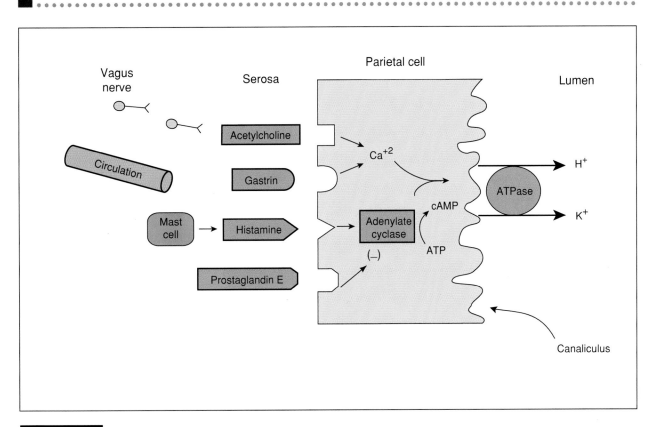

FIGURE 7-2.

The parietal cell and gastric acid secretion. Gastric acid secretion is a highly regulated process involving paracrine, neurocrine, and endocrine mechanisms. Three receptors on the serosal side of the parietal cell are involved with acid secretion. Binding of histamine, released locally from tissue mast cells, to the histamine$_2$ receptor augments acid secretion by increasing intracellular cyclic AMP (cAMP) (paracrine) levels. Acetylcholine released from the vagus nerve stimulates gastric acid secretion by increasing intracellular calcium concentration (neurocrine). After release from the gastrin-producing cells of the gastric antrum, circulating gastrin binds to its receptor, resulting in an increase in intracellular calcium concentrations (endocrine).

Ultimately, increases in cAMP and intracellular calcium concentrations trigger the hydrogen potassium ATPase to pump hydrogen against a steep concentration gradient into the lumen with potassium brought into the cell. This proton pump (H, K, ATPase) is on the cannalicular membrane. A prostaglandin receptor appears to exist on the serosal surface of the parietal cell. Prostaglandins exert a negative feedback on acid secretion through a G protein on adenylate cyclase causing a decrease in cAMP. An appreciation of the physiology of gastric acid secretion has importance when discussing treatments of peptic ulcer. ECL—enterochromaffin-like cell.

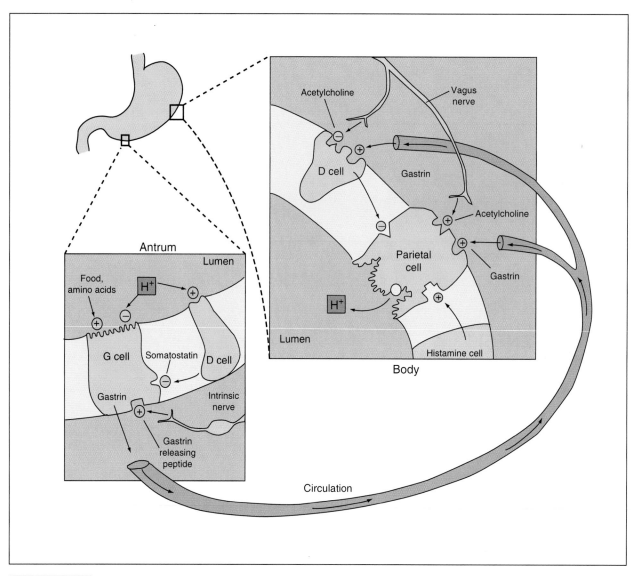

FIGURE 7-3.

Feedback regulation of acid secretion. The D cell (somatostatin cell) plays an important role in feedback regulation of gastric acid secretion. It has a negative feedback on the gastrin cell in the antrum as well as the parietal cell. Diverse stimuli result in somatostatin secretion. Recent evidence suggests that *Helicobacter pylori* antritis affects somatostatin cell function. (*From* Daugherty *et al.* [4]; with permission.)

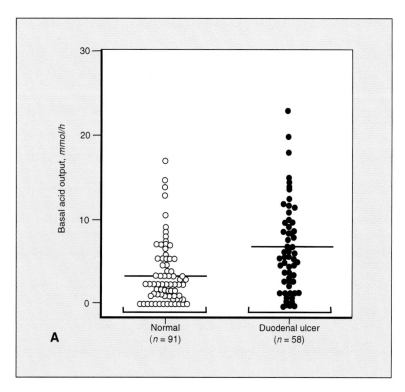

FIGURE 7-4.

Gastric acid secretion in patients with duodenal ulcer compared with normal patients. **A,** Overall, basal acid output is roughly twice as high in patients with duodenal ulcer as that found in normal patients (7.1 mmol/hr versus 3.3 mmol/hr); however, significant overlap does exist between these groups.

(Continued on next page)

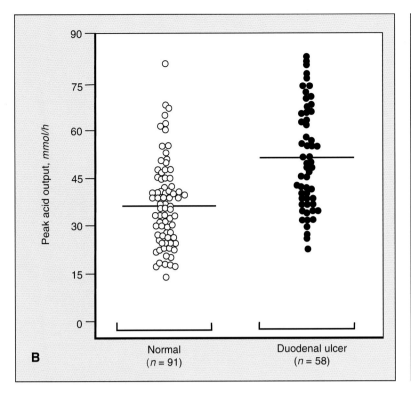

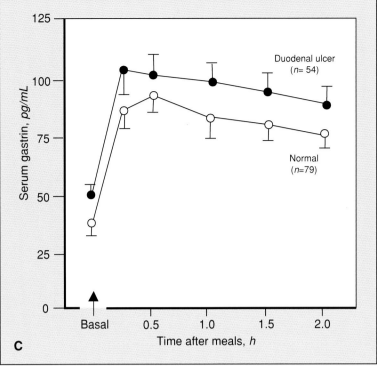

FIGURE 7-4. (CONTINUED)

B, Similarly, patients with duodenal ulcer have a higher peak acid output. **C**, Serum gastrin concentration is also higher in patients with duodenal ulcer than in normal subjects, although the gastrin response to a meal is similar. (*From* Blair *et al.* [5]; with permission.)

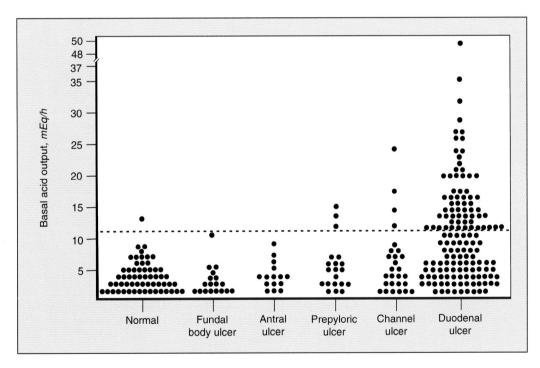

FIGURE 7-5.

Gastric acid secretion in patients with gastric ulcer. Regardless of location, patients with gastric ulcer have basal acid outputs more closely approximating those found in normal subjects. Some patients with prepyloric or pyloric channel ulcers have acid outputs similar to those found in patients with duodenal ulcer. As demonstrated in the findings of other studies, duodenal ulcer patients have higher basal acid outputs than those seen in normal subjects. (*From* Collen and Sheridan [6]; with permission.)

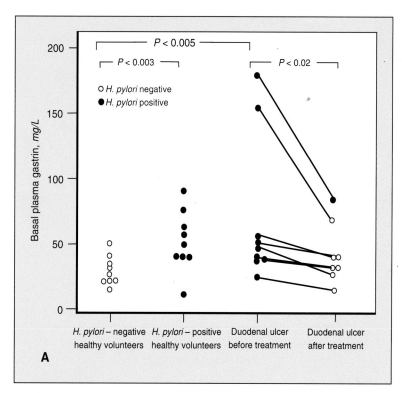

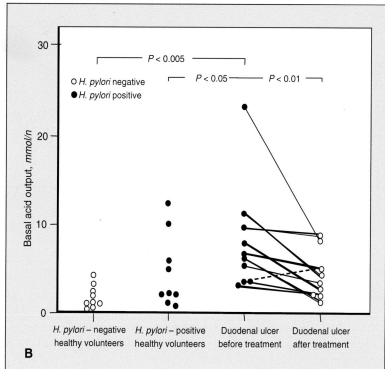

FIGURE 7-6.

Alterations in serum gastrin and gastric acid secretion after eradication of *Helicobacter pylori*. With effective eradication of *H. pylori* and antral gastritis, serum gastrin levels (**A**) and basal acid output (**B**) return to normal in patients with duodenal ulcer. (*From* El-Omar *et al.* [7]; with permission.)

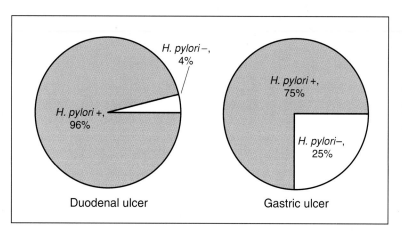

FIGURE 7-7.

Prevalence of *Helicobacter pylori* in peptic ulcer. It has been recognized for many years that antral gastritis was almost uniformly present in patients with duodenal ulcer and in many patients with gastric ulcer as well. It is now known that *H. pylori* causes this gastritis. The lower frequency of *H. pylori* in patients with gastric ulcer may relate to the ingestion of nonsteroidal anti-inflammatory drugs as the primary cause of ulcer. (*Adapted from* Bayerdorffer and Mannes [8]; with permission.)

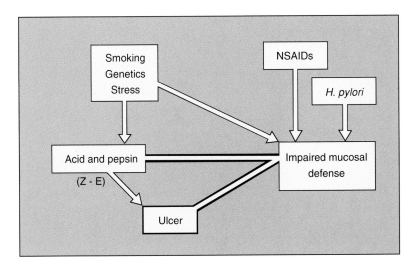

FIGURE 7-8.

Summary of pathogenic mechanisms in ulcer disease. Several factors may alone or in combination cause peptic ulcer. Non-steroidal anti-inflammatory drugs and *Helicobacter pylori* impair mucosal defense. Exogenous factors, such as smoking, also impair mucosal defense. Genetic factors play a role in predisposing to ulcer disease. The role of stress in the genesis of ulcer remains controversial. In Zollinger-Ellison (Z-E) syndrome, acid and pepsin alone cause ulceration. (*Adapted from* Soll [9]; with permission.)

CLINICAL FEATURES

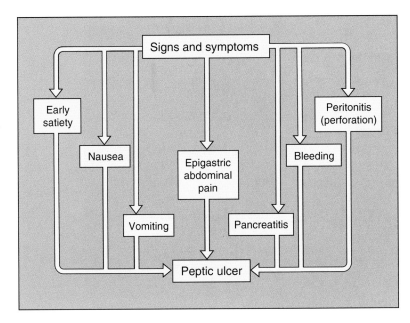

FIGURE 7-9.

Clinical manifestations of ulcer disease. The most common finding on presentation of both gastric and duodenal ulcers is abdominal pain. The pain is usually localized to the epigastrium, although it may be located in the right upper quadrant (duodenal ulcer) or the left upper quadrant (gastric ulcer). Pain typically occurs between meals or at night in patients with duodenal ulcer but can be seen in gastric ulcer as well. Nausea and vomiting may be a prominent feature in the absence of outlet obstruction and occurs with or without food ingestion. The index manifestation of either gastric or duodenal ulcer may be a complication such as gastrointestinal bleeding, gastric outlet obstruction manifested by nausea and vomiting, or an acute abdomen caused by perforation. Unusual presentations of ulcers include chest or back pain or pancreatitis.

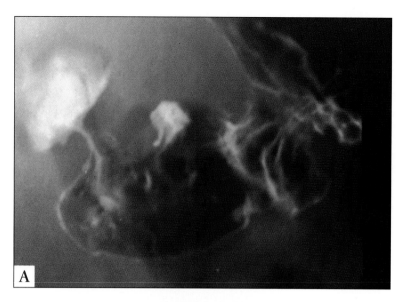

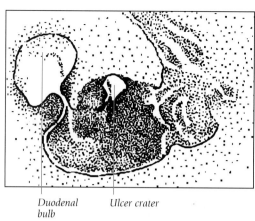

Duodenal bulb   Ulcer crater

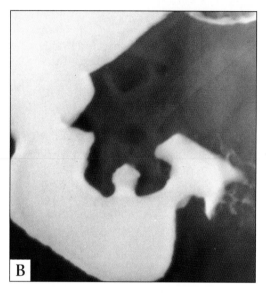

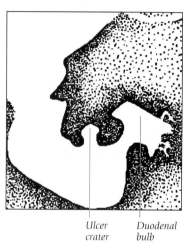

Ulcer crater   Duodenal bulb

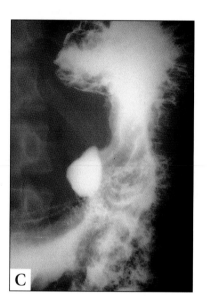

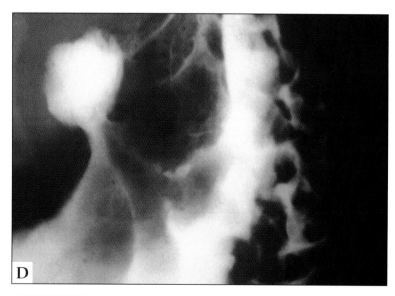

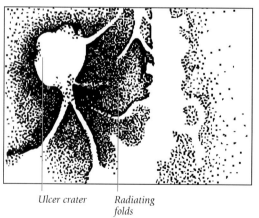

Ulcer crater   Radiating folds

Typical radiographic features of a benign gastric ulcer. This ulcer on the distal lesser curvature in the antrum is well circumscribed (**A**) and lateral views (**B**) demonstrate projection of the crater away from the lumen. A large well-circumscribed ulcer is seen on the angularis (**C**). Rugal folds can be seen radiating to the crater (**D**).

(Continued on next page)

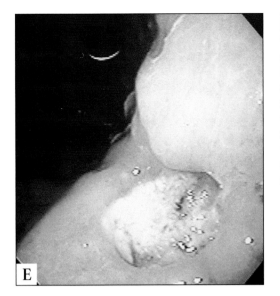

FIGURE 7-10. (CONTINUED)

The ulcer crater at endoscopy is shown in **E**. The lesion is large and well circumscribed with a symmetrical appearance. Multiple biopsies did not demonstrate carcinoma and the ulcer was demonstated to heal on follow-up endoscopy. Radiographic features suggestive of a benign ulcer include projection of the ulcer away from the lumen, abscence of mass effect or mucosal nodularity, and rugal folds of normal appearance, which extend to the ulcer crater. The sensitivity of barium radiography for the diagnosis of gastric ulcer is approximately 65% to 90%; the sensitivity increases with the size of the lesion.

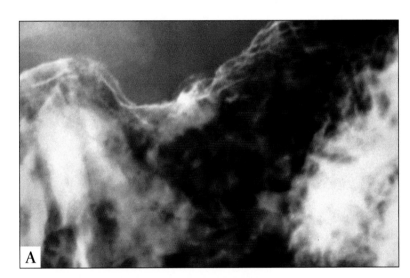

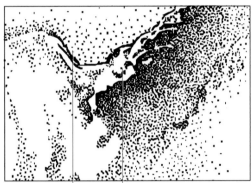

Retraction   Ulcer crater

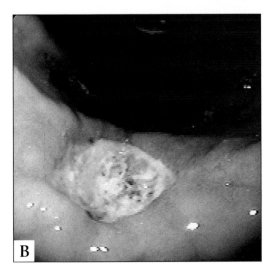

FIGURE 7-11.

Benign gastric ulcer. **A**, Barium radiograph demonstrates a lesion on the angularis atypical for a benign lesion because the angularis is retracted. The ulcer margin is also not well demarcated. No abnormal rugal folds surround the lesion. Radiographically, a malignant lesion could not be excluded. **B**, Typical endoscopic appearance of a benign gastric ulcer. The ulcer is on the angularis—the most common location for a gastric ulcer—and is well circumscribed without any associated mass effect. The surrounding mucosa is mildly erythematous and without nodularity.

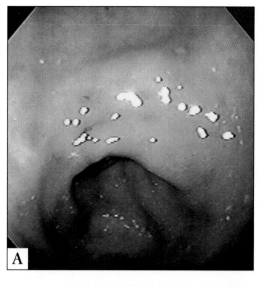

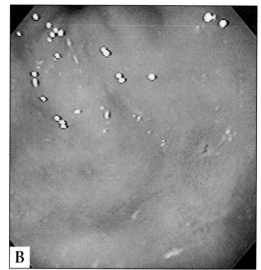

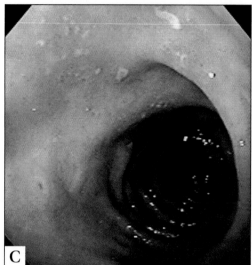

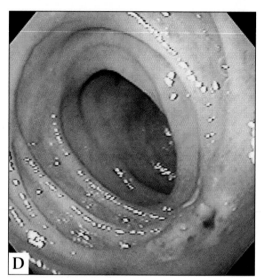

FIGURE 7-12.

Nonsteroidal anti-inflammatory drug (NSAID)–induced disease. Although NSAID–induced lesions may occur anywhere in the stomach or duodenum, the most common location is the antrum. In this patient, subepithelial hemorrhage, erosions and small ulcers are seen in the antrum (A–B). Erosions in the duodenal bulb (C) and a posterior duodenal ulcer (D) are also present.

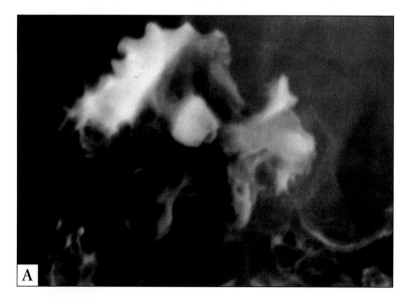

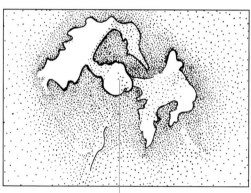

Ulcer crater

FIGURE 7-13.

Typical radiographic features of duodenal ulcer. A, This duodenal bulb ulcer is associated with marked edema, resulting in the appearance of radiating folds to the ulcer crater. The bulb is also distored secondary to previously existing ulceration.

(Continued on next page)

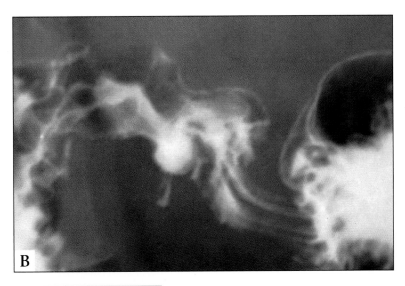

B

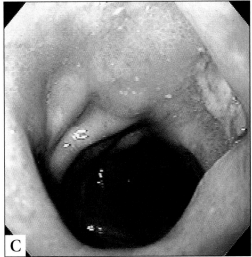

C

FIGURE 7-13. (CONTINUED)

B, A posterior bulbar ulcer is seen associated with distortion of the bulb. C, The duodenal ulcer as seen during endoscopy. The bulb is edematous and hemorrhagic with diffuse erosions. The sensitivity of barium studies for duodenal ulcer is 50% with the single-contrast technique but increases to between 80% and 90% when the double-contrast technique is performed.

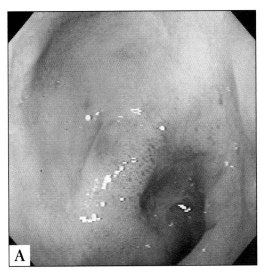

A

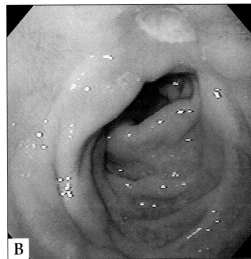

B

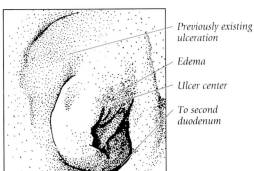

Previously existing ulceration

Edema

Ulcer center

To second duodenum

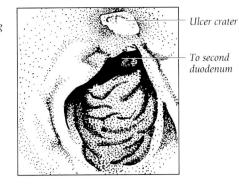

Ulcer crater

To second duodenum

FIGURE 7-14.

Duodenal ulcer. A, An ulcer is seen from an anterior view. Such ulcers are associated with deformity and a large depression secondary to previously existing ulceration. B, A well-circumscribed lesion as seen in a superior view. The remaining portion of the bulb is mildly edematous but without any associated subepithelial hemorrhage or erosions.

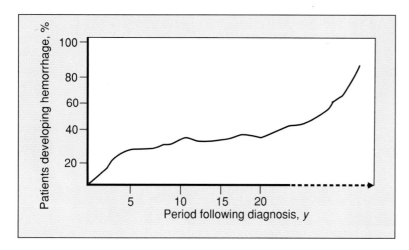

FIGURE 7-15.

Gastrointestinal bleeding represents the most common complication of peptic ulcer. Longitudinal studies of patients with uncomplicated peptic ulcer document a variable incidence of hemorrhage. Depending on the length of follow-up, the proportion of patients ultimately developing hemorrhage varies from 10% to almost 80%. (*Adapted from* Penston and Wormsley [10]; with permission.)

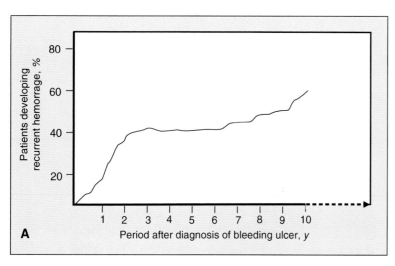

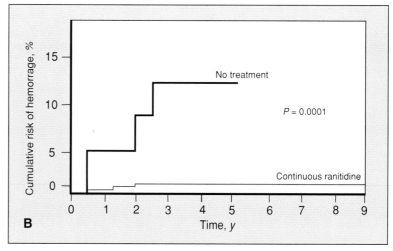

FIGURE 7-16.

Incidence of recurrent bleeding in patients with previously existing peptic ulcer bleeding. Long-term follow-up observation without maintenance antiacid therapy documents a significant proportion with recurrent bleeding. **A,** Depending on the length of follow-up, the incidence of recurrent hemorrhage is variable, although over 50% of patients may have recurrent bleeding. **B,** If a patient remains on maintenance therapy with H_2-receptor antagonists, recurrent bleeding is dramatically reduced. (**A,** *Adapted from* Penston and Wormsley [10]; with permission.) (**B,** *From* Penston [11]; with permission.)

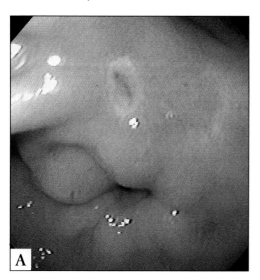

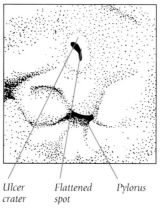

Ulcer crater   Flattened spot   Pylorus

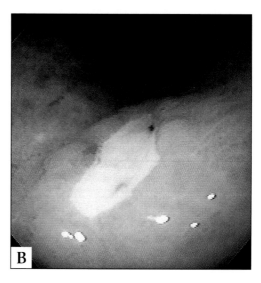

FIGURE 7-17.

Stigmata of recent hemorrhage in patients with bleeding ulcer. **A,** A linear, flat, red spot in the base of a small peripyloric ulcer. **B,** Two flat black spots in the base of a benign-appearing ulcer on the angularis. *(Continued on next page)*

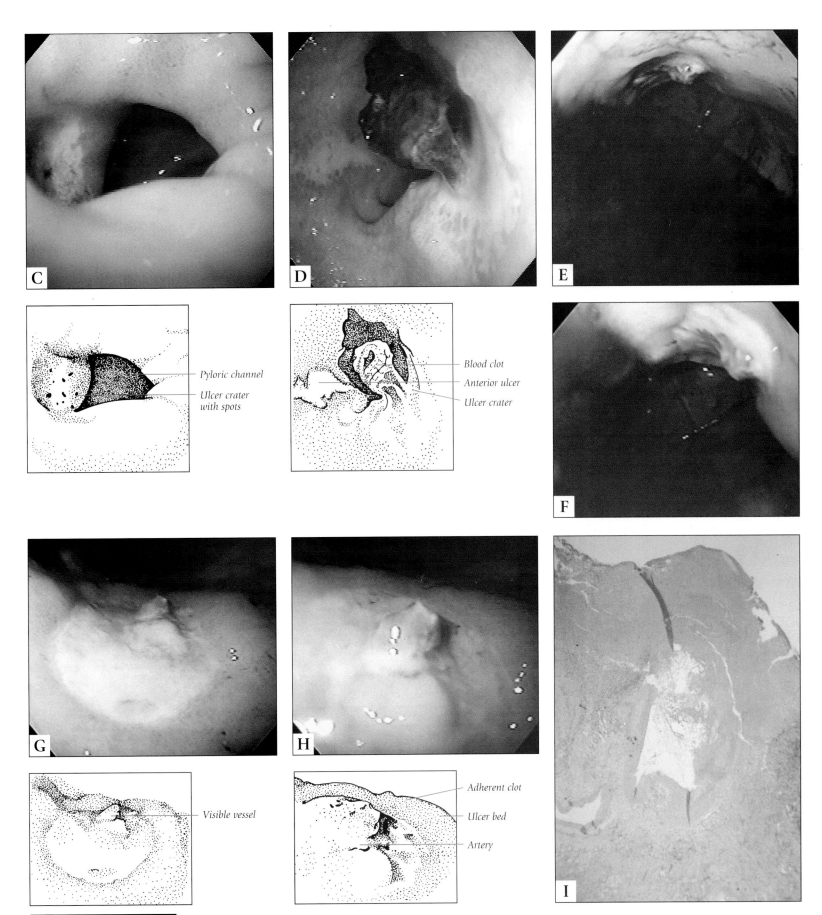

FIGURE 7-17. (CONTINUED)

C, Multiple black spots in the base of a pyloric channel ulcer. The risk of recurrent bleeding with spots in an ulcer base is very low, approximately 5%. D, Two ulcers in the duodenal bulb. A large blood clot is seen overlying the posterior bulbar ulcer (*right*). There is some increase in bleeding with a blood clot in an ulcer base. E, Nonbleeding visible vessel. A gastric ulcer high on the lesser curve with a protuberance from the center of the lesion (*E*). F, Close-up of the lesion demonstrates a visible vessel. G, A benign-appearing gastric ulcer located on the

angularis has a protruberance in the center of the crater characteristic of a visible vessel (**G**) (*bottom* [**H, close up view**]). This stigmata has approximately 50% chance of rebleeding. Certain colors of the visible vessel may increase the chance of rebleeding to 90%. (In this patient, hemorrhage recurred and gastric ulcer resection was performed.) I, The histopathologic equivalent of the visible vessel is shown. In this patient, a large artery is seen in the base of the ulcer with clot resulting in a nipplelike projection from the ulcer base.

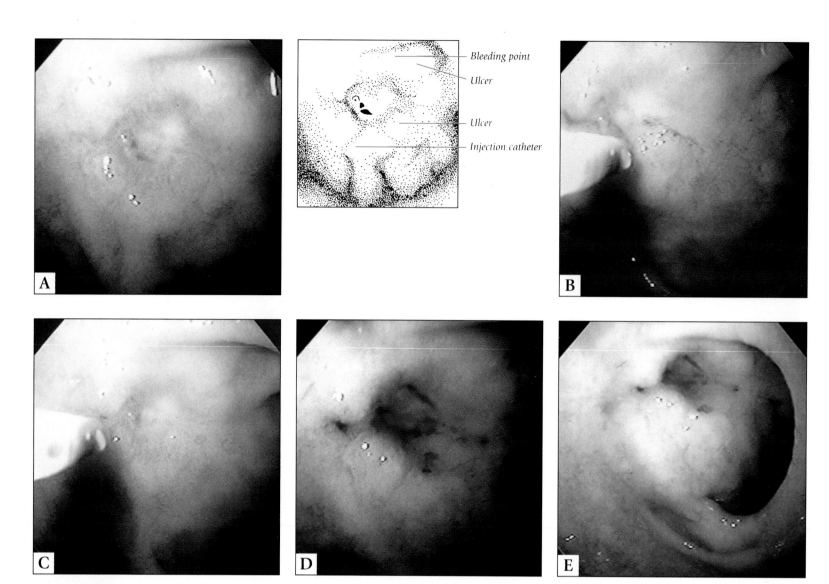

Bleeding point
Ulcer
Ulcer
Injection catheter

FIGURE 7-18.

Endoscopic therapy of bleeding ulcer. Endoscopic therapy has produced significant advancements in the diagnosis and treatment of bleeding ulcer. At the time of endoscopy, endoscopic therapy may be applied to bleeding lesions to arrest the bleeding and to prevent rebleeding. **A–C,** In this patient with an oozing duodenal ulcer, a standard injection needle was placed into the base of the ulcer nearest the area of bleeding with injection of epinephrine (concentration of 1:10,000). **D** and **E,** The ulcer bed and surrounding duodenal mucosa is then seen to blanch.

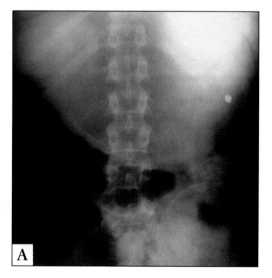

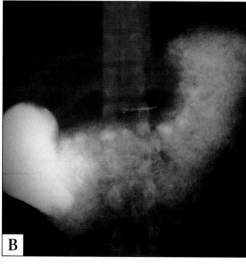

FIGURE 7-19.

Pyloric outlet obstruction related to peripyloric ulcer disease is uncommon. Acutely, obstruction may result from edema. In some patients, however, chronic disease results in fixed fibrosis and outlet obstruction. **A,** Plain film of the abdomen in a patient presenting with nausea and vomiting and a succussion splash on physical examination demonstrates a massively enlarged stomach with inferior displacement of the transverse colon; a nasogastric tube is seen in the stomach. **B,** Barium upper gastrointestinal study demonstrates the size of the stomach.

(Continued on next page)

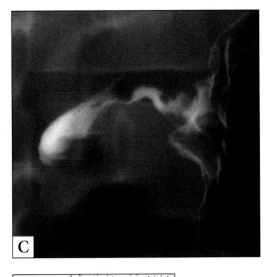

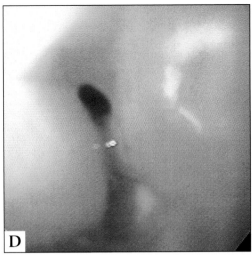

FIGURE 7-19. (CONTINUED)

C, Edema, spasm, and a small ulcer crater are present in the pyloric channel area. **D**, Endoscopy demonstrates the pyloric obstruction with an active ulcer crater seen in the pyloric channel. Nasogastric suction and intravenous H_2-receptor antagonists resulted in a clinical cure. In some patients, surgery may be required. Endoscopic balloon dilation has been useful in some patients with fixed obstruction without active ulcer disease.

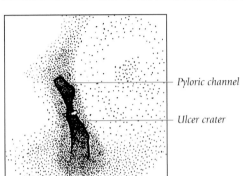

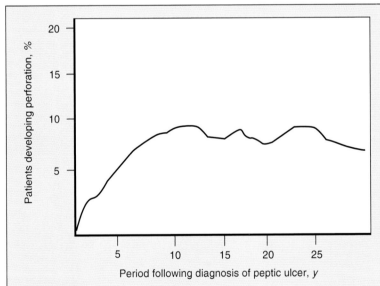

FIGURE 7-20.

Peptic ulcer perforation The incidence of perforation in patients with uncomplicated peptic ulcer is less than with bleeding, approaching 10%. (*Adapted from* Penston and Wormsley [10]; with permission.)

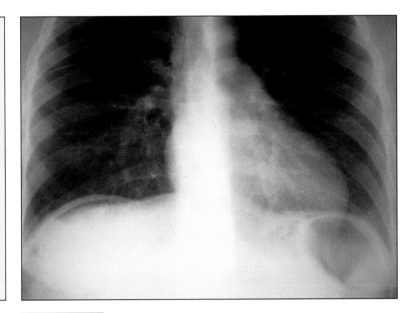

FIGURE 7-21.

Perforated peptic ulcer. Air is present under the right hemidiaphragm in a patient with acute severe abdominal pain. This patient had Zollinger-Ellison syndrome and a perforated anterior duodenal bulbar ulcer. Perforated ulcer has also been associated with non-steroidal anti-inflammatory drug ingestion and cocaine use.

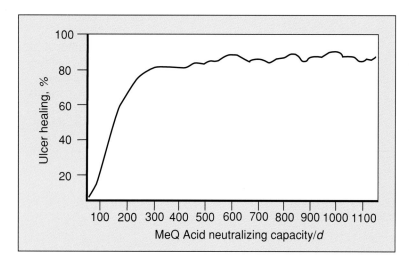

FIGURE 7-22.

Healing rates of duodenal ulcer with varying doses of antacids. Antacids have been employed for many years to treat peptic ulcer. In the treatment of duodenal ulcer, if at least 200 mEq per day of acid-neutralizing capacity of an antacid are used, the healing rate at 4 weeks approaches 80% or better. The acid-neutralizing capacity of these lower-dose regimens suggests that mechanisms other than buffering of acid alone result in healing.

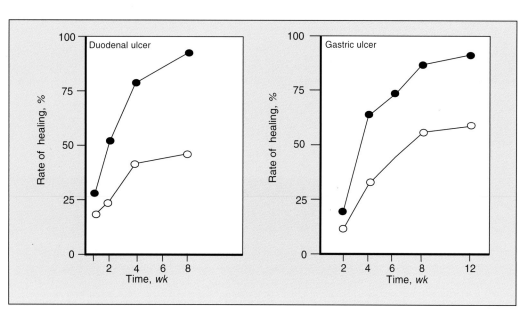

FIGURE 7-23.

Healing rates for gastric and duodenal ulcer with H_2-receptor antagonists. The healing rate of duodenal ulcers with standard doses of any H_2-receptor antagonist increases consistently until 8 weeks, when approximately 90% of ulcers are healed. Prolonging therapy for an additional 2 to 4 weeks may further increase healing, although in approximately 5% of patients, ulcers will still remain unhealed. Placebo healing rates at 8 weeks are approximately 40%. In patients with gastric ulcer, healing rates are similar, although 12 weeks of therapy may be required to obtain approximately 90% ulcer healing. (*From* Feldman and Burton [12]; with permission.)

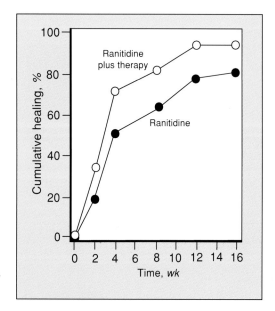

FIGURE 7-24.

Rate of duodenal ulcer healing with *Helicobacter pylori* treatment. With the addition of antibiotic therapy to eradicate *H. pylori*, duodenal ulcer healing rates at 8 and 12 weeks are significantly higher than with standard H_2-receptor antagonists, further suggesting a role for *H. pylori* in duodenal ulcer disease. (*From* Graham *et al.* [13]; with permission.)

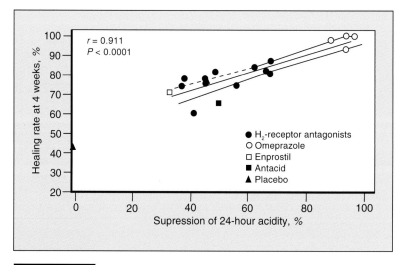

FIGURE 7-25.

Relationship of degree of acid suppression to rate of duodenal ulcer healing. A significant relation exists between the degree of acid suppression and rate of duodenal ulcer healing. If 24-hour acid suppression is 90% or greater, 4-week healing rates approach 100%. In patients with gastric ulcer, profound acid suppression will also result in more rapid healing, although not as striking as seen with duodenal ulcer. (*From* Dobrilla *et al.* [14]; with permission.)

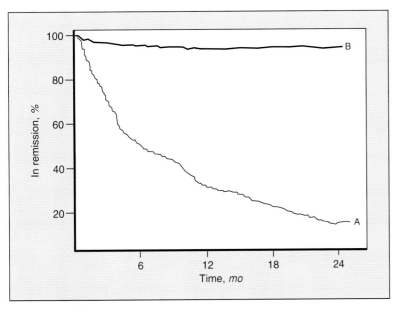

FIGURE 7-26.

Natural history of duodenal ulcer. The natural history of duodenal ulcer is one of recurrence. Depending on the length of follow-up and the intervals at which endoscopy is performed, duodenal ulcer may recur in over 90% of patients at 1 to 2 years (**A**). The rate of gastric ulcer recurrence is less, although significant. With effective eradication of *Helicobacter pylori*, the 1-year reinfection rate is less than 1%, and the relapse rate for ulcer is dramatically reduced in comparison with standard treatments (**B**). In some studies with 7 or more years of follow-up, almost all patients in whom *H. pylori* is eradicated remained free of ulcer relapse. Thus, eradication of *H. pylori* affects the natural history of ulcer disease and offers the possibility of cure. Similar results have been found in the treatment of *H. pylori*–associated gastric ulcer.

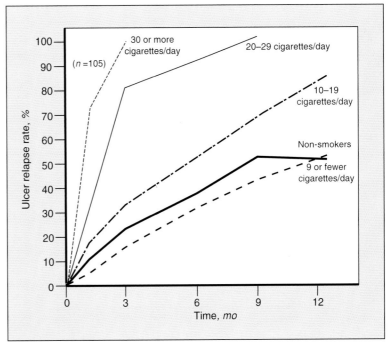

FIGURE 7-27.

The effect of cigarette smoking on ulcer recurrence. Cigarette smoking has an important influence on the rate of duodenal ulcer relapse. When comparing nonsmokers with those smoking 30 cigarettes a day, the recurrence rate varies from 45% to nearly 100%. Ulcers recur more rapidly as the number of cigarettes smoked per day increases. Recent evidence suggests, however, that if *Helicobacter pylori* is eradicated, smoking does not increase the rate of recurrence. (*From* Dammann and Walter [15]; with permission.)

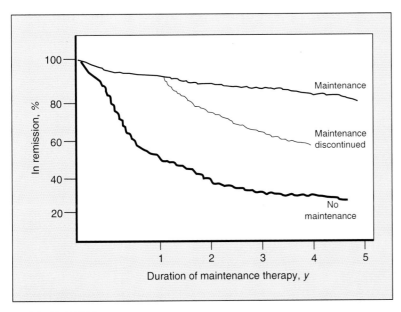

FIGURE 7-28.

Ulcer recurrence on long-term H$_2$-receptor antagonist maintenance treatment. Long-term therapy with any H$_2$-receptor antagonist dramatically reduces the rate of ulcer recurrence. In studies to 9 years, ulcer remission is approximately 80% in the treated groups as compared with 10% in untreated patients. For those patients in the treated group in whom H$_2$-receptor antagonists are discontinued, the recurrence of ulcer will then approach the untreated group. Thus, in contrast to *Helicobacter pylori* eradication, H$_2$-receptor antagonists do not alter the natural history of duodenal ulcer. Similar results have been found with gastric ulcer as well.

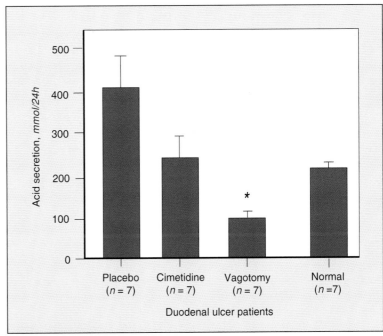

FIGURE 7-29.

Effect of antiulcer therapy and highly selective vagotomy on acid secretion. In duodenal ulcer patients, highly selective vagotomy reduces 24-hour gastric acid secretion to levels below H$_2$-receptor antagonists and significantly less than placebo. Depending on the length of follow-up, the long-term recurrence rate of 10% to 30% after highly selective vagotomy is slightly higher than long-term H$_2$-receptor antagonist therapy where recurrence rates over 9 years approximate 10% to 20%. Truncal vagotomy and antrectomy with vagotomy have recurrence rates of 10% and 2%, respectively, given their greater reductions in acid secretion. (*From* Feldman and Richardson [16]; with permission.)

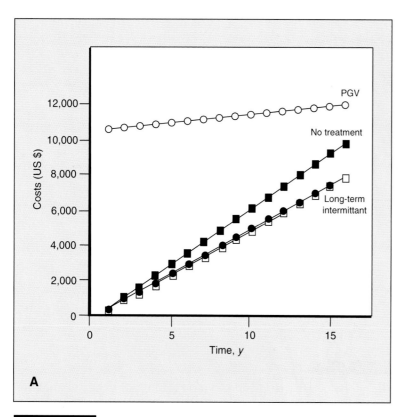

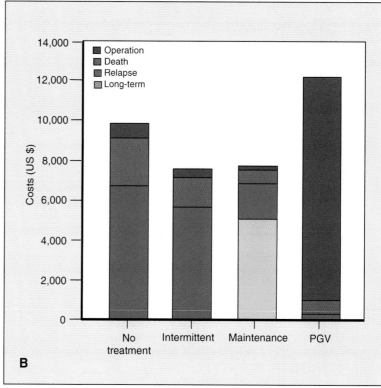

FIGURE 7-30.

Comparison of three treatment strategies for the long-term management of duodenal ulcer. **A,** Proximal gastric vagotomy (PGV) has the highest initial treatment cost. The use of no treatment approaches the cost of parietal cell vagotomy at 15 years. Strategies employing no treatment had an intermediate cost. Long-term maintenance treatment or intermittent H$_2$-receptor therapy were associated with the lowest cost at 15 years. **B,** For

both the no treatment and intermittent treatment groups, the major costs related to use of therapy for relapse. These treatment strategies do not evaluate the cost effectiveness of initial *Helicobacter pylori* eradication. Given the efficacy of currently available regimens, one might anticipate the long-term costs employing an eradication strategy would be significantly reduced. (*From* Ruszniewski [17]; with permission.)

▌REFERENCES AND RECOMMENDED READING

1. Bloom BS: Cross-national changes in the effects of peptic ulcer disease. *Ann Intern Med* 1991, 114:558–562.

2. Kurata JH, Haile BM: Epidemiology of peptic ulcer disease. *Clin Gastroenterol* 1984, 13:289–307.

3. Christensen A, Bousfield R, Christensen J: Incidence of perforated and bleeding peptic ulcers before and after the introduction of H$_2$ receptor antagonists. *Ann Surg* 1988, 207:4–6.

4. Daugherty DF, Lucey MR, Yamada T: Gastric secretion. In *Textbook of Gastroenterology.* Edited by Yamada T, Alpers DH, Owyang C, *et al*: Philadelphia: JB Lippincott; 1991:233–264.

5. Blair AJ III, Feldman M, Barnett C, *et al.*: Detailed comparisons of basal and food-stimulated gastric acid secretion rates and serum gastrin concentrations in duodenal ulcer patients and normal subjects. *J Clin Invest* 1987, 79:582–587.

6. Collen MJ, Sheridan MJ: Gastric ulcers differ from duodenal ulcers: Evaluation of basal acid output. *Dig Dis Sci* 1993, 38:2281–2286.

7. El-Omar E, Penman CA, Ardill JES, McColl KEL: Eradicating *Helicobacter pylori* infection lowers gastrin mediated acid secretion by two thirds in patients with duodenal ulcer. *Gut* 1993, 34:1060–1065.

8. Bayerdorffer E, Mannes GA: The effect of eradication of *Helicobacter pylori* on peptic ulcer disease. *Prac Gastroenterol* 1993, 17(suppl):S10–15.

9. Soll AH: Pathogenesis of peptic ulcer and implications for therapy. *N Engl J Med* 1990, 322:909–916.

10. Penston JG, Wormsley KG: Maintenance treatment with H$_2$ receptor antagonists for peptic ulcer. *Aliment Pharmacol Ther* 1992, 6:3–29.

11. Penston JG: A decade of experience with long-term continuous treatment of peptic ulcers with H$_2$ antagonists. *Aliment Pharmacol Ther* 1993, 7(suppl 2);27–33.

12. Feldman M, Burton ME: Histamine 2 receptor antagonists: Standard therapy for acid-peptioc diseases. *N Engl J Med* 1990, 323:1749–1755.

13. Graham DY, Lew GM, Evans DG, *et al:* Effect of triple therapy (antibiotics plus bismuth) on duodenal ulcer healing: A randomized controlled trial. *Ann Intern Med* 1991, 115:266– 269.

14. Dobrilla G, Zancanella L, Amplatz S: The need for long-term treatment of peptic ulcer. *Aliment Pharmacol Ther* 1993, 7(suppl 2):3–15.

15. Dammann HG, Walter TA: Efficacy of continuous therapy for peptic ulcer in controlled clinical trials. *Aliment Pharmacol Ther* 1993, 7(suppl 2):17–25.

16. Feldman M, Richardson CT: Total 24 hour gastric acid secretion in patients with duodenal ulcer: Comparison with normal subjects and effects of cimetidine and parietal cell vagotomy. *Gastroenterology* 1986, 90:540–544.

17. Ruszniewski P: Pharmaco-economic considerations in the long-term management of peptic ulcer disease. *Aliment Pharmacol Ther* 1993, 7(suppl 2):41–48.

Chapter 8

Zollinger-Ellison Syndrome

ROBERT T. JENSEN

Zollinger-Ellison syndrome is characterized by marked gastric acid hypersecretion that results in refractory peptic ulcer disease, owing to autonomous release of gastrin by a gastroduodenalpancreatic endocrine tumor (a gastrinoma). Almost all (>95%) gastrinomas are located in the pancreas or duodenum. Treatment of the Zollinger-Ellison syndrome requires treatment of both the gastric acid hypersecretion and treatment directed against the gastrinomas itself, because 60% to 90% are malignant in older studies. Twenty percent of patients with Zollinger-Ellison syndrome have the syndrome as part of multiple endocrine neoplasia type 1 (MEN-I), an autosomal dominant disease, and because they differ in treatment required and natural history, it is important these patients be identified.

Proper treatment of Zollinger-Ellison syndrome requires proper diagnosis, adequate control of the gastric acid hypersecretion, both acutely and long term, identification of which patients have MEN-I, detailed tumor localization studies to identify the primary tumor location and the extent of the disease, surgery for possible cure in certain patients, and therapy directed against the tumor itself in patients with metastatic disease.

Zollinger-Ellison syndrome is the most common malignant, symptomatic pancreatic endocrine tumor and closely resembles the other less common pancreatic endocrine tumors in its pathology, immunohistochemical characteristics, growth patterns, malignancy spread, natural history, localization methods and results, surgical approach, and treatment of advanced disease. Zollinger-Ellison syndrome therefore is a good model, because of its frequency, to study various clinical aspects that are likely applicable to the other less common pancreatic endocrine tumoral syndromes (ie, vasoactive intestinal peptide-releasing tumors (VIPomas), glucagonomas, growth hormone releasing factor tumors (GRFomas), somatostatinomas).

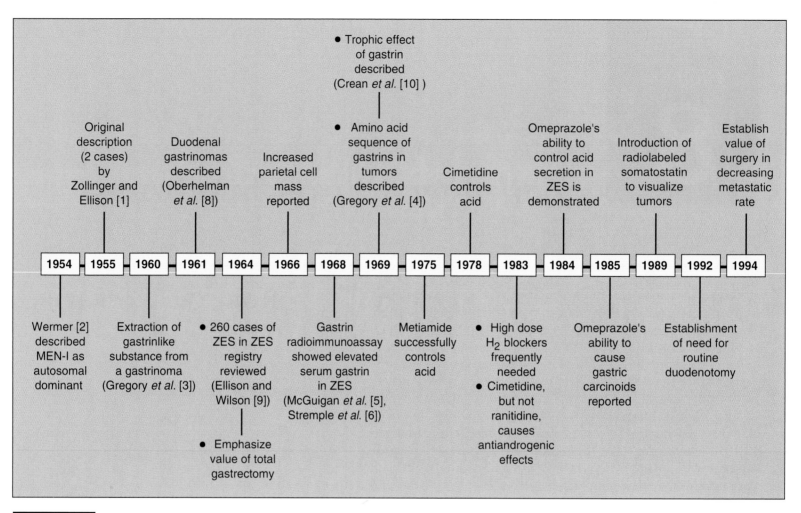

FIGURE 8-1.

Major developments in the history of Zollinger-Ellison syndrome (ZES). ZES, as characterized by severe peptic ulcer disease caused by extreme gastric acid hypersection resulting from a non-beta islet cell tumor of the pancreas, was first described in 1955 [1]. This syndrome was discovered at approximately the same time Wermer [2] was proposing the autosomal dominance inheritance of the familial syndrome of occurrence of tumors involving the pituitary gland, parathyroid glands, and the endocrine pancreas (multiple endocrine neoplasia type I (MEN-I) syndrome). It was later recognized that MEN-I causes 20% of all cases of ZES. The period from the 1950s to the 1970s was characterized by a recognition that the causative hormone secreted in ZES is gastrin [3,4], the development of serum RIAs to diagnose it [5,6], defining other clinical features such as increase parietal cell number due to the trophic action of gastrin [7] or that gastrinomas were frequently duodenal in location [8], and establishing that total gastrectomy was the only effective surgical treatment [9]. The period from 1975 to 1985 was characterized by the description of the trophic effects of gastrin [10], the development of effective medical therapies for hypersection including histamine H_2 blockers (metamide [11], cimetidine [12], ranitidine [13,14], and later the H^+-K^+ ATPase inhibitor, omeprazole [15]. Recently, with the improved ability to control acid hypersecretion medically in all patients [16], the most significant advances have been the recognition of the possible long-term risks of hypergastrinemia (gastric carcinoids [17]) and descriptions of increasingly effective means of finding gastrinomas (imaging modalities [16], radiolabeled somatostatin scanning [18]) and the use of intraoperative ultrasound [19,20] and routine duodenotomy [21] at surgery. The most important recent advance is the demonstration for the first time that routine surgery and tumor excision reduce the rate of development of liver metastases by Fraker and coworkers [22].

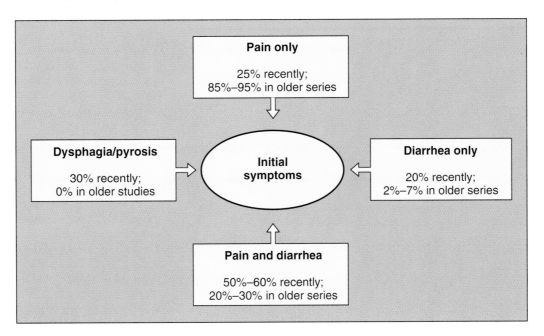

FIGURE 8-2.

Clinical features of Zollinger-Ellison syndrome (ZES). The results in this figure are based on data from two recently published large series of patients with ZES involving 165 [23] and 144 [24] patients analyzed in a recent review [25], and from other earlier studies involving 34 [26], 40 [27], 26 [28], and 260 [9] patients with ZES. The percentages given in the figure refer to the percentages of all patients with the indicated symptom as the initial presenting symptom. Abdominal pain remains the most common initial feature of the disease, either alone or with diarrhea. Increasingly, however, diarrhea and esophageal reflux disease symptoms are being recognized. In the past, patients frequently presented with complications of severe peptic disease, however, at present, a typical patient first has symptoms indistinguishable from those seen in a patient with routine peptic ulcer disease, resulting in an average delay of 6 years in making the diagnosis of ZES [25]. At present, bleeding, severe nausea and vomiting, or perforation occur in 10%, 30%, and 7% of patients with ZES [25,29,30].

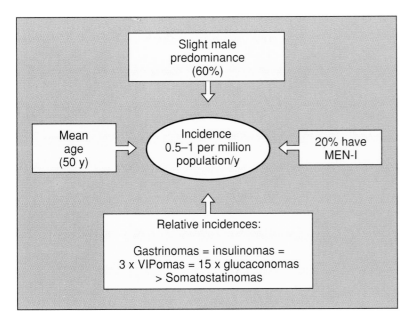

FIGURE 8-3.

Epidemiologic features of Zollinger-Ellison syndrome (ZES). These data are based on epidemiologic studies in Ireland [31], Sweden [32], Denmark [26], and on several recent reviews of series in the United States [25,33]. The multiple endocrine neoplasia type I (MEN-I) syndrome is an autosomal dominant disorder characterized by endocrine tumors or hyperplasia of multiple organs. Hyperparathyroidism, resulting from parathyroid hyperplasia, is the most common feature in patients with MEN-I and is present in 95% to 98%, functional endocrine tumors are the second most common (82%), pituitary adenomas develop in 54% to 65%, and adrenal abnormalities in 26% to 36% [34,35]. Of patients with MEN-I, 100% develop pancreatic polypeptide-producing tumors and 54% develop gastrinomas, whereas insulinomas, glucagonomas, and vasoactive intestinal polypeptide–secreting tumors (VIPomas) occur in 21%, 3%, and 1% [25,35,36]. Most patients with ZES are between 45 to 51 years of age; however, ZES does also occur, if rarely, in children [37,38] and in the elderly.

TABLE 8-1. CLINICAL FEATURES OR LABORATORY TESTS THAT SHOULD LEAD TO A SUSPICION OF ZES

I. Clinical features
  A. In a patient with duodenal ulcers
    1. No *Helicobacter pylori* present
    2. Presence of diarrhea
    3. Failure of the duodenal ulcer to heal with *H. pylori* eradication or with standard doses of histamine H$_2$ blockers
  B. Multiple duodenal ulcers or ulcers in unusual locations
  C. Severe peptic ulcer disease leading to a complication (*eg*, bleeding perforation, intractability)
  D. Severe or resistant peptic esophageal disease
  E. History of nephrolithiasis or endocrinopathies
  F. Family history of nephrolithiasis, endocrinopathies, or peptic ulcer disease
II. Laboratory features in a patient with peptic ulcer that should suggest ZES
  A. Hypergastrinemia
  B. Hypercalcemia
  C. Endocrinopathy
  D. Prominent gastric folds on upper gastrointestinal tract radiograph or at upper gastrointestinal endoscopy

TABLE 8-1.

Clinical features or laboratory results that should lead to a suspicion of Zollinger-Ellison syndrome (ZES). Because most patients with ZES present with pain that is indistinguishable from pain observed in patients with routine peptic ulcer disease, resulting in a mean delay in diagnosis of 6 years [25,39], it is important to have a high index of suspicion for this disease. Diarrhea particularly should suggest the diagnosis, because even in patients with routine peptic ulcer disease who are gastric acid hypersecreters, diarrhea is rare [40]. *Helicobacter pylori* is found in 90% to 98% of patients with duodenal ulcers with routine peptic ulcer disease [25,39,41] but is found in less than 50% of patients with ZES [42–44]. *H. pylori* eradication results in healing in 90% of patients with routine peptic ulcer disease, but it will not result in ulcer healing in ZES. Any feature suggesting multiple endocrine neoplasia type 1 syndrome (associated endocrinopathy) or a family history of peptic ulcer disease should raise the suspicion of ZES in a patient with peptic ulcer disease.

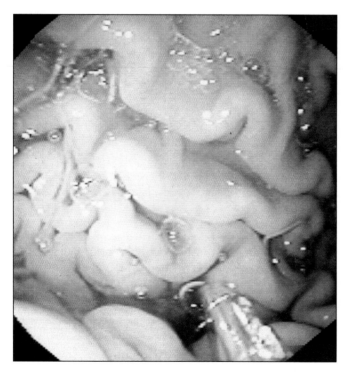

FIGURE 8-4.

Prominent gastric folds in a patient with Zollinger-Ellison syndrome (ZES) on gastroscopy. Gastrin has trophic effects on the gastric mucosa [10,17,45,46] resulting in prominent gastric folds, increased numbers of parietal cells, and increased numbers of enterochromaffin-like (ECL) cells. This figure shows the prominent gastric folds in a 17-year-old patient who presented with peptic ulcer disease (NIH #2663004), who was eventually diagnosed to have ZES. The presence of prominent folds such as this should lead to a possible suspicion of ZES in the patient.

DIAGNOSIS

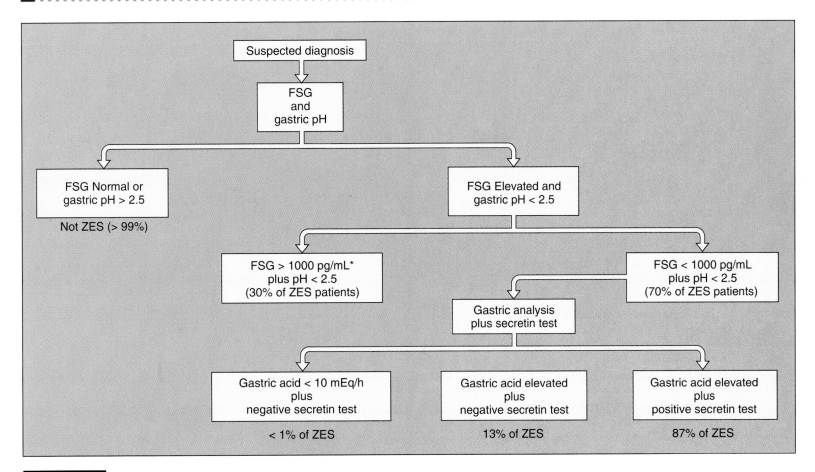

FIGURE 8-5.

Algorithm for diagnosis of Zollinger-Ellison syndrome (ZES). More than 99% of patients with ZES will have an elevated fasting gastrin level and gastric pH below 2.5 [25,44,48,49]. Except for ZES and the retained gastric antrum syndrome [25,44,48,49], no diseases give a pH below 2.5 and fasting serum gastrin (FSG) greater than 1000 pg/mL [25,44,48,49] (normal <100); therefore, if a patient has this combination and has not had a previous partial gastrectomy with gastrojejunostomy, the diagnosis of ZES can be made without additional tests. Several diseases including antral G hyperplasia/hyperfunction, *Helicobacter pylori* infection, chronic renal failure, short bowel syndrome, and chronic gastric outlet obstruction can result in gastric elevations from 100 to 1000 pg/mL and pH below 2.5; they can be confused with ZES and will need to be excluded by performing a secretin-provocative test [25,44,50–52].

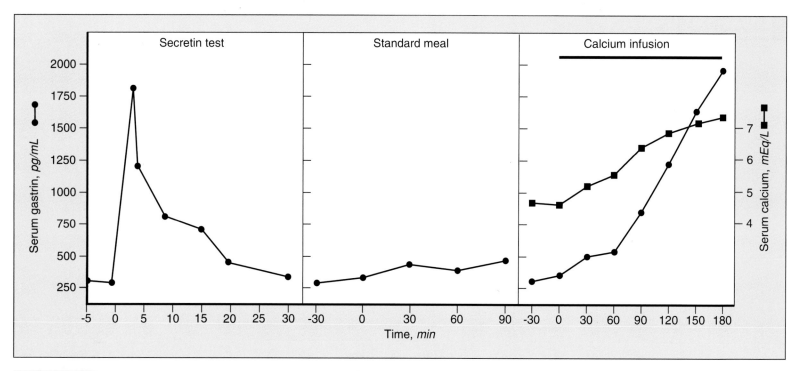

FIGURE 8-6.

Typical gastrin provocative test results in a patient with Zollinger-Ellison syndrome (ZES). Three provocative tests are reported useful in differentiating ZES from other conditions causing gastric acid hypersecretion and elevated gastrins between 100 to 1000 pg/mL. It is now recommended [53,54] that in the secretin test (*left panel*), the serum gastrin response be measured before and at 2, 5, 10, 15, and 20 minutes after the bolus injection of secretin (two clinical units Kabi Secretin/kg of body weight), in the calcium infusion test (*right panel*), the serum gastrin and calcium be measured before and at 120, 160, and 180 minutes after starting a continuous infusion of 10% calcium gluconate (5 mg Ca^{2+}/kg/h x 3 h), and in the standard meal test (*center panel*), the gastrin levels should be measured before and at 30, 60, and 90 minutes after eating a standard meal [53,55,56]. The secretin test will be positive (> 200 pg/mL increase) [54] in 87% of patients with ZES with fasting gastrin levels of 100 to 1000 pg/mL. There are no false positives except in patients with achlorhydria [57] who would not have a pH below 2.5 (*see* Fig. 8-5). The calcium infusion test will be positive (above 395 pg/mL increase) [54,58] in 56% of patients with fasting serum gastrin levels between 100 to 1000 pg/mL and a gastric pH below 2.5 and is positive in 20% of the patients with ZES with negative secretin tests [54]. The characteristic response to standard meal testing, which has been proposed to distinguish ZES from antral G-cell syndromes [53,56], in patients with ZES is an increase in serum gastrin level after the meal of less than 50% over the premeal value. Some 30% of ZES patients have a positive response (> 100% increase) that overlaps with the characteristic exaggerated response in antral syndromes [54]. Measuring secretin is the provocative test of choice for patients with fasting gastrin levels between 100 to 1000 pg/mL and generally only it should be used [53–55].

MANAGEMENT

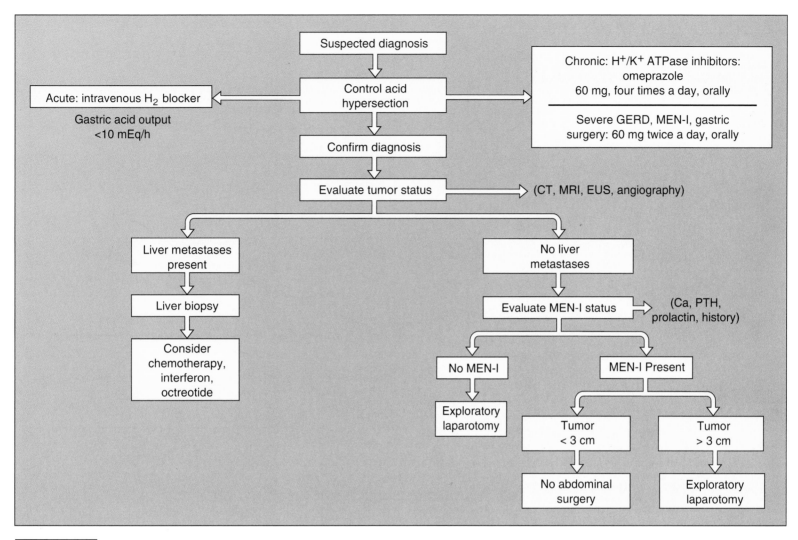

FIGURE 8-7.

Algorithm for management of Zollinger-Ellison syndrome (ZES). As soon as ZES is suspected, even before the diagnosis is fully established, it is important to control acutely the gastric acid hypersecretion either with oral gastric-acid antisecretory drugs (histamine H_2-receptor antagonists, H^+-K^+ ATPase inhibitors) or by using an intravenous infusion of histamine H_2 blockers [25,59,60]. The diagnosis can be confirmed later, followed by tumor localization with various imaging studies. Patients without hepatic metastases lacking medical conditions limiting life expectancy without multiple endocrine neoplasia type I (MEN-I) should be considered for exploratory laparotomy for possible curative resection [61,62]. Ca—calcium; CT—computed tomography; EUS—endoscopic ultrasound; GERD—gastroesophageal reflux disease; MRI—magnetic resonance imaging.

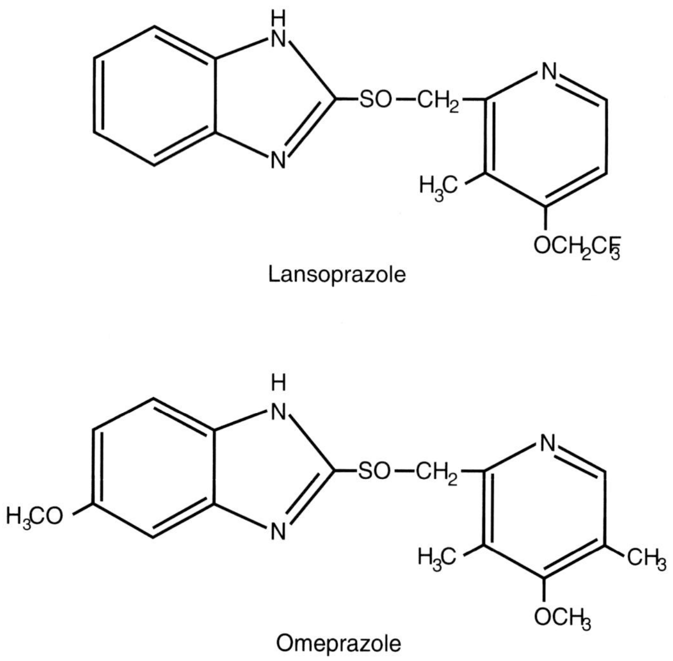

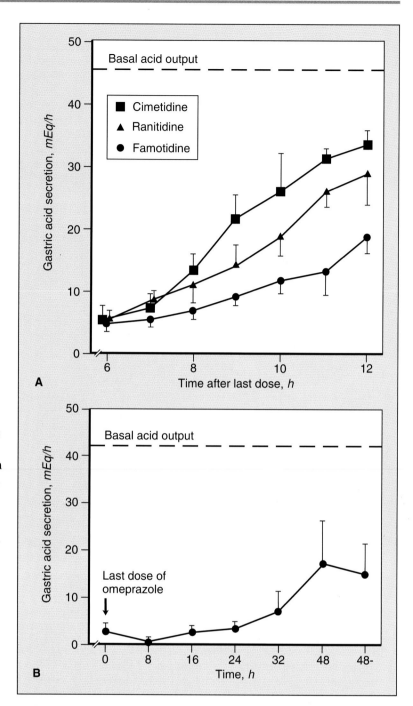

FIGURE 8-8.

Structure of the two H^+-K^+ ATPase inhibitors shown to be effective in Zollinger-Ellison syndrome (ZES). H^+-K^+ ATPase inhibitors are now the drugs of choice in ZES for inhibiting gastric hypersecretion [16,25,49] because of their long duration of action, which result in once a day dosing in 80% of patients [63–66]. Studies show both omeprazole and lansoprazole [67,68] are effective both short term and long term in patients with ZES. Patients have been treated with omeprazole up to 9 years [64] without developing either tachyphylaxis or toxicity.

FIGURE 8-9.

Duration of action of histamine H_2 blockers and omeprazole in Zollinger-Ellison syndrome (ZES). For each class of drugs, the minimum dose that reduced gastric acid secretion to less than 10 mEq/h for the hour before the next dose was determined in a group of patients with ZES. This level of control, which will result in healing of peptic ulcers and prevent their reappearance [69,70], has been demonstrated to be the acceptable safe level. For histamine H_2 blockers, this level was at 6 hours after drug therapy for omeprazole, and this time was 24 hours after drug therapy. No additional drug was given and the duration of the acid suppressive action determined. The *dotted line* labeled basal acid output represents the basal acid output when no drug effect is present. **A,** No difference in the mean duration of action of ranitidine or cimetidine existed, however, famotidine had duration of action a third longer in the five patients studied [71]. **B,** In five patients, the duration of action of omeprazole was determined [69]. Both omeprazole and lansoprazole have a similar duration of action for a single dose (*ie,* time to reach half the acid output without drug equals 37 hours), which is at least three times longer than any histamine H_2 blocker [49,60,67,72].

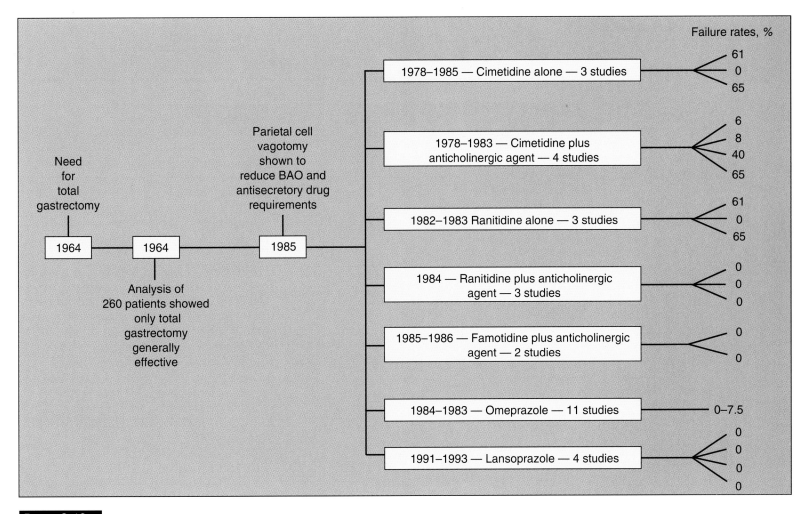

Failure rates, %

	Failure rates, %
1978–1985 — Cimetidine alone — 3 studies	61 0 65
1978–1983 — Cimetidine plus anticholinergic agent — 4 studies	6 8 40 65
1982–1983 Ranitidine alone — 3 studies	61 0 65
1984 — Ranitidine plus anticholinergic agent — 3 studies	0 0 0
1985–1986 — Famotidine plus anticholinergic agent — 2 studies	0 0
1984–1983 — Omeprazole — 11 studies	0–7.5
1991–1993 — Lansoprazole — 4 studies	0 0 0 0

Left timeline: Need for total gastrectomy — 1964 — 1964 (Analysis of 260 patients showed only total gastrectomy generally effective) — 1985 (Parietal cell vagotomy shown to reduce BAO and antisecretory drug requirements)

FIGURE 8-10.

Chronology of the development of treatments for the gastric acid hypersecretion in Zollinger-Ellison syndrome (ZES). Initially only total gastrectomy was effective [1,9,73]. With the availability of histamine H_2 blockers in the 1980s, highly selective vagotomy was shown to be effective if combined with continued low doses of histamine H_2 blockers [74]. Three studies showed cimetidine alone had a failure rate from 0% to 65%, four studies showed cimetidine plus an anticholinergic agent had a failure rate of 0% to 65%, one study showed ranitidine alone and one study showed ranitidine plus an anticholinergic agent had a 0% to 40% failure rate, and famotidine alone or with an anticholinergic agent had 0% failure rate [25,49]. It has been pointed out that these widely varying failure rates in different series resulted from a failure in many cases to use an acceptable criterion for control of acid secretion which resulted in inadequate control of the acid hypersecretion [70]. If sufficiently high doses of histamine H_2 blockers are used, acid secretion can be controlled in almost every patient [25,48]. Recently, 10 studies have shown omeprazole and three studies have shown lansoprazole generally have a 0% failure rate (25,49,60]. At present, it is recommended that patients with uncomplicated ZES (ie, no previous gastric surgery, severe reflux disease, or absence of multiple endocrine neoplasia type I) should be started on 60 mg/d of omeprazole, and over time the dosage can be reduced to 20 mg/d in more than 80% of patients. In patients with complicated disease, the initial dose should be 60 mg twice a day [25,49,63,64]. BAO—basal acid output.

Computed tomography

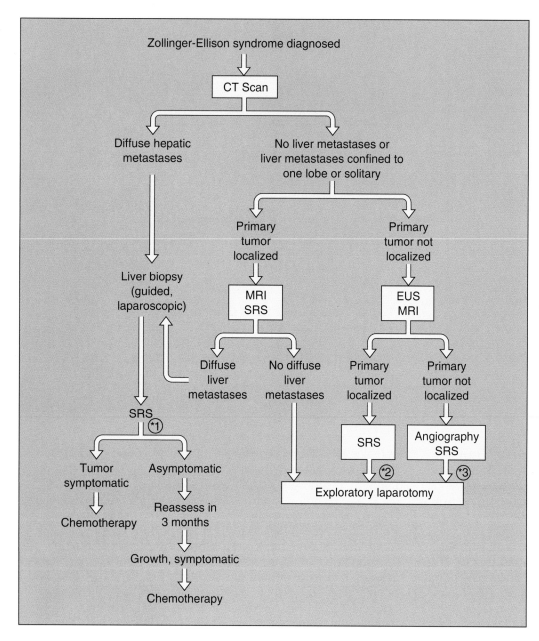

FIGURE 8-11.

Algorithm for tumor localization in a patient with Zollinger-Ellison syndrome (ZES). After ZES is diagnosed, a computed tomographic (CT) scan is recommended as the initial localization study because it is widely available and has a good overall sensitivity [25,29,75]. If presence of liver metastases is predicted (30% of patients) [25], somatostatin receptor scintigraphy (SRS) using [^{111}In-DTPA-DPhe^1]-octreotide is recommended to identify distal metastases [18] and a percutaneous liver biopsy can be performed for histologic confirmation. If, after CT scanning, the disease is potentially resectable, additional localization studies are needed. Recent studies using magnetic resonance imaging (MRI) report a marked increase over the past few years in the sensitivity of this modality for identifying liver metastases. It is now the imaging study of choice for this condition [76–78]. If a primary tumor is not localized, endoscopic ultrasound is indicated because recent studies report that this study is more sensitive than SRS for localizing primary pancreatic endocrine tumors [79–81]. The *asterisk* indicates that if a patient has multiple endocrine neoplasia type I and gastrinoma, it remains unclear whether surgery should be done routinely [62,82,83]. EUS—endoscopic ultrasound.

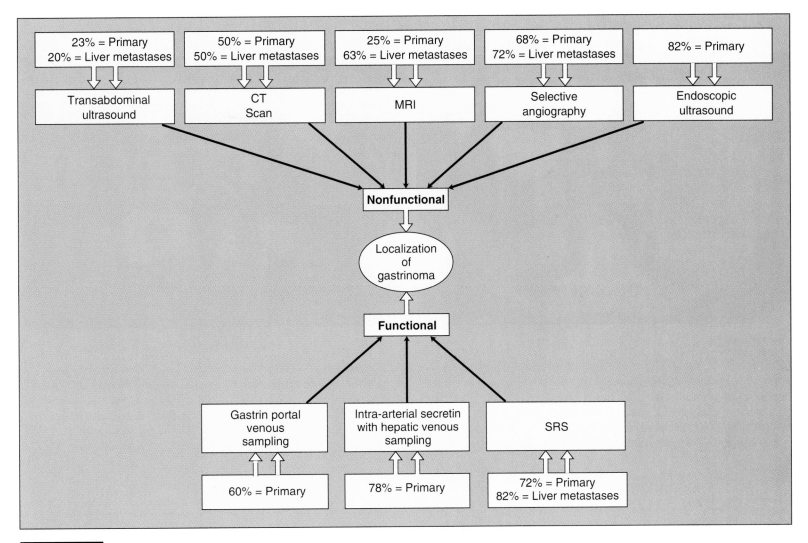

FIGURE 8-12.

Results of localization of primary and metastatic gastrinoma in the liver. Localization of the primary refers to the correct identification of the primary site and identification of liver metastases refers to identification of metastatic gastrinoma in the liver [25,78,84]. Somatostatin receptor scintigraphy (SRS) uses either [^{125}I-Tyr^3]-octreotide or [^{111}In DTPA-DPhe^1]-octreotide [80,81,85]. The numbers refer to the mean sensitivity for detecting either the primary tumor or metastatic tumor in the liver from various series. The current recommended order of using these various studies is shown in Figure 8-11. CT—computed tomography, MRI—magnetic resonance imaging.

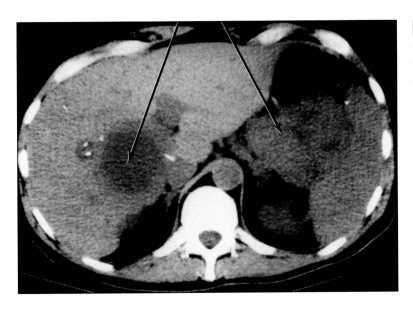

FIGURE 8-13.

Computed tomographic scan of patients with Zollinger-Ellison syndrome. A primary pancreatic gastrinoma with metastases to the liver is shown. The primary tumor and largest hepatic metastases are indicated by the *arrows*. Recent studies show that pancreatic gastrinomas much more frequently metastasize to the liver than duodenal gastrinomas do, whereas the rate of metastases of duodenal and pancreatic gastrinoma to lymph nodes is equal [21,86–88]. The ability of the computed tomographic scan to detect primary gastrinomas is dependent on tumor size. It will identify 0% to 10% of primary tumors smaller than 1 cm in diameter, 30% of tumors 1 to 3 cm in diameter, and 95% of those larger than 3 cm [75].

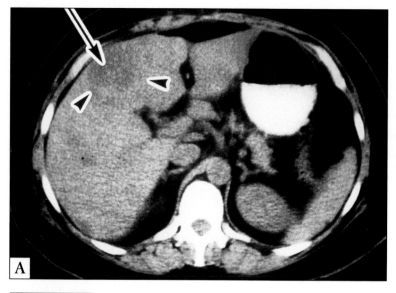

FIGURE 8-14.

Comparison of the ability of computed tomography (*panel A*) and magnetic resonance imaging (MRI) (*panel B*) to localize liver metastases in a patient with Zollinger-Ellison syndrome. Recent studies show that MRI is now the noninvasive procedure of choice to localize liver metastases [76–78]. The reason the MRI is superior to the computed tomographic scan is clearly illustrated in this case.

A, The patient appears to have a single large liver metastasis by computed tomographic scan, the margins of which are poorly seen and shown by the *arrows*. On the short T1 inversion-recovery image of the MRI (**B**), the metastasis is clearly seen as well as other smaller foci in the left lobe indicated by the *arrow*.

Angiography

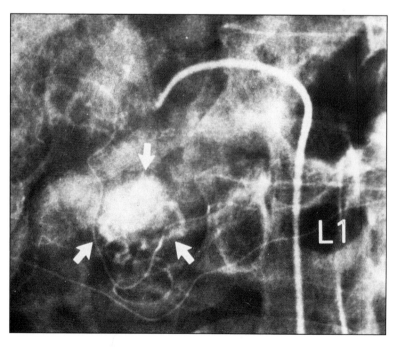

FIGURE 8-15.

Localization of a primary gastrinoma by selective angiography. A primary gastrinoma in the duodenum (*arrows*) is shown on this selective injection of the gastroduodenal artery in this patient with Zollinger-Ellison syndrome. Selective angiography remains the most sensitive test of the older, standard localization tests (ultrasound, angiography, computed tomography, magnetic resonance imaging) usually advocated to localize primary gastrinomas [25,78,84,89]. Recent studies suggest, especially for pancreatic gastrinomas, that endoscopic ultrasound and perhaps somatostatin receptor scintigraphy may be more sensitive. Whether either of the newer methods is more sensitive than angiography remains unclear, especially in the case of duodenal gastrinomas [90].

Somatostatin receptor scintigraphy

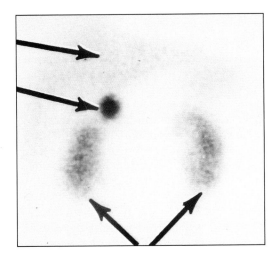

FIGURE 8-16.

Somatostatin receptor scintigraphy (SRS) localization of a gastrinoma in the pancreatic head area in a patient with Zollinger-Ellison syndrome (ZES). This figure shows the localization of a gastrinoma (*lower arrow at left*) in a patient with ZES using SRS with [^{111}In-DTPA-DPhe^1]-octreotide. As this figure shows [^{111}In-DTPA-DPhe^1]-octreotide is primarily excreted in the urine (kidneys [*arrows at bottom*]), however, a small amount also is taken up by the liver (*upper arrow at left*). Recent data suggest SRS will be particularly helpful in diagnosis of gastrinomas [18,78,85,91]. Nearly 100% of gastrinomas are reported to possess increased numbers of somatostatin receptors [92]. Another advantage of SRS is its ability of also frequently detecting previously unrecognized distal metastases [18]. The false-positive rate, whether SRS will detect small duodenal gastrinomas, and whether it is more sensitive than angiography remain unclear [78,93].

Selective intra-arterial injection

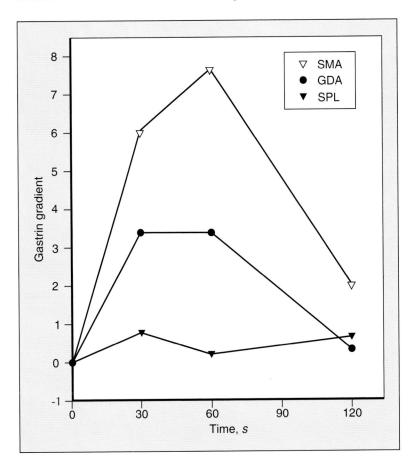

FIGURE 8-17.

Results of selective intra-arterial injection of secretin and hepatic venous gastrin sampling in a patient with Zollinger-Ellison syndrome. In this study, secretin was injected into various abdominal arteries selectively and the gastrin level determined in venous block sampled from the hepatic veins. The gastrinoma was found during surgery in the duodenal wall in this patient. The venous gastrin increase was highest with injection of the superior mesenteric artery (SMA) and the gastroduodenal artery (GDA), which supply the area of the pancreatic head where the gastrinoma was found. The splenic (SPL) artery supplying the pancreatic tail demonstrated no change. This localization method has the advantage of functionally localizing the tumor and is not dependent on tumor size [84,88,94,95]. The intra-arterial secretin test X, because of the ease of performing it, greater sensitivity, and the lack of need for a separate procedure from angiography, is now the procedure of choice and has replaced the other method of portal venous gastrin sampling shown in Figure 8-19 [84,88].

Selective percutaneous venous sampling

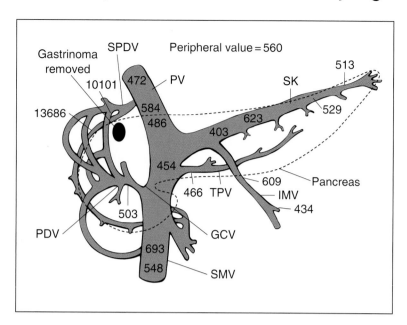

FIGURE 8-18.

Results of selective percutaneous venous sampling for gastrin from portal venous tributaries (PVS) in a patient with Zollinger-Ellison syndrome. This PVS was performed on the same patient that the intra-arterial secretin (IAS) test shown in Figure 8-18 was done on. In PVS a catheter is inserted across the liver into various portal vein (PV) tributaries and venous samples taken for gastrin determinations at various locations. The gastrinoma was found at surgery in the duodenal wall in this patient. The serum venous gastrin concentration at various portal venous locations is shown. The simultaneous peripheral venous value from the antecubital vein was 560 pg/mL. In the pancreatic head area there was a marked increase in serum gastrin resulting in a gastrin gradient of 2344% (positive is > 50%). The site of the gastrinoma is indicated. This localization method, as is the IAS shown in Figure 8-18, has the advantage of functionally localizing the tumor and are not dependent on tumor size [84,88,94,95]. PVS has now been replaced by IAS [84,88]. GCV—gastrocolic vein; IMV—inferior mesenteric vein; PDV—pancreaticoduodenal vein; SMV—superior mesenteric vein; SPDV—superior PDV; SV—splenic view; TPV—transverse pancreatic vein.

Intraoperative detection

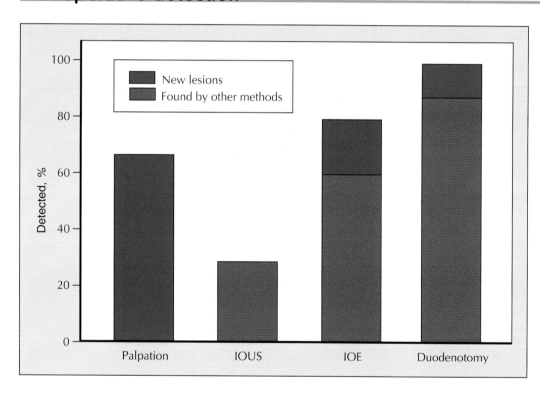

FIGURE 8-19.

Intraoperative detection of duodenal gastrinomas. These data are derived from 42 patients with Zollinger-Ellison syndrome who underwent exploratory laparotomy for cure at the National Institutes of Health. At surgery each patient had palpation of the duodenum to localize duodenal gastrinomas, followed by intraoperative ultrasound (IOUS), intraoperative endoscopy (IOE) with transillumination of the duodenum, and finally, a duodenotomy as described previously [16,21,96]. Biopsies were performed on all possible tumors localized by any method. In a total of 30 patients, 36 duodenal gastrinomas were found. Results are expressed as the percentage of duodenal tumors found by the indicated method. The *green bars* represent the percentage of new duodenal tumors found by using that method, and the *pink bars* the percentage supplied found by using other methods. Palpation detected 65% of all duodenal tumors and IOUS supplied no additional cases. Duodenotomy and IOE detected 15% and 20% more cases, respectively. These data demonstrate the necessity of duodenotomy being performed on all patients to detect small duodenal tumors [96]. The IOE frequently assists in localizing the site to perform the duodenotomy and therefore is recommended [96,97].

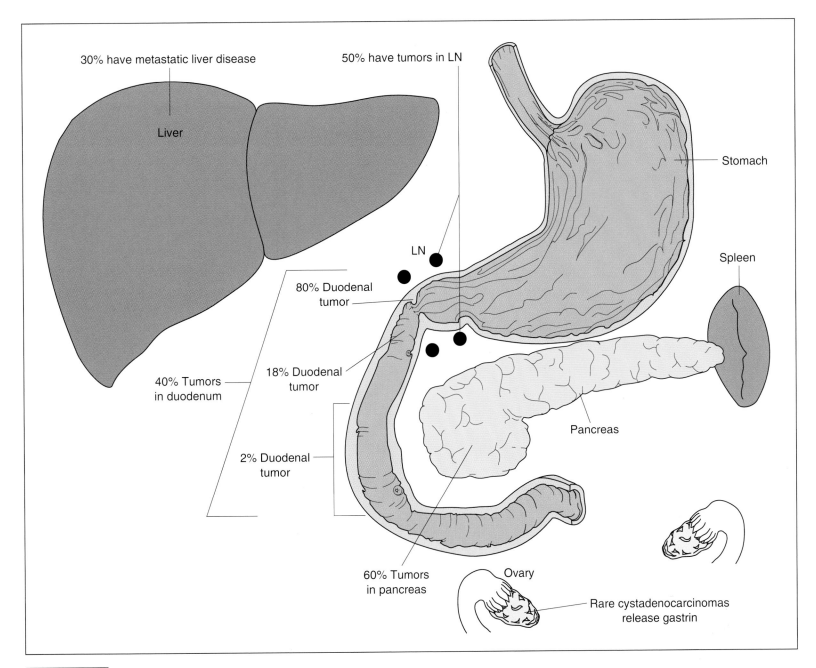

FIGURE 8-20.

Location of gastrinomas. Data are summarized from recent studies from the National Institutes of Health and reviews of various smaller series [21,25,98,99] and involve data from more than 400 patients with Zollinger-Ellison syndrome. At present, 30% of patients present with metastatic disease in the liver. For the primary tumor location, the percentage of tumors in the pancreas or duodenum varies markedly in different series. Currently, if careful duodenal exploration is done [100,101], at least 40% of the patients have duodenal gastrinomas and almost all remaining patients have the gastrinoma discovered either in the pancreas or only in the lymph nodes (*LN*). Within the duodenum, 80% of the gastrinomas are in the first part, 18% in the second, and 2% in the third. In recent studies, tumors are found in 95% of all patients at surgery [21,96,102]. Up to 20% to 30% of patients have gastrinomas found only in lymph nodes, some of whom are cured by surgical resection, and it remains controversial whether lymph node primary gastrinomas exist [103].

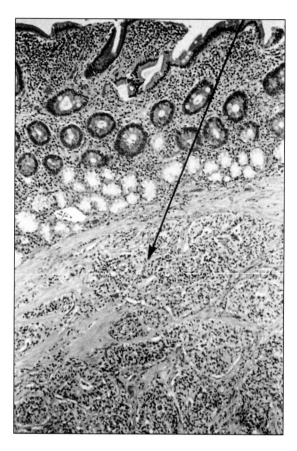

FIGURE 8-21.

Pathology of duodenal gastrinomas. Duodenal gastrinoma are characteristically submucosal [101] as shown in this figure with the tumor location indicated by the *arrow*. Hematoxylin/eosin stain.

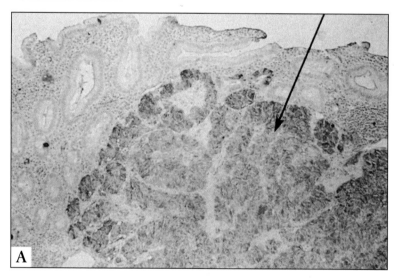

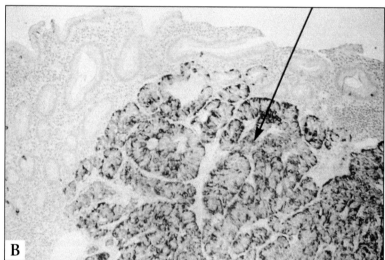

FIGURE 8-22.

Gastrin and chromogranin A staining of duodenal gastrinoma. This tumor (*arrows*) is from the same patient shown in Figure 8-21. More than 95% of gastrinomas stain for gastrin (**A**) [25,51]. Chromogranin A (**B**) is a 48-kD protein that is costored and coreleased with peptide hormones from gut endocrine cell tumors [25,104,105]. Thus, it is a marker for the endocrine nature of the tumor when other peptides may not be present.

■ PROGNOSIS

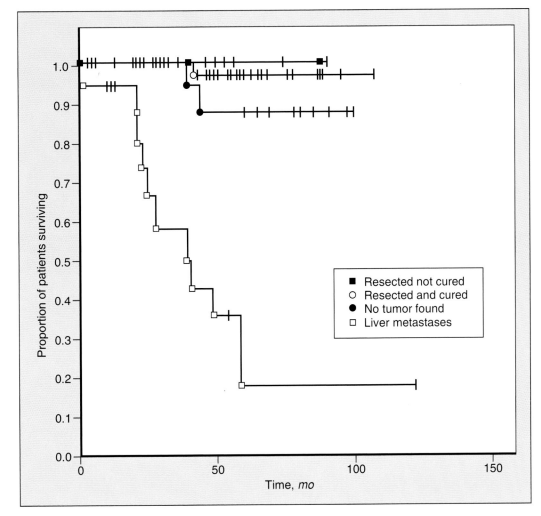

FIGURE 8-23.

Prognosis in Zollinger-Ellison syndrome. Prognosis is related to tumor extent [21,25,34,98,106]. These data are from National Institutes of Health studies. All patients had histologic confirmation of the tumor location either at surgery, by autopsy, or by percutaneous biopsy. Eighteen patients had metastatic gastrinomas to the liver, 42 patients were rendered disease free (negative secretin test, normal gastrins, negative imaging studies) [96,107], 15 patients had all visible disease removed but were biochemically not cured, and 20 patients had no tumor found at surgery. (*Data from* Norton *et al.* [21], Norton *et al.* [34], and Norton *et al.* [98]; with permission.)

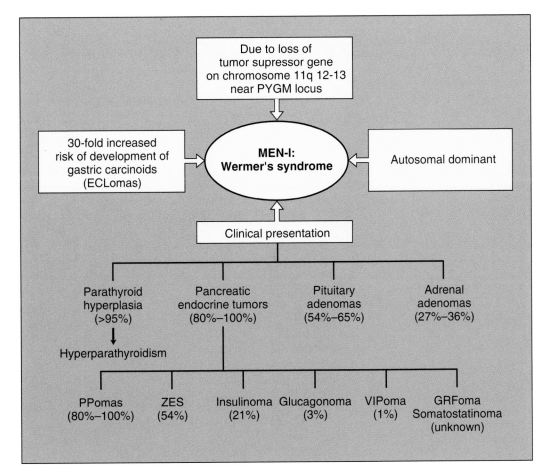

FIGURE 8-24.

Multiple endocrine neoplasia type I (MEN-I) syndrome. Of the three types of multiple endocrine neoplasia syndromes, only patients with MEN-I routinely develop pancreatic endocrine tumors [34,35]. This syndrome is an autosomal dominant disorder, resulting from a genetic alteration on chromosome 11 q12–13 area near the skeletal muscle glycogen phosphorylase locus (PYGM) [34,108]. It is clinically characterized by hyperplasia or tumors of multiple endocrine organs with a relative frequency of: (1) parathyroid, (2) endocrine pancreas, (3) pituitary, and (4) adrenal [34,35]. The most common functional endocrine tumor is a gastrinoma although pancreatic polypeptide-producing tumor (PPomas) are the most frequently seen tumor type. PPomas cause symptoms resulting only from the bulk of the tumor itself [33,109]. Patients with MEN-I with Zollinger-Ellison syndrome (ZES) also have an increased risk of developing gastric carcinoid tumors of the stomach compared with patients with ZES but without MEN-I [110–112]. ECLomas—gastric carcinoid tumor arising from enterochromaffin-like cells; GRFoma—growth hormone releasing factor–releasing tumor; VIPoma—vasoactive intestinal peptide–releasing tumor.

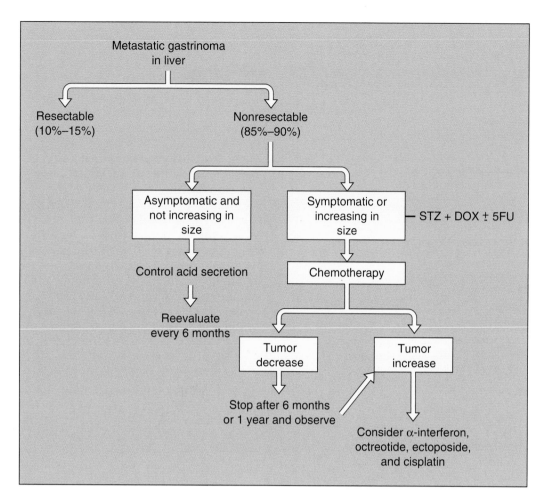

FIGURE 8-25.

Treatment of metastatic gastrinoma. Up to 15% of metastatic gastrinomas found in the liver may be resectable [113]. Most patients have diffuse metastases involving both hepatic lobes, however, the decision needs to be made whether chemotherapy or some other treatment should be instituted because of the patients poor prognosis (*see* Fig. 8-20). A small percentage of patients do not demonstrate progressive disease and after acid secretion is controlled, are asymptomatic, and thus no further treatment is required [114]. If the tumor progresses in size or becomes symptomatic, chemotherapy with streptozotocin (STZ) and doxorubicin (DOX) with or without 5-fluorouracil (5FU) is recommended. Approximately 50% will respond with a decrease in tumor size, but with time the tumor usually begins to grow again [115–117]. Subsequent treatment with interferon, octreotide, or possibly ectoposide and cisplatin might be considered [34,115,118–120].

REFERENCES AND RECOMMENDED READING

1. Zollinger RM, Ellison EH: Primary peptic ulcerations of the jejunum associated with islet cell tumors of the pancreas. *Ann Surg* 1955, 142:709–728.

2. Wermer P:Genetic aspects of adenomatosis of endocrine glands. *Am J Med* 1954, 16:363–371.

3. Gregory RA, Tracy HJ, French JM, Sircus W: Extraction of a gastrin-like substance from a pancreatic tumour in a case of Zollinger-Ellison syndrome. *Lancet* 1960, 1:1045–1048.

4. Gregory RA, Tracy HJ, Agarwal KL, Grossman MI: Amino acid constitution of two gastrins isolated from Zollinger-Ellison tumor tissue. *Gut* 1969, 10:603–608.

5. McGuigan JE, Trudeau WL: Immunochemical measurement of elevated levels of gastrin in the serum of patients with pancreatic tumors of the Zollinger-Ellison variety. *N Engl J Med* 1968, 278:1308–1313.

6. Stremple JF, Meade RC: Production of antibodies to synthetic human gastrin I and radioimmunoassay of gastrin in the serum of patients with the Zollinger-Ellison syndrome. *Surgery* 1968, 64:165–174.

7. Polacek MA, Ellison EH: Parietal cell mass and gastric acid secretion in the Zollinger-Ellison syndrome. *Surgery* 1966, 60:606–614.

8. Oberhelman HA Jr, Nelsen TS, Johnson AN, Dragstedt LR: Ulcerogenic tumors of the duodenum. *Ann Surg* 1961, 153:214–227.

9. Ellison EH, Wilson SD: The Zollinger-Ellison syndrome: Re-appraisal and evaluation of 260 registered cases. *Ann Surg* 1964, 160:512–530.

10. Crean GP, Marshall MW, Ramsey RD: Parietal cell hyperplasia induced by the administration of pentagastrin (ICI-50,123) to rats. *Gastroenterology* 1969, 57:147–155.

11. McCarthy DM, Olinger EJ, May RJ, *et al.*: H$_2$-histamine receptor blocking agents in the Zollinger-Ellison syndrome. Experience in seven cases and implications for long-term therapy. *Ann Intern Med* 1977, 87:668–675.

12. McCarthy DM: Report on the United States experience with cimetidine in Zollinger-Ellison syndrome and other hypersecretory states. *Gastroenterology* 1978, 74:453–458.

13. Collen MJ, Howard JM, McArthur KE, *et al.*: Comparison of ranitidine and cimetidine in the treatment of gastric hypersecretion. *Ann Intern Med* 1984, 100:52–58.

14. Jensen RT, Collen MJ, McArthur KE, *et al.*: Comparison of the effectiveness of ranitidine and cimetidine in inhibiting acid secretion in patients with gastric acid hypersecretory states. *Am J Med* 1984, 77:90–105.

15. Lamers CBHW, Lind T, Moberg S, *et al.*: Omeprazole in Zollinger-Ellison syndrome: Effects of a single dose and of long term treatment in patients resistant to histamine H$_2$-receptor antagonists. *N Engl J Med* 1984, 310:758–761.

16. Jensen RT, Fraker DL: Zollinger-Ellison syndrome: Advances in treatment of the gastric hypersecretion and the gastrinoma. *JAMA* 1994, 271:1–7.

17. Ekman L, Hansson E, Havu N, *et al.*: Toxicological studies on omeprazole. *Scand J Gastroenterol* 1985, 20(suppl 108):53–69.

18. Lamberts SW, Bakker WH, Reubi JC, Krenning EP: Somatostatin-receptor imaging in the localization of endocrine tumors. *N Engl J Med* 1990, 323:1246–1249.

19. Norton JA, Cromack DT, Shawker TH, *et al.*: Intraoperative ultrasonographic localization of islet cell tumors. A prospective comparison to palpation. *Ann Surg* 1988, 207:160–168.

20. Norton JA: Surgical treatment of islet cell tumors with special emphasis on operative ultrasound. In *Endocrine Tumors of the Pancreas: Recent advances in research and management.* Edited by Mignon M, Jensen RT. Basel; Karger; 1995:309–332.

21. Norton JA, Doppman JL, Jensen RT: Curative resection in Zollinger-Ellison syndrome: Results of a 10-year prospective study. *Ann Surg* 1992, 215:8–18.

22. Fraker DL, Norton JA, Alexander HR, *et al.*: Surgery in Zollinger-Ellison syndrome alters the natural history of gastrinoma. *Ann Surg* 1994, 220:320–330.

23. Jensen RT, Gardner JD: Zollinger-Ellison syndrome: Clinical presentation, pathology, diagnosis and treatment. In *Peptic Ulcer and Other Acid-Related Diseases.* Edited by Dannenberg A, Zakim D. Armonk: Academic Research Associates; 1991:117–212.

24. Bonfils S, Landor JH, Mignon M, Hervoir P: Results of surgical management in 92 consecutive patients with Zollinger-Ellison syndrome. *Ann Surg* 1981, 194:692–697.

25. Jensen RT, Gardner JD: Gastrinoma. In *The Pancreas: Biology, Pathobiology and Disease,* edn 2. Edited by Go VLW, DiMagno EP, Gardner JD, *et al.*: New York: Raven Press, 1993:931–978.

26. Stage JG, Stadil F: The clinical diagnosis of the Zollinger-Ellison syndrome. *Scand J Gastroenterol* 1979; 53(suppl):79–91.

27. Regan PT, Malagelada JR: A reappraisal of clinical, roentgenographic, and endoscopic features of the Zollinger-Ellison syndrome. *Mayo Clin Proc* 1978, 53:19–23.

28. Cameron AJ, Hoffman HN: Zollinger-Ellison syndrome: Clinical features and long-term follow-up. *Mayo Clin Proc* 1974, 49:44–51.

29. Jensen RT, Maton PN: Zollinger-Ellison syndrome. In *The Stomach.* Edited by Gustavsson S, Kumar D, Graham DY. London: Churchill Livingstone; 1992:341–374.

30. Waxman I, Gardner JD, Jensen RT, Maton PN: Peptic ulcer perforation as the presentation of Zollinger-Ellison syndrome. *Dig Dis Sci* 1991, 16:19–24.

31. Buchanan KD, Johnston CF, O'Hare MM, *et al.*: Neuroendocrine tumors: A European view. *Am J Med* 1986, 81(suppl 6B):14–22.

32. Eriksson B, Oberg K, Skogseid B: Neuroendocrine pancreatic endocrine tumors. Clinical findings in a prospective study of 84 patients. *Acta Oncologia* 1989, 28:373–377.

33. Jensen RT, Norton JA: Pancreatic endocrine neoplasms. In *Gastrointestinal Diseases: Pathophysiology, Diagnosis and Management,* edn 5. Edited by Fordtran JS, Sleisenger MH, Feldman M, Scharschmidt BF. Philadelphia: WB Saunders; 1993:1695–1721.

34. Norton JA, Levin B, Jensen RT: Cancer of the endocrine system. In *Cancer: Principles and Practice of Oncology,* edn 4. Edited by DeVita VT Jr, Hellman S, Rosenberg SA. Philadelphia: JB Lippincott; 1993:1333–1435.

35. Metz DC, Jensen RT, Bale AE, *et al.*: Multiple endocrine neoplasia type 1: Clinical features and management. In *The Parathyroids.* Edited by Bilezekian JP, Levine MA, Marcus R. New York: Raven Press; 1994:591–646.

36. Eberle F, Grun R: Multiple endocrine neoplasia, type I (MEN I). *Erbeg Inn Med Kinderheilkd* 1981, 46:76–149.

37. Wilson SD: The role of surgery in children with the Zollinger-Ellison syndrome. *Surgery* 1982, 92:682–692.

38. Wilson SD: Zollinger-Ellison syndrome in children: 1 25-year follow-up. *Surgery* 1991, 110:696–702.

39. Isenberg JI, Walsh JH, Grossman MI: Zollinger-Ellison syndrome. *Gastroenterology* 1973, 65:140–165.

40. Collen MJ, Jensen RT: Idiopathic gastric acid hypersecretion: Comparison with Zollinger-Ellison syndrome. *Dig Dis Sci* 1994, 39:1434–1440.

41. Tytgat GNJ, Noach LA, Rauws EAJ: *Helicobacter pylori* infection and duodenal ulcer disease. *Gastroenterol Clin North Am* 1993, 22:127–139.

42. Saeed ZA, Evans DJ Jr, Evans DG, *et al.*: *Helicobacter pylori* and the Zollinger-Ellison syndrome. *Dig Dis Sci* 1991, 36:15–18.

43. Fich A, Talley NJ, Shorter RG, Philips SF: Zollinger-Ellison syndrome. Relation to *Helicobacter pylori*-associated chronic gastritis and gastric acid secretion. *Dig Dis Sci* 1991, 36:10–14.

44. Weber HC, Orbuch M, Jensen RT: Diagnosis and treatment of the gastric and hypersecretion in patients with Zollinger-Ellison syndrome. In *Pancreatic Endocrine Tumors. Seminars in Gastrointestinal Diseases.* Edited by Jensen RT. Duluth: WB Saunders; 1995:79–89.

45. Willems G: Trophic action of gastrin on specific target cells in the gut. In *Endocrine Tumors of the Pancreas: Recent Advances in Research and Management.* Edited by Mignon M, Jensen RT. Basel: Karger; 1995:30–44.

46. Helander HF, Bordi C: Morphology of gastric mucosa during prolonged hypergastrinemia. In *Endocrine Tumors of the Pancreas: Recent Advances in Research and Management.* Edited by Mignon M, Jensen RT. Basel: Karger; 1995:372–384.

47. Neuburger P, Lewin M, Recherche CD, Bonfils S: Parietal and chief cell population in four cases of the Zollinger-Ellison syndrome. *Gastroenterology* 1972, 63:937–942.

48. Wolfe MM, Jensen RT: Zollinger-Ellison syndrome: Current concepts in diagnosis and management. *N Engl J Med* 1987, 317:1200–1209.

49. Metz DC, Jensen RT: Advances in gastric antisecretory therapy in Zollinger-Ellison syndrome. In *Endocrine Tumors of the Pancreas: Recent Advances in Research and Management.* Edited by Mignon M, Jensen RT. Basel: Karger; 1995, 240–257.

50. Metz DC, Weber HC, Orbuch M, *et al.*: *Helicobacter pylori* infection: A reversible cause of hypergastrinemia and hypercholrhydria which can mimic Zollinger-Ellison syndrome. *Dig Dis Sci* 1995, 40:153–159.

51. Jensen RT, Doppman JL, Gardner JD: Gastrinoma. In *The Exocrine Pancreas: Biology, Pathobiology and Disease.* Edited by Go VLW, Brooks FA, DiMagno EP, *et al.* New York: Raven Press; 1986:727–744.

52. Doppman JL, Miller DL, Chang R, *et al.*: Insulinomas: Localization with selective intraarterial injection of calcium. *Radiology* 1991, 178:237–241. [published erratum appears in *Radiology* 1993, 187:880].

53. Frucht H, Howard JM, Stark HA, *et al.*: Prospective study of the standard meal provocative test in Zollinger-Ellison syndrome. *Am J Med* 1989, 87:528–536.

54. Frucht H, Howard JM, Slaff JI, *et al.*: Secretin and calcium provocative tests in the Zollinger-Ellison syndrome: A prospective study. *Ann Intern Med* 1989, 111:713–722.

55. Wolfe MM: Diagnosis of gastrinoma: Much ado about nothing [Comment]. *Ann Intern Med* 1989, 111:697–699.

56. Lamers CB, Van Tongeren JHM: Comparative study of the value of calcium, secretin, and meal stimulated increase in serum gastrin in the diagnosis of the Zollinger-Ellison syndrome. *Gut* 1977, 18:128–134.

57. Feldman M, Schiller LR, Walsh JH, *et al.*: Positive intravenous secretin test in patients with achlorhydria-related hypergastrinemia. *Gastroenterology* 1987, 93:59–62.

58. Deveney CW, Deveney KS, Jaffe BM, *et al.*: Use of calcium and secretin in the diagnosis of gastrinoma (Zollinger-Ellison syndrome). *Ann Intern Med* 1977, 87:680–686.

59. London J, Frucht H, Doppman JL, *et al.*: Zollinger-Ellison syndrome in the acute care setting. *J Intensive Care Med* 1989, 4:272–283.

60. Metz DC, Pisegna JR, Fishbeyn VA, *et al.*: Control of gastric acid hypersecretion in the management of patients with Zollinger-Ellison syndrome. *World J Surg* 1993, 17:468–480.

61. Norton JA: Advances in the management of Zollinger-Ellison syndrome. *Adv Surg* 1994, 27:129–159.

62. Norton JA, Jensen RT: Unresolved surgical issues in the management of patients with the Zollinger-Ellison syndrome. *World J Surg* 1991, 15:151–159.

63. Metz DC, Pisegna JR, Fishbeyn VA, *et al.*: Currently used doses of omeprazole in Zollinger-Ellison syndrome are too high. *Gastroenterology* 1992, 103:1498–1508.

64. Metz DC, Strader DB, Orbuch M, *et al.*: Use of omeprazole in Zollinger-Ellison: A prospective nine-year study of efficacy and safety. *Aliment Pharmacol Ther* 1993, 7:597–610.

65. Frucht H, Maton PN, Jensen RT: Use of omeprazole in patients with the Zollinger-Ellison syndrome. *Dig Dis Sci* 1991, 36:394–404.

66. Lloyd-Davies KA, Rutgersson K, Solvell L: Omeprazole in the treatment of Zollinger-Ellison syndrome: A 4-year international study. *Aliment Pharmacol Ther* 1988, 2:13–32.

67. Metz DC, Pisegna JR, Ringham GL, *et al.*: Prospective study of efficacy and safety of lansoprazole in Zollinger-Ellison syndrome. *Dig Dis Sci* 1993, 38:245–256.

68. Jensen RT, Metz DC, Koviack PD, Feigenbaum KM: Prospective study of the long-term efficacy and safety of lansprazole in patients with Zollinger-Ellison syndrome. *Aliment Pharmacol Ther* 1993, 7 (suppl 1):41–50.

69. McArthur KE, Collen MJ, Maton PN, *et al.*: Omeprazole: Effective, convenient therapy for Zollinger-Ellison syndrome. *Gastroenterology* 1985, 88:939–944.

70. Jensen RT: Basis of failure of cimetidine in patients with Zollinger-Ellison syndrome. *Dig Dis Sci* 1984, 29:363–366.

71. Howard JM, Chremos AN, Collen MJ, *et al.*: Famotidine, a new, potent, long-acting histamine H_2-receptor antagonist: Comparison with cimetidine and ranitidine in the treatment of Zollinger-Ellison syndrome. *Gastroenterology* 1985, 88:1026–1033.

72. Vinayek R, Amantea MA, Maton PN, *et al.*: Pharmacokinetics of oral and intravenous omeprazole in patients with the Zollinger-Ellison syndrome. *Gastroenterology* 1991, 101:138–147.

73. Zollinger RM, Ellison EC, Fabri PJ, *et al.*: Primary peptic ulcerations of the jejunum associated with islet cell tumors. Twenty-five-year appraisal. *Ann Surg* 1980, 192:422–430.

74. Richardson CT, Peters MN, Feldman M, *et al.*: Treatment of Zollinger-Ellison syndrome with exploratory laparotomy, proximal gastric vagotomy, and H_2-receptor antagonists. A prospective study. *Gastroenterology* 1985, 89:357–367.

75. Wank SA, Doppman JL, Miller DL, *et al.*: Prospective study of the ability of computerized axial tomography to localize gastrinomas in patients with Zollinger-Ellison syndrome. *Gastroenterology* 1987, 92:905–912.

76. Frucht H, Doppman JL, Norton JA, *et al*: Gastrinomas: Comparison of MR Imaging with CT, angiography and US. *Radiology* 1989, 171:713–717.

77. Pisegna JR, Doppman JL, Norton JA, *et al.*: Prospective comparative study of ability of MR imaging and other imaging modalities to localize tumors in patients with Zollinger-Ellison syndrome. *Dig Dis Sci* 1993, 38:1318–1328.

78. Orbuch M, Doppman JL, Strader DB, *et al.*: Imaging for pancreatic endocrine tumor localization: Recent advances. In *Endocrine Tumors of the Pancreas: Recent Advances in Research and Management.* Edited by Mignon M, Jensen RT. Basel: Karger; 1995:268–281.

79. Ruszniewski P, Amouyal P, Amouyal G, *et al.*: Endocrine tumors of the pancreatic area: Localization by endoscopic ultrasonography. In *Endocrine Tumors of the Pancreas: Recent Advances in Research and Management.* Edited by Mignon M, Jensen RT. Basel; Karger: 1995:258–267.

80. Zimmer T, Ziegler K, Bader M, *et al.*: Localisation of neuroendocrine tumours of the upper gastrointestinal tract. *Gut* 1994, 35:471–475.

81. Rôosch T, Lightdale CJ, Botet JF, *et al.*: Localization of pancreatic endocrine tumors by endoscopic ultrasonography. *N Engl J Med* 1992, 326:1721–1726.

82. Mignon M, Cadiot G, Rigaud D, *et al.*: Management of islet cell tumors in patients with multiple endocrine neoplasia type I. In *Endocrine Tumors of the Pancreas: Recent Advances in Research and Management.* Edited by Mignon M, Jensen RT. Basel: Karger; 1995:342–359.

83. Jensen RT. Zollinger-Ellison syndrome: Past, present, and future controversies. *Yale J Biol Med* 1994; 67:195–214.

84. Strader DB, Doppman JL, Orbuch M, *et al.*: Functional localization of pancreatic endocrine tumors. In *Frontiers of Gastrointestinal Research.* Edited by Mignon M, Jense RT. Basel; Karger; 1995:282–297.

85. Kwekkeboom DJ, Krenning EP, Oei HY, *et al.*: Use of radiolabeled somatostatin to localize islet cell tumors. In *Endocrine Tumors of the Pancreas: Recent Advances in Research and Management.* Edited by Mignon M, Jensen RT. Basel: Karger; 1995:298–308.

86. Weber HC, Venzon DJ, Fishbein VA, *et al*: Determinants of metastatic rate and survival in patients with Zollinger-Ellison syndrome (ZES): Results of a prospective long-term study [Abstract]. *Gastroenterology* 1994, 106:A330.

87. Donow C, Pipeleers-Marichal M, Schroder S, *et al.*: Surgical pathology of gastrinoma: Site, size, multicentricity, association with multiple endocrine neoplasia type 1, and malignancy. *Cancer* 1991, 68:1329–1334.

88. Thom AK, Norton JA, Doppman JL, *et al.*: Prospective study of the use of intraarterial secretin injection and portal venous sampling to localize duodenal gastrinomas. *Surgery* 1992, 112:1002–1008.

89. Maton PN, Miller DL, Doppman JL, *et al.*: Role of selective angiography in the management of Zollinger-Ellison syndrome. *Gastroenterology* 1987, 92:913–918.

90. Orbuch M, Doppman JL, Jensen RT: Recent advances in the localization of pancreatic endocrine tumors. In *Pancreatic endocrine tumors.* Edited by Sleisenger MH, Fordtran JS. Edited by Jensen RT. In *Seminars in Gastrointestinal Diseases. 6.* Duluth; WB Saunders; 1995:90–101.

91. Lamberts SWJ, Chayvialle JA, Krenning EP: The visualization of gastro-enteropancreatic endocrine tumors. *Digestion* 1993; 54(suppl 1):92–97.

92. Krenning EP, Kwekkeboom DJ, Bakker WH, *et al.*: Somatostatin receptor scintigraphy with [^{111}In-DTPA-D-Phe^1]- and [^{123}I-Tyr^3]-octreotide: The Rotterdam experience with more than 1000 patients. *Eur J Nucl Med* 1993, 20:716–731.

93. Nakamura Y, Larsson C, Julier C, *et al.*: Localization of the genetic defect in multiple endocrine neoplasia type I within a small region of chromosome 11. *Am J Hum Genet* 1989, 44:751–755.

94. Cherner JA, Doppman JL, Norton JA, *et al.*: Selective venous sampling for gastrin to localize gastrinomas. A prospective study. *Ann Intern Med* 1986; 105:841–847.

95. Imamura M, Takahashi K, Adachi H, *et al.*: Usefulness of selective arterial secretin injection test for localization of gastrinoma in the Zollinger-Ellison syndrome. *Ann Surg* 1987, 205:230–239.

96. Sugg SL, Norton JA, Fraker DL, *et al.*: A prospective study of intraoperative methods to diagnose and resect duodenal gastrinomas. *Ann Surg* 1993; 218:138–144.

97. Frucht H, Norton JA, London JF, *et al.*: Detection of duodenal gastrinomas by operative endoscopic transillumination: A prospective study. *Gastroenterology* 1990, 99:1622–1627.

98. Norton JA, Doppman JL, Collen MJ, *et al.*: Prospective study of gastrinoma localization and resection in patients with Zollinger-Ellison syndrome. *Ann Surg* 1986, 204:468–479.

99. Weber HC, Venzon DJ, Lin JT, *et al.*: Determinants of metastatic rate and survival in Zollinger-Ellison syndrome: A prospective long-term study. *Gastroenterology* 1995, 108:1637–1649.

100. Delcore R Jr, Cheung LY, Friesen SR: Characteristics of duodenal wall gastrinomas. *Am J Surg* 1990, 160:621–623.

101. Thom AK, Norton JA, Axiotis CA, Jensen RT: Location, incidence and malignant potential of duodenal gastrinomas. *Surgery* 1991, 110:1086–1093.

102. Howard TJ, Zinner MJ, Stabile BE, Passaro E Jr: Gastrinoma excision for cure. A prospective analysis. *Ann Surg* 1990, 211:9–14.

103. Arnold WS, Fraker DL, Alexander HR, *et al.*: Apparent lymph node primary gastrinoma. *Surgery* 1994, 116:1123–1130.

104. Lloyd RV, Mervak T, Schmidt K, *et al.*: Immunohistochemical detection of chromogranin and neurospecific enolase in pancreatic endocrine tumors. *Am J Surg Pathol* 1984; 8:607–614.

105. Sobol R, Memoli V, Deftos LJ: Hormone-negative, chromogranin A-positive endocrine tumors. *N Engl J Med* 1989, 320:444–447.

106. Stabile BE, Passaro E Jr: Benign and malignant gastrinoma. *Am J Surg* 1985, 49:144–150.

107. Fishbeyn VA, Norton JA, Benya RV, *et al.*: Assessment and prediction of long-term cure in patients with Zollinger-Ellison syndrome: The best approach. *Ann Intern Med* 1993; 119:199–206.

108. Skogseid B, Oberg K: Genetics of multiple endocrine neoplasia type 1. In *Endocrine Tumors of the Pancreas: Recent Advances in Research and Management.* Edited by Mignon N; Jensen RT. Basel: Karger; 1995:60–69.

109. Eriksson B, Oberg K: PPomas and nonfunctioning endocrine pancreatic tumors: Clinical presentation, diagnosis, and advances in management. In *Endocrine Tumors of the Pancreas: Recent Advances in Research and Management.* Edited by Mignon M, Jensen RT. Basel: Karger; 1995:208–222.

110. Jensen RT: Gastrinoma as a model for prolonged hypergastrinemia in man. In *Gastrin.* Edited by Walsh JH. New York: Raven Press; 1993:373–393.

111. Solcia E, Capella C, Fiocca R, *et al.*: Gastric argyrophil carcinoidosis in patients with Zollinger-Ellison syndrome due to type 1 multiple endocrine neoplasia. A newly recognized association. *Am J Surg Pathol* 1990, 14:503–513.

112. Solcia E, Capella C, Fiocca R, *et al.*: The gastroenteropancreatic endocrine system and related tumors. *Gastroenterol Clin North Am* 1989; 18:671–693.

113. Norton JA, Sugarbaker PH, Doppman JL, *et al.*: Aggressive resection of metastatic disease in selected patients with malignant gastrinoma. *Ann Surg* 1986; 203:352–359.

114. Arnold R, Neuhaus C, Benning R, *et al.*: Somatostatin analog sandostatin and inhibition of tumor growth in patients with metastatic endocrine gastroenteropancreatic tumors. *World J Surg* 1993, 17:511–519.

115. Gibril F, Doppman JL, Jensen RT: Treatment of metastatic pancreatic endocrine tumors. In *Pancreatic Endocrine Tumors. Seminars in Gastrointestinal Disease*. Edited by Jensen RT. Duluth: WB Saunders; 1995:114–121.

116. von Schrenck T, Howard JM, Doppman JL, *et al.*: Prospective study of chemotherapy in patients with metastatic gastrinoma. *Gastroenterology* 1988; 94:1326–1334.

117. Moertel CG, Lefkopoulo M, Lipsitz S, *et al.*: Streptozotocin-doxorubicin, streptozotocin-fluorouracil or chlorozotocin in the treatment of advanced islet cell carcinoma. *N Engl J Med* 1992, 326:519–523.

118. Moertel CG, Kvols LK, O'Connell MJ, Rubin J: Treatment of neuroendocrine carcinomas with combined etoposide and cisplatin. Evidence of major therapeutic activity in the anaplastic variants of these neoplasms. *Cancer* 1991, 68:227–232.

119. Pisegna JR, Slimak GG, Doppman JL, *et al.*: An evaluation of human recombinant alpha interferon in patients with metastatic gastrinoma. *Gastroenterology* 1993, 105:1179–1183.

120. Arnold R, Frank M: Systemic chemotherapy for endocrine tumors of the pancreas: Recent advances. In *Endocrine Tumors of the Pancreas: Recent Advances in Research and Management*. Edited by Mignon M, Jensen RT. Basel: Karger; 1995:431–438.

Chapter 9

Bleeding Lesions of the Stomach and Duodenum

Karl Fukunaga

Russell Yang

Upper gastrointestinal tract hemorrhage is a major health problem accounting for more than 300,000 hospital admissions per year [1]. With the introduction and widespread application of video endoscopy, evaluation of the upper gastrointestinal tract has become superior to that seen using barium radiographic studies (*ie*, upper gastrointestinal series) for several reasons. First, endoscopy is more accurate in establishing the site of bleeding [1]. Second, endoscopy offers potential therapeutic intervention. Finally, endoscopic diagnosis can provide prognostic information to assist the clinician in further management decisions. For example, peptic ulcers, which are *clean-based*, and Mallory-Weiss tears have less than a 5% chance of recurrent hemorrhage. On the other hand, peptic ulcers with a visible vessel are associated with a 43% to 55% chance of rebleeding [2]. Those lesions, which have a high risk of recurrent hemorrhage, are ideal targets for endoscopic intervention.

Most cases of upper gastrointestinal hemorrhage result from bleeding peptic ulcers (>50%) [3]. Despite development of potent antisecretory agents for peptic ulcer, no therapy has proven beneficial in reducing the morbidity, mortality, or recurrence of bleeding peptic ulcer [3,4]. Thus, the lack of effective medical therapy is reflected in the fact that bleeding ulcer mortality and need for surgical intervention have not changed in 3 decades [5]. With the advent of therapeutic endoscopy and hemostatic techniques, however, nonsurgical treatment of high-risk bleeding lesions do result in significant reduction of recurrent hemorrhage, blood transfusion requirement, length of hospital stay, need for urgent surgery, and perhaps, hospital mortality rate [3,6].

In this chapter, we demonstrate a variety of bleeding lesions of the stomach and duodenum observed at Los Angeles County General Hospital, Los Angeles, CA. In doing so, we hope to familiarize clinicians with the endoscopic appearance, clinical significance, and, in some cases, therapeutic hemostatic intervention to treat these lesions.

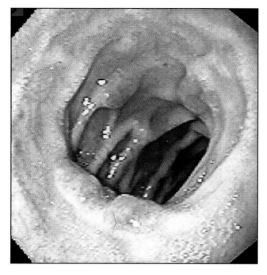
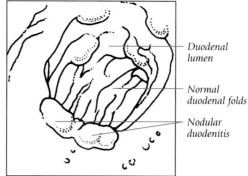

FIGURE 9-1.

Nodular duodenitis. Esophagogastroduodenoscopy in stable hemodialysis patients reveals a mucosal abnormality as often as 50% of the time. Nodular duodenitis—raised areas of erythema and erosions in the duodenum—is commonly seen in patients with dialysis-dependent end-stage renal disease. These lesions appear to be reversible after renal transplantation [7].

Duodenal lumen

Normal duodenal folds

Nodular duodenitis

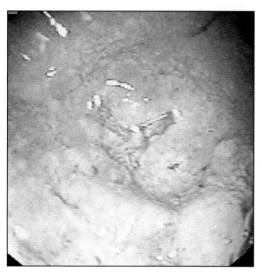
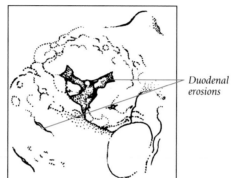

FIGURE 9-2.

Erosive duodenitis. Diffuse mucosal superficial defects, with or without subepithelial hemorrhages, may be associated with upper gastrointestinal bleeding. The subjective lack of depth in the mucosal defect distinguishes this lesion from an actual duodenal ulcer. This erosive duodenitis was present in a patient with Zollinger-Ellison syndrome; however, it can occur in patients without a hypersecretory state [8].

Duodenal erosions

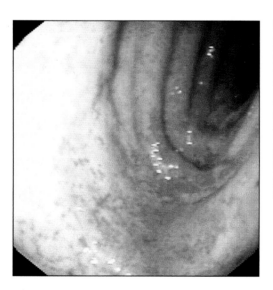
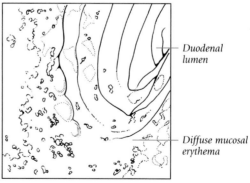

FIGURE 9-3.

Duodenal *Strongyloides*. *Strongyloides stercoralis* is a nematode capable of invading the small intestinal mucosa. The infective larvae—filariform—invade the host through the skin or buccal mucosa. They eventually reach the lungs where they develop into adolescent worms. They are subsequently swallowed and invade the small bowel mucosa. Patients with *S. stercoralis* usually present with epigastric pain, nausea, vomiting, weight loss, or even malabsorption. This parasitic infestation can occur in immigrants from developing countries, patients on immunosuppressive medications, or in patients with AIDS. The endoscopic appearance is that of a diffuse mucosal abnormality resembling an infiltrative process. The mucosa contains confluent areas of punctate erythema superimposed on a diffusely eroded mucosal surface.

Duodenal lumen

Diffuse mucosal erythema

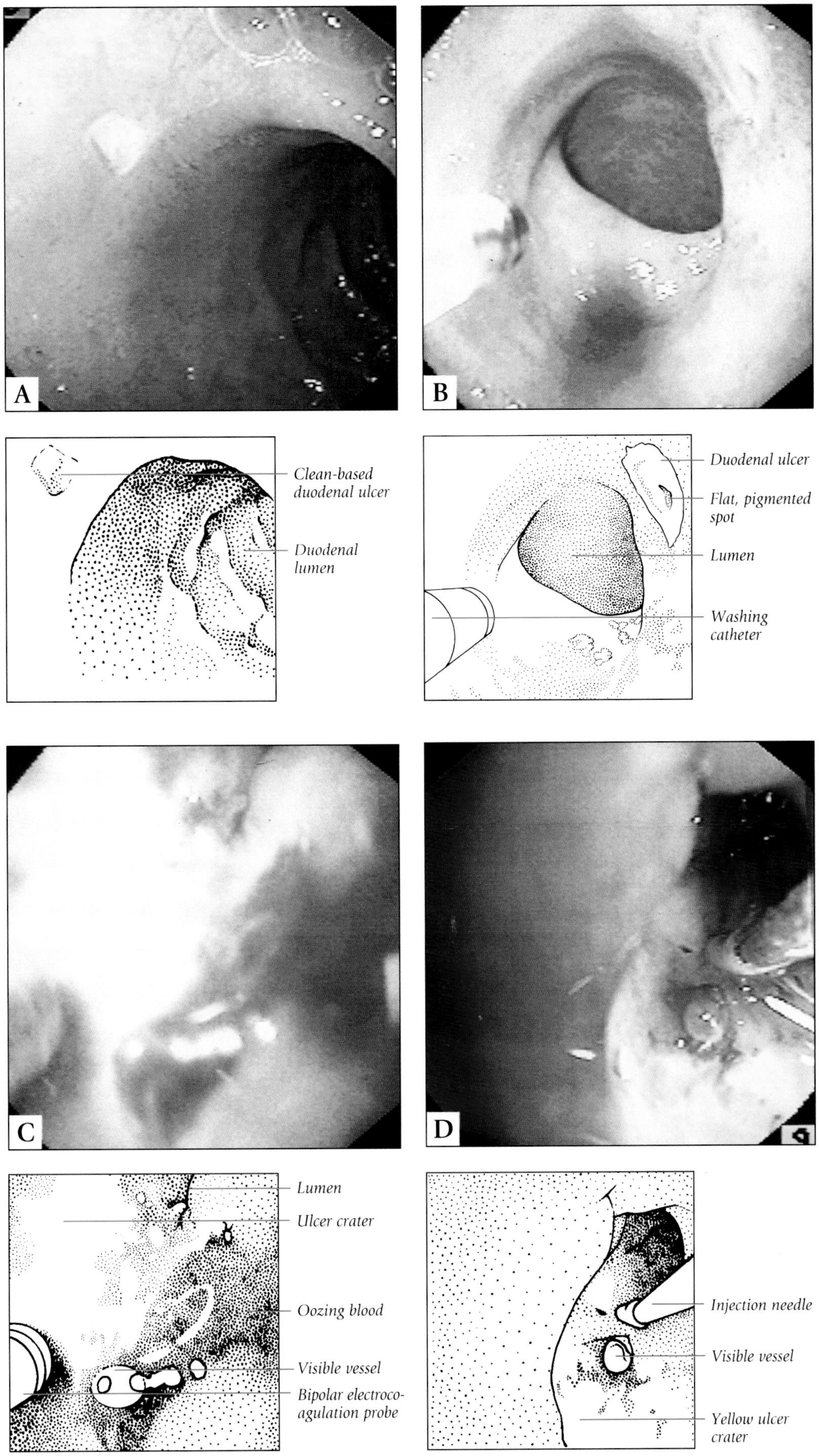

A

Clean-based
duodenal ulcer

Duodenal
lumen

B

Duodenal ulcer

Flat, pigmented
spot

Lumen

Washing
catheter

C

Lumen

Ulcer crater

Oozing blood

Visible vessel

Bipolar electroco-
agulation probe

D

Injection needle

Visible vessel

Yellow ulcer
crater

FIGURE 9-4.

Duodenal ulcer. Approximately 50% of patients with upper gastrointestinal hemorrhage have experienced bleeding from a peptic ulcer. Bleeding duodenal ulcers are twice as common as gastric ulcers. Endoscopic appearance of an ulcer, that is, the presence or absence of stigmata predicting recurrent bleeding, is of value in assessing prognosis. **A**, A clean-based ulcer carries a 1% risk of recurrent hemorrhage. Some authors have advocated discharging from the hospital a patient with such a lesion immediately after replenishing intravascular volume. **B**, A flat, pigmented spot carries a 7% risk of recurrent bleeding. Notice that on tangential view there is no appearance of elevation in such a lesion. **C**, A visible vessel is a well-circumscribed, glistening, and raised area within the ulcer crater. A visible vessel carries a 43% to 55% risk of recurrent bleeding and a 30% chance of requiring urgent surgical intervention. Therefore, an ulcer with a visible vessel should be treated with endoscopic therapy in order to affect patient outcome. This ulcer crater (yellow mucosa) has a nonbleeding visible vessel (red protuberance). Endoscopic therapy is being applied using an injection catheter. **D**, This visible vessel was seen in an edematous duodenal bulb (hence the close-up view). It is actively oozing. A bipolar electrocoagulation probe is poised in the lower left corner before therapy.

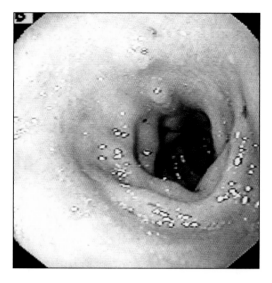

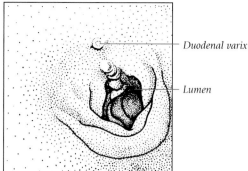

Duodenal varix

Lumen

FIGURE 9-5.

Duodenal varices. Duodenal varices are a rare manifestation of portal hypertension. Hemorrhage from duodenal varices does not typically respond to conventional forms of endoscopic therapy such as sclerotherapy and ligation. Cyanoacrylate injection—an adhesive tissue glue—may play a role in therapy. Refractory hemorrhage from duodenal varices is, however, an indication for portosystemic shunting, performed either radiologically or surgically.

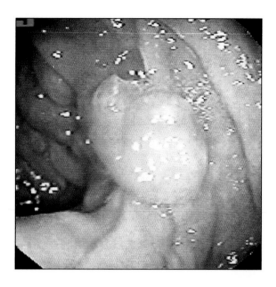

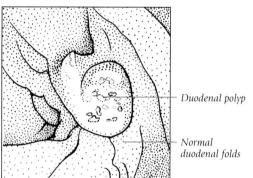

Duodenal polyp

Normal duodenal folds

FIGURE 9-6.

Duodenal polyp. Duodenal polyps may occur sporadically as they did in this patient. They also occur in patients with colonic polyposis syndromes. If they are located near the ampulla of Vater, they may present a challenge during endoscopic polypectomy.

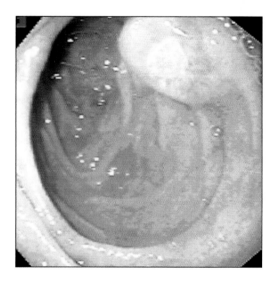

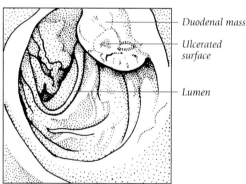

Duodenal mass

Ulcerated surface

Lumen

FIGURE 9-7.

Duodenal mass. The differential diagnosis for a duodenal mass is broad. Neoplastic causes include both benign and malignant types. Of the benign tumors, one must consider benign adenomatous polyp, villous adenoma, leiomyoma, carcinoid tumor, and benign inflammatory masses. Malignant causes include primary adeno-carcinoma, metastatic tumor, leiomyosar-coma, carcinoid tumor, or lymphoma. This patient, who carried a diagnosis of AIDS, had a duodenal lymphoma. Notice that the surface of the tumor is ulcerated.

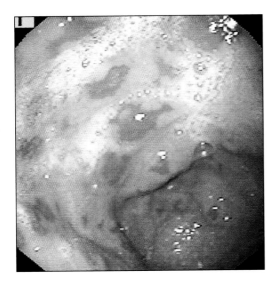
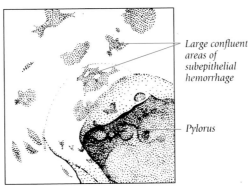

Large confluent
areas of
subepithelial
hemorrhage

Pylorus

FIGURE 9-8.

Hemorrhagic gastritis. *Gastritis* is a histologic term that does not necessarily correlate with the endoscopic appearance. Gastritis or more precisely, gastropathy, usually occurs in the setting of stress, alcohol abuse, or nonsteroidal anti-inflammatory drug use. This figure is an extreme example of hemorrhagic gastritis. There are several areas of confluent subepithelial hemorrhage (with an appearance of blood under plastic wrap) separated by areas of eroded mucosa.

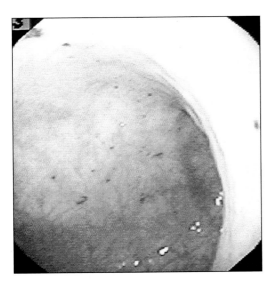
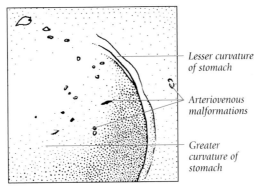

Lesser curvature
of stomach

Arteriovenous
malformations

Greater
curvature of
stomach

FIGURE 9-9.

Osler-Weber-Rendu disease. Osler-Weber-Rendu disease (*ie*, hereditary hemorrhagic telangiectasia), an autosomal dominant disorder, may present with diffuse arteriovenous malformations throughout the gastrointestinal tract. If sufficiently localized, endoscopic ablation is the treatment of choice. If the lesions are diffuse, however, estrogen-progesterone therapy may be helpful [9]. Oral aminocaproic acid has also been reported to be of prophylactic benefit [10].

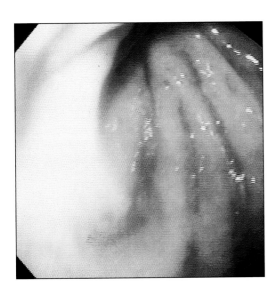
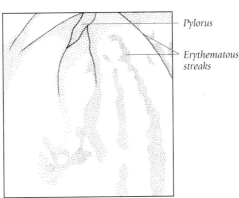

Pylorus

Erythematous
streaks

FIGURE 9-10.

Watermelon stomach [11]. This lesion results from multiple antral vascular ectasias formed in a pattern of linear streaks radiating from the pylorus. Histologically, it consists of multiple dilated venules with focal thrombosis and fibromuscular hyperplasia. The cause of watermelon stomach is not known but it occurs primarily in older women. It presents with iron-deficient anemia, which is usually manageable with iron supplementation. In extreme cases, endoscopic thermal therapy or surgical antrectomy may be necessary.

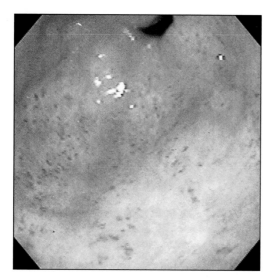

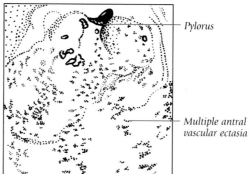

FIGURE 9-11.

Antral vascular ectasia. Multiple antral vascular ectasia have been described in primary biliary cirrhosis usually when associated with the CREST (calcinosis, Raynaud's phenomenon, esophageal dysfunction, sclerodactyly, and telangiectasia) syndrome. The ectasia appears as multiple punctate areas of erythema on the antral mucosa.

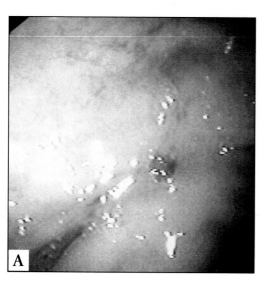

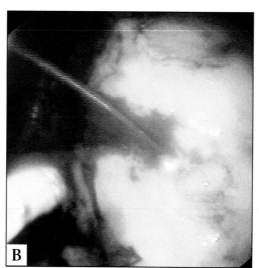

FIGURE 9-12.

Dieulafoy's lesion. Dieulafoy's lesion is a rare cause of massive and recurrent upper gastrointestinal hemorrhage. The lesion is an extramural caliber artery present in the submucosa. Bleeding probably results from pressure exerted by such a blood vessel on the overlying mucosa so that it is ultimately exposed to the lumen. Dieulafoy's lesion is most common in the gastric cardia, 6 cm from the gastroesophageal junction. Mortality is high because the bleeding site is often difficult to identify. A, Rarely Dieulafoy's lesion may have the appearance of a visible blood vessel in the absence of an ulcer crater. B, When exposed to the lumen, the vessel's wall may actually break down and lead to dramatic bleeding [12].

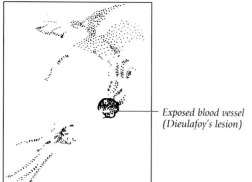

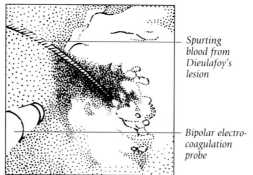

Exposed blood vessel
(Dieulafoy's lesion)

Spurting
blood from
Dieulafoy's
lesion

Bipolar electro-
coagulation
probe

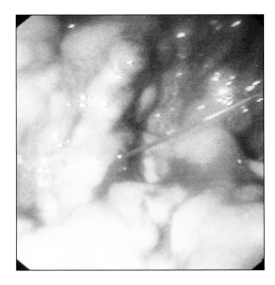

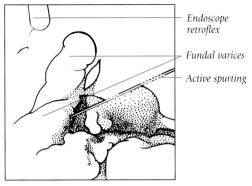

Endoscope retroflex

Fundal varices

Active spurting

FIGURE 9-13.

Fundal varices. Gastric varices usually occur in the fundus of the stomach. These fundal varices are best seen on retroflex view; they have the classic appearance of a submucosal *cluster of grapes*. These fundal varices, which are demonstrating active bleeding, occurred in a patient with hepatocellular carcinoma with sinistral portal hypertension secondary to tumor invasion of the portal vein. It is believed that up to 10% of variceal bleeds result from bleeding fundal varices [13]. Bleeding fundal varices are associated with a higher mortality rate than bleeding esophageal varices. In addition, conventional sclerotherapy has produced disappointing results with high rebleeding rates, often secondary to sclerotherapy-induced ulceration. There is some evidence that injection of fundal varices with a tissue adhesive, histoacryl, may be successful in controlling hemorrhage [14].

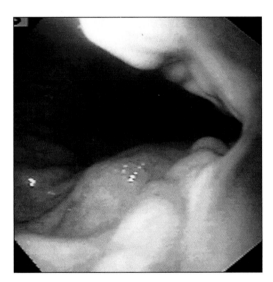

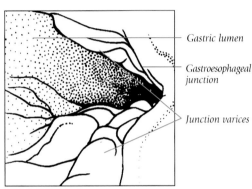

Gastric lumen

Gastroesophageal junction

Junction varices

FIGURE 9-14.

Junctional varices. Junctional varices are defined as gastric (distal to gastroesophageal junction) varices that arise no more than 2 cm below the gastroesophageal junction [15]. These junctional varices can be seen projecting just distal to the gastroesophageal junction. Junctional varices are believed to be a subset of gastric varices distinct from fundal varices; during follow-up, 37% of patients with junctional varices develop significant bleeding compared with nearly 100% of patients with fundal varices.

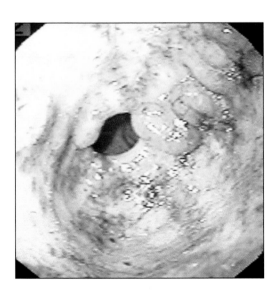

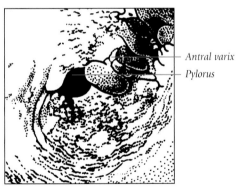

Antral varix

Pylorus

FIGURE 9-15.

Antral varices. This antral varix has the appearance of a tortuous cord radiating from the pylorus. This patient, who had a history of alcoholic liver disease, presented with actively bleeding esophageal varices that responded well to conventional sclerotherapy. Little is known about the natural history of antral varices because they are a very rare manifestation of portal hypertension.

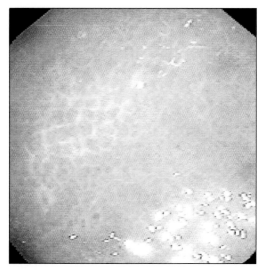
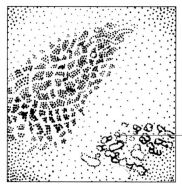

FIGURE 9-16.

Mosaic pattern of portal hypertensive gastropathy

Portal hypertensive gastropathy. Typically portal hypertensive gastropathy has the appearance of a mucosal mosaic pattern with a speckling of subepithelial hemorrhages superimposed upon it. Histologically, it consists of vascular dilation and ectasia. Despite being very common in patients with portal hypertension, it is not clear if portal hypertensive gastropathy by itself is responsible for significant upper gastrointestinal hemorrhaging.

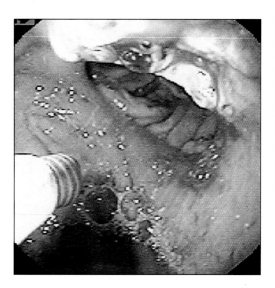
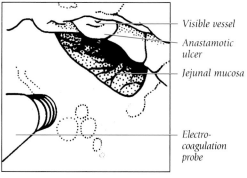

Visible vessel

Anastamotic ulcer

Jejunal mucosa

Electro-coagulation probe

FIGURE 9-17.

Anastomotic ulcer. This anastomotic ulcer is seen as a mucosal defect adjacent to a Billroth II gastrojejunostomy. A visible vessel (red, well-circumscribed nodule within ulcer) is present and a electrocoagulation therapeutic probe is poised for intervention. An endoscopic evaluation is mandatory in a patient with upper gastrointestinal bleeding after having gastric surgery. The differential diagnosis includes anastomotic ulcer versus recurrent gastric ulcer which may be secondary to underlying carcinoma, hypersecretory state, or incomplete surgical vagotomy.

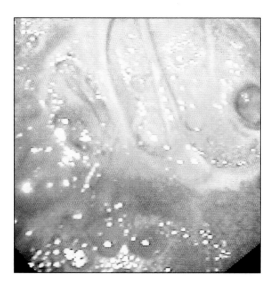
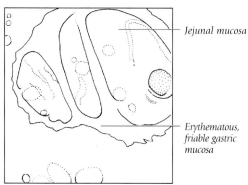

Jejunal mucosa

Erythematous, friable gastric mucosa

FIGURE 9-18.

Bile reflux gastropathy. Bile reflux gastropathy has the endoscopic appearance of erythema and friability of the mucosa adjacent to a gastrojejunostomy anastamosis. Patients with bile reflux gastropathy, or alkaline "gastritis," present with post prandial abdominal pain and bilious vomiting. However, as the mucosa is typically friable, it can present with upper gastrointestinal bleeding or iron deficiency. It is believed that exposure of the gastric mucosa to duodenal contents leads to this irritation.

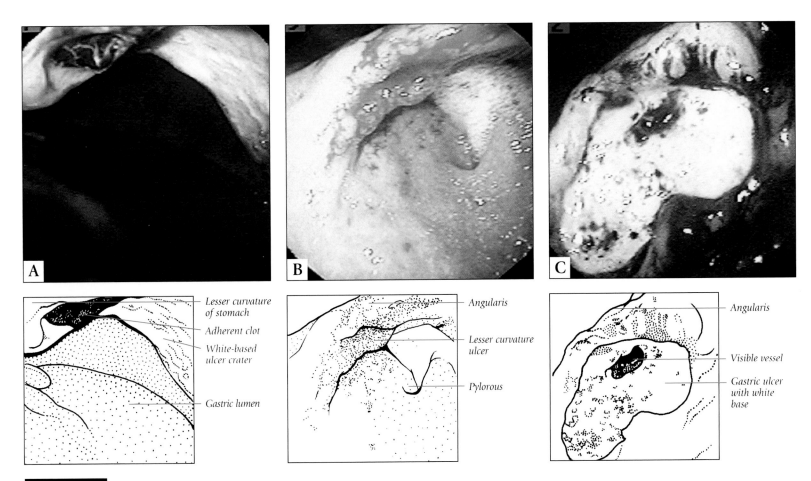

FIGURE 9-19.

Gastric ulcer (*See* Figure 9-4). **A**, Gastric ulcer with adherent clot. This patient presented with massive upper gastrointestinal bleeding. This gastric ulcer lies on the lesser curvature in close proximity to the gastroesophageal junction (as evidenced by the endoscope seen on retroflexion view). Notice adherent clot within the ulcer crater—a diffuse, poorly organized collection of blood—that did not wash off the ulcer base with a jet of water from the endoscope. **B**, Gastric ulcer with active bleeding. This gastric ulcer lies on the incisura angularis of the lesser curvature, which is the most common location for gastric ulcers. Although there is no visible vessel within the ulcer crater, blood actively oozes from the margin of the ulcer. **C**, Gastric ulcer with visible vessel. This gastric ulcer also lies along the lesser curvature and is so large that it occupies almost the entire angularis. Within the crater of the ulcer is a visible vessel—a well-circumscribed and glistening nodule.

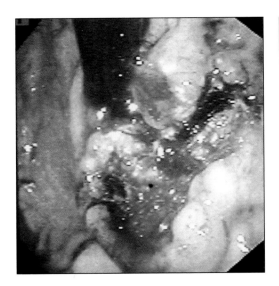
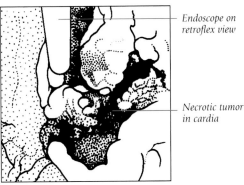

FIGURE 9-20.

Cardia carcinoma. The gastric cardia is that portion of the stomach immediately adjoining the esophagus. Because of the proximity to the esophagus, carcinoma of the gastric cardia can result in dysphagia. This carcinoma is seen on retroflexion view and has a friable, necrotic appearance. Surgical resection of such a tumor is challenging because it may require an esophagectomy in addition to a partial gastrectomy.

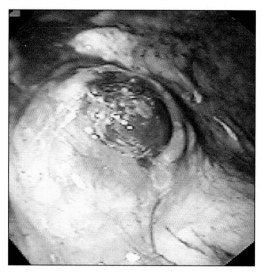

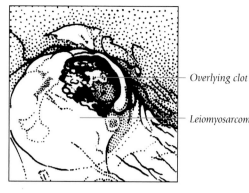

Overlying clot

Leiomyosarcoma

FIGURE 9-21.

Gastric leiomyosarcoma. Gastric leiomyosarcoma accounts for 1% of malignant tumors of the stomach. This leiomyosarcoma presented with hematemesis; notice that the tumor appears as a submucosal nodule within the gastric lumen. However, there is a clot overlying the lesion where the tumor had ulcerated and hemorrhaged. Although curative resection can be attempted, the 5-year survival rate is 25% to 30% [16].

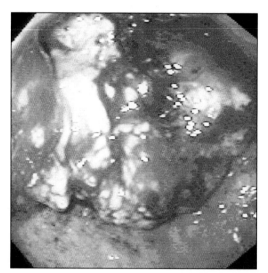

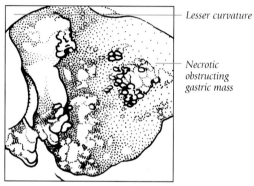

Lesser curvature

Necrotic obstructing gastric mass

FIGURE 9-22.

Gastric carcinoma. Gastric adenocarcinoma accounts for more than 95% of the malignant tumors of the stomach. This lesion was discovered in a patient who presented with melenic stools and progressive anemia. This carcinoma is a fungating and friable mass, which could easily account for gastrointestinal bleeding. Unfortunately, most gastric carcinomas present as this one did and are not resectable at the time of diagnosis.

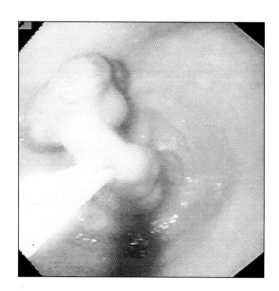

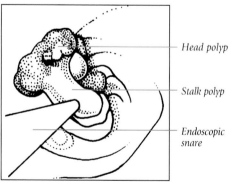

Head polyp

Stalk polyp

Endoscopic snare

FIGURE 9-23.

Gastric polyp. Gastric polyps have a prevalence of 0.4% in autopsy series [17]. The vast majority are symptomatic; however, when they are a large enough, surface ulceration and bleeding may occur. Polyps are most commonly hyperplastic, which are not premalignant; polyps are less commonly adenomatous, which are premalignant. This particular polyp was a 2-cm pedunculated polyp that was removed using an endoscopic coagulation snare.

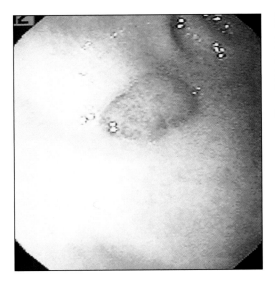

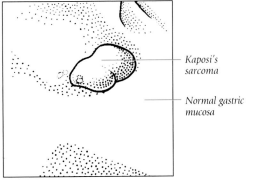

Kaposi's sarcoma

Normal gastric mucosa

Figure 9-24.

Gastric Kaposi's sarcoma. In the area of AIDS, a variety of bleeding gastrointestinal lesions have been noted. Kaposi's sarcoma is a spindle cell tumor that often has a submucosal location histologically; hence the yield of biopsy is low, 23%, despite a typical endoscopic appearance [18]. Although gastrointestinal Kaposi's sarcoma can occur in the absence of cutaneous lesions, increasing numbers of skin lesions predict a higher incidence of gastrointestinal lesions. The lesion is typically a well-circumscribed, submucosal, erythematous or violaceous mass lesion. Bleeding gastrointestinal Kaposi's sarcoma lesions are a reflection of advanced immunosuppression and poor long-term survival. Some authors have, however, reported good acute control of active bleeding with endoscopic sclerotherapy [19].

■ REFERENCES

1. Laine L: Upper gastrointestinal hemorrhage. *West J Med* 1991, 155:274–279.

2. Laine L: Rolling review: Upper gastrointestinal bleeding. *Aliment Pharmacol Ther* 1993, 7:207–232.

3. Laine L, Peterson W: Medical progress: Bleeding peptic ulcer. *N Engl J Med* 1994, 331:717–727.

4. Daneshmend T, Hawkey C, Laugman M, *et al.*: Omeprazole versus placebo for acute upper gastrointestinal bleeding: Randomized double blind controlled trial. *BMJ* 1992, 304:143–147.

5. NIH Consensus Conference: Therapeutic endoscopy and bleeding ulcers. *JAMA* 1989, 262:1369–1372.

6. Chalmers T: Meta-analysis and its role in evaluating endoscopic therapies for bleeding peptic ulcer. *Masters in Gastroenterology* 1994, 6:12–17.

7. Musola R, Franzin G, Mora R, Manfrini C: Prevalence of gastroduodenal lesions in uremic patients undergoing dialysis and after renal transplantation. *Gastrointest Endosc* 1984, 30:343–346.

8. Silverstein F, Gilbert D, Tedesco F, *et al.*: The national ASGE survey on upper gastrointestinal bleeding. *Gastrointest Endosc* 1981, 27:80–93.

9. Van Cutsem E, Rutgeerts P, Vantrappen G: Treatment of bleeding gastrointestinal vascular malformations with oestrogen-progesterone. *Lancet* 1990, 335:953–955.

10. Saba H, Morelli G, Logrono L: Treatement of bleeding in hereditary hemorrhagic telangiectasia with aminocaproic acid. *N Engl J Med* 1994, 330:1789–1790.

11. Jabbari J, Cherry R, Lough J, *et al.*: Gastric antral vascular ectasia: The watermelon stomach. *Gastroenterology* 1984, 87:1165–1170.

12. Eidus L, Rasuli P, Manion D, Heringer R: Caliber-persistent artery of the stomach. *Gastroenterology* 1990, 99:1507–1510.

13. Trudeau W, Prindiville T: Endoscopic injection sclerosis of bleeding gastric varices. *Gastrointest Endosc* 1986, 32:264–268.

14. Grimm H, Maydeo A, Noar M, Soehendra N: Bleeding esophagogastric varices: Is endoscopic treatment with cyanoacrylate the final answer? *Gastrointest Endosc* 1991, :A174.

15. Korula J, Chin K, Ko Y, Yamada S: Demonstration of two distinct subsets of gastric varices. *Dig Dis Sci* 1991, 36:303–309.

16. Bedikian A, Khankhanian N, Valdivieso M, *et al.*: Sarcoma of the stomach: Clinicopathologic study of 43 cases. *J Surg Oncol* 1980, 13:121–127.

17. Bentivenga S, Panagopoulos P: Adenomatous gastric polyps. *Am J Gastroenterol* 1965, 44:138–148.

18. Friedman S, Wright T, Altman D: Gastrointestinal Kaposi's sarcoma in patients with acquired immunodeficiency syndrome: Endoscopic and autopsy findings. *Gastroenterology* 1985, 89:102–108.

19. Lew E, Dieterich D: Severe hemorrhage caused by gastrointestinal Kaposi's syndrome in patients with the acquired immunodeficiency syndrome. *Am J Gastroenterol* 1992, 87:1471–1474.

Chapter 10

Neoplasms of the Stomach and Duodenum

DANIEL C. DEMARCO

Neoplasia of the stomach and duodenum involve a vast array of entities that are accompanied with very different prognoses. Thorough workup and evaluation of these abnormalities are essential if patients are to be well informed regarding their possible choices of necessary therapy, both curative or palliative. Multiple diagnostic modalities are widely available to the clinician. Not every modality, however, should be considered for use on every patient, whether in the interest of maximum efficiency or to satisfy the needs of cost-containment programs predicted by insurers and Health Maintenance Organizations (HMOs). Quite often, endoscopic biopsies (even those done with large biopsy techniques) will reveal ambiguous findings. Such lesions can be further evaluated with endoscopic sonography [1], computed tomography, or magnetic resonance imaging. The presence of serologic markers is rarely helpful diagnostically. Finally, intraoperative sonography may be helpful in staging the disease.

Treatment of the various types of neoplasms of the stomach and small bowel must be individualized. Many lesions will remain asymptomatic and will thus require no further treatment. Other types of malignant lesions may require therapy with combined modalities in an attempt at palliation, whereas many lesions may be curable by using therapy of both single and combined modalities. The aggressiveness of the treatment selected must take into consideration the prognosis of the lesion as well as the physiologic age of the affected patient.

MALIGNANT GASTRIC NEOPLASMS

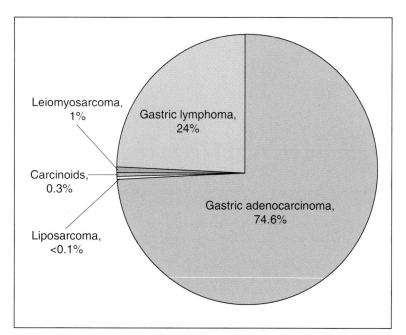

FIGURE 10-1.

Malignant gastric neoplasms. Pie chart demonstrating the relative incidence of malignant tumors of the stomach. The vast majority of these malignancies and neoplasms are gastric adenocarcinomas [2].

Gastric carcinoma

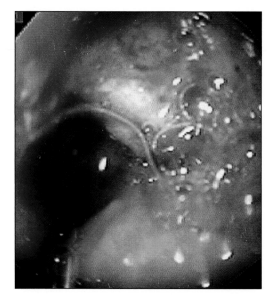

FIGURE 10-2.

Gastric carcinoma. The most common type of all malignant gastric neoplasms is the gastric adenocarcinoma. Squamous cell carcinomas of the stomach, as well as the hepatoid adeno-carcinomas, are both very rare forms of gastric carcinomas. The 5-year survival rate for patients with gastric adenocarcinoma is 15%. It should be noted, however, that this percentage represents an average survival rate. Survival rates are thought to be considerably lower in younger patients than middle-aged and elderly patients. Treatment includes local resection for patients with "early gastric cancer", extensive resection and lymph node dissection for patients with advanced gastric cancer, and the addition of chemotherapeutic modalities for those patients in whom there is evidence of widespread metastatic disease. The possible role of adjuvant, neoadjuvant, hormonal, or radiographic therapy in the treatment of patients with advanced gastric cancer remains uncertain. Certain groups of patients are at significantly higher risk than others, including postpartial gastrectomy patients, patients with pernicious anemia, patients of lower socioeconomic status, and patients whose diet includes intake of large amounts of salted fish, starches, pickled vegetables, meat, smoked foods, nitrates, and nitrites. Even for such patients, routine endoscopic screening is not warranted. When a person from such a high-risk group develops symptoms, however, the patient should have upper gastrointestinal endoscopy. The possible endoscopic features seen can include such an ulcerated mass as shown in this figure.

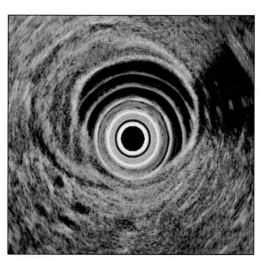

FIGURE 10-3.

Use of endoscopic ultrasound confirms the depth of invasion of this lesion as seen in Figure 10-2. Involvement is to the fourth layer, which is composed of the muscularis mucosae. The serosa is not involved. No lymphadenopathy is seen. No adjacent organs are involved. This is classified as a $T_2 N_0 M_0$ lesion [3].

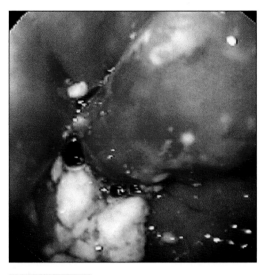

FIGURE 10-4.

The appearance of the lesions is sometimes more subtle, as is demonstrated here in a view from another patient who has a lesion present at the gastroesophageal junction.

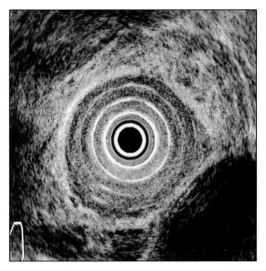

FIGURE 10-5.

In this figure, the patient has evidence of a more subtle lesion, the presence of which is confirmed by the use of endoscopic ultrasonography.

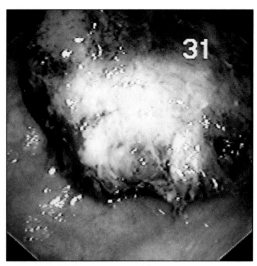

FIGURE 10-6.

This endoscopic view reveals the presence of an obviously ulcerated mass. Biopsy is one type of modality frequently used to reveal the presence of adenocarcinoma.

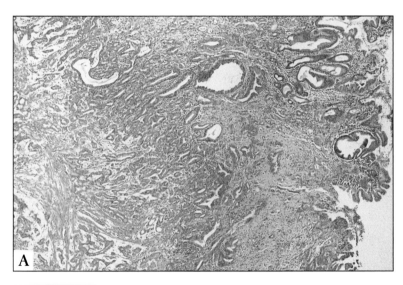

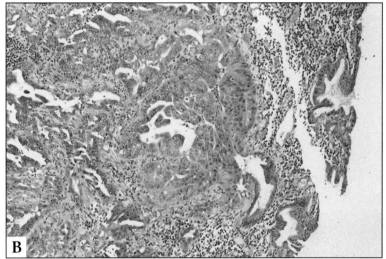

FIGURE 10-7.

A, Gastric mucosa showing infiltrating, moderately differentiated adenocarcinoma of the intestinal type. The tumor partially involves the surface and then infiltrates the underlying submucosa. Tumor cells form tubular glands of varying sizes and shapes with surrounding stromal desmoplasia (hematoxylin and eosin stain; original magnification × 40). B, Same view as A, although at different magnification (hematoxylin and eosin stain; original magnification × 100).

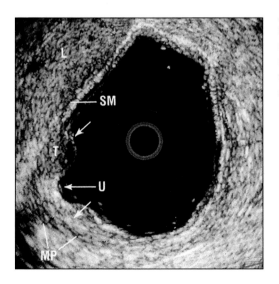

FIGURE 10-8.

Carcinoma in the body of the stomach. A 68-year-old man with a carcinoma in the body of the stomach was referred for preoperative staging. Endoscopic ultrasound shows an ulcer with nodular margins (*arrows*) containing an intrasubmucosal carcinoma (T). SM—submucosa. (*From* Tio [4]; with permission.)

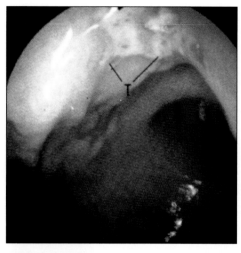

FIGURE 10-9.

In the same patient as shown in Figure 10-8, endoscopy shows an ulcerative carcinoma (T) located at the lesser curvature of the stomach. (*From* Tio [4]; with permission.)

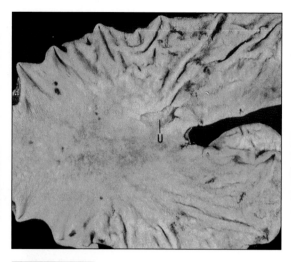

FIGURE 10-10.

Macroscopically, the resected specimen shows an ulcer (U) at the lesser curvature of the stomach. It was subsequently proven during additional analysis to be an early gastric carcinoma of submucosal type. (*From* Tio [4]; with permission.)

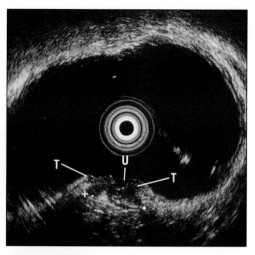

FIGURE 10-11.

A 79-year-old man with recurrent abdominal pain was referred for gastroscopy. A malignant ulcer was found at the junction between the fundus and body of the stomach. Endoscopic ultrasound testing revealed a hypoechoic intrasubmucosal carcinoma (T) adjacent to an ulcer (U). (*From* Tio [4]; with permission.)

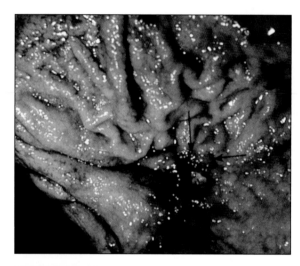

FIGURE 10-12.

Macroscopically, the resected specimen shows an ulcer (U) at the lesser curvature of the stomach with some divergent gastric folds (*arrows*). This view is from the same patient shown in Figure 10-11. (*From* Tio [4]; with permission.)

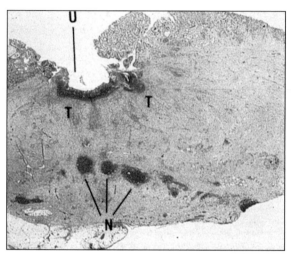

FIGURE 10-13.

Histology of the resected specimen shown in Figure 10-12 confirms the diagnosis of the intrasubmucosal early gastric cancer (T). Three small nonmetastatic lymph nodes (N) also exist. U—ulcer. (*From* Tio [4]; with permission.)

TABLE 10-1. EARLY VERSUS ADVANCED GASTRIC CANCER

DEPTH OF INVASION	LYMPH NODE INVOLVEMENT, %	5-YEAR SURVIVAL, %
Early gastric cancer	7	91
Mucosa	14	81
Submucosa	45	36
Advanced gastric cancer	66	4
Muscularis	24	78
Serosa	68	21

TABLE 10-1.

TABLE 10-1.

Neoplasms of the stomach. Early gastric cancer is considered by many to be a separate entity from advanced gastric cancer. (*From* Davis [2]; with permission.)

GASTRIC LYMPHOMA

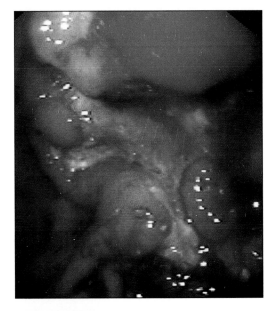

FIGURE 10-14.

Gastric lymphoma. Gastric lymphoma represents less than 5% of the gastric malignant neoplasms seen. The stomach remains the most common site of involvement for extranodal non-Hodgkin's lymphoma. Using only endoscopy and radiographic barium studies, lymphoma may be difficult to differentiate from gastric adenocarcinoma. Biopsies also are not particularly helpful in making the diagnosis. The 5-year survival rate for patients who have gastric lymphoma is approximately 50% when all combinations of patients and therapeutic modalities are considered. This endoscopic view reveals thickened folds. The differential diagnosis of thickened gastric folds includes many entities such as Zollinger-Ellison syndrome, Ménétrier's disease, varices lues, idiopathic hypertrophic gastrophy, eosinophilic gastritis, pseudolymphoma, and lymphoma.

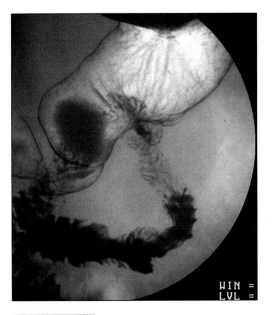

FIGURE 10-15.

Thickened gastric folds and a mass noted involving the stomach. Often such deformities can extend into the duodenum. Such lesions are often difficult to distinguish from those present resulting from gastric adenocarcinoma.

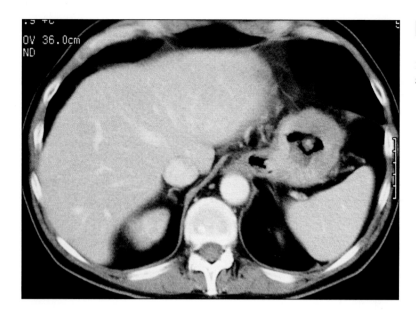

FIGURE 10-16.

Image from a computed tomographic scan demonstrating gastric involvement with lymphoma. The duodenum, pancreas, liver, spleen, and retroperitoneum remain uninvolved.

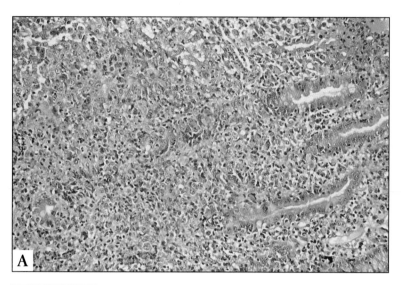

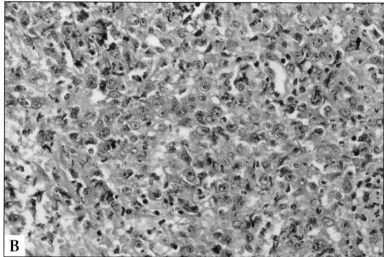

FIGURE 10-17.

A, Gastric mucosa with involvement by lymphoma. Infiltration of the lamina propria with destruction of glands by a diffuse infiltrate of large atypical lymphoid cells (hematoxylin and eosin stain; original magnification × 100). B, Same condition as shown in A, although at a different magnification (hematoxylin and eosin stain; original magnification × 200).

Maltoma

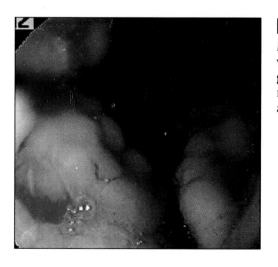

FIGURE 10-18.

Maltoma. Endoscopic view of an edematous gastric mucosa with marked erythema and friability.

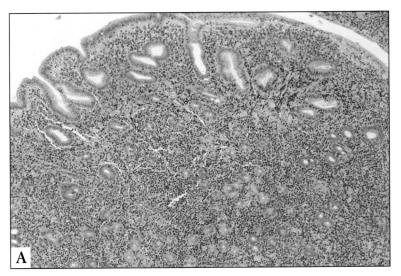
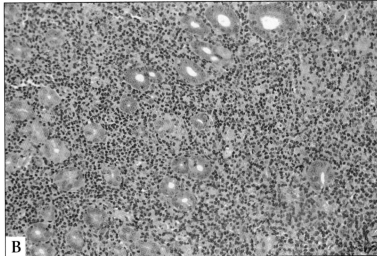

FIGURE 10-19.

A, View of gastric mucosa showing diffuse infiltration and expansion of the lamina propria of small atypical lymphocytes. Infiltration and destruction of gastric glands forming so-called lymphoepithelial lesions (hematoxylin and eosin stain; original magnification × 40). B, Same view as in A, although at a different magnification (hematoxylin and eosin stain; original magnification × 100).

LEIOMYOMAS AND LEIOMYOSARCOMAS

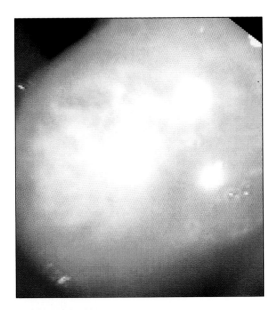

FIGURE 10-20.

Leiomyomas and leiomyosarcomas are usually asymptomatic. Leiomyomas are the most common type of benign tumor of the stomach. Quite often, the benign leiomyoma and the malignant leiomyosarcoma are difficult to distinguish endoscopically, endosonographically, or even histologically. The leiomyosarcoma does, however, tend to be larger and more frequently ulcerated. Leiomyoma in a 62-year-old man with dyspepsia is depicted. Multiple, deep endoscopic biopsies were negative, however, because the lesion is submucosal and endoscopic biopsies are primarily biopsies of the mucosa.

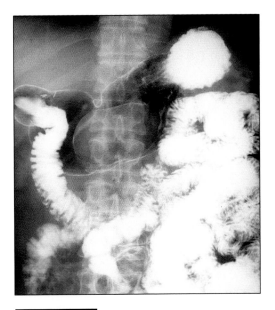

FIGURE 10-21.

A series of tests of the upper gastrointestinal tract proved to be confirmative. Note the presence of a large submucosal, intramural mass and its effect on the gastric lumen. The existence of a hiatal hernia is noted, but the remainder of the study is unremarkable except for the evident mass.

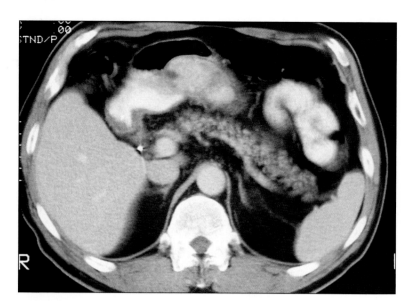

FIGURE 10-22.

Computed tomographic scan shows no evidence of extragastric disease but very clearly demonstrates the presence of the tumor. The liver, pancreas, and biliary tree are free of involvement.

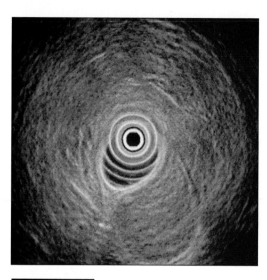

FIGURE 10-23.

Endoscopic ultrasound imagery shows the lesion arising from the muscularis propria (layer 4) without extension to the serosa. No lymphadenopathy or adjacent organ involvement is evident. The mucosa and submucosa are displaced but remain uninvolved by the mass.

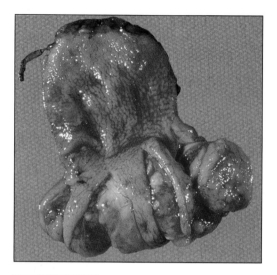

FIGURE 10-24.

Diagnosis of lesion arising from the muscularis propria. This diagnosis was confirmed at the time of resection. The gross photograph shows the submucosal placement of the tumor. There is no extragastric involvement.

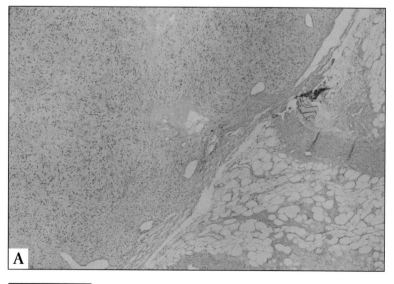

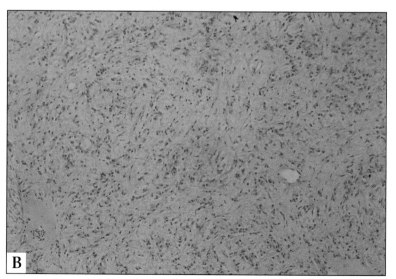

FIGURE 10-25.

A, Gastric leiomyoma forming a well-circumscribed mass. Tumor is composed of spindle-shaped cells forming irregular fascicles (hematoxylin and eosin stain; original magnification × 100).

B, Same view as seen in A, although at a different magnification (hematoxylin and eosin stain; original magnification × 200).

GASTRIC POLYP

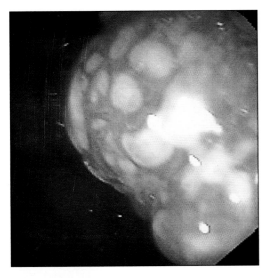

FIGURE 10-26.

Hyperplastic gastric polyp. Gastric polyps are made up of hyperplastic or adenomatous tissues. Those formed by hyperplastic polyps are by far the most common, accounting for 75% to 90% of all gastric polyps. They have no potential for malignancy. Removal or resection is mandated only by symptoms or hemorrhage if present. Adenomatous polyps of the stomach are thought to have potential for malignant development and should be removed if the size of the polyp and condition of the patient permit such therapy. In this figure, an asymptomatic pedunculated benign gastric polyp as seen on upper gastrointestinal endoscopy is shown. Note the "malignant appearance."

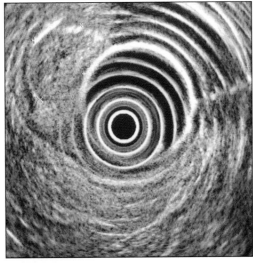

FIGURE 10-27.

Hyperplastic gastric polyp. View of the same lesion in Figure 10-26 imaged through use of endoscopic ultrasound. The muscularis propria (layer 4) is intact. No evidence of invasion is present. The neoplastic or hyperplastic tissue is hypoechoic. The sonographic appearance suggests that the polyp has multiple cystic areas.

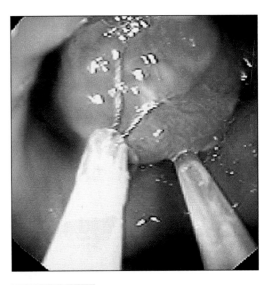

FIGURE 10-28.

Snare removal of the polyp shown in Figure 10-26. A two-channel endoscope is used in combination with a basket and with snare electrocautery so that the polyp would not be lost should it migrate out of the stomach after polypectomy. The patient should be placed on antipeptic therapy after the polypectomy procedure.

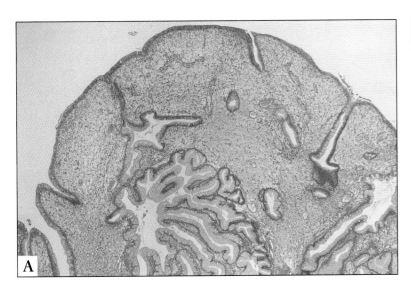 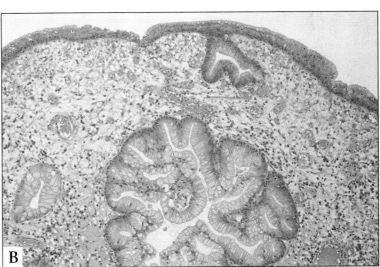

FIGURE 10-29.

A, Gastric hyperplastic polyp showing dilated, branching, hyperplastic glands. The surrounding stroma is edematous and inflamed (hematoxylin and eosin stain; original magnification × 40).

B, Same view as seen in A, although at a different magnification (hematoxylin and eosin stain; original magnification × 100).

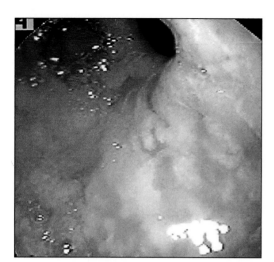

FIGURE 10-30.

Intestinal metaplasia. This endoscopic view reveals multiple raised plaque-like areas. This can occur in any area of the stomach. It is thought to be a reaction to mucosal injury where epithelial cells develop the features of intestinal epithelia.

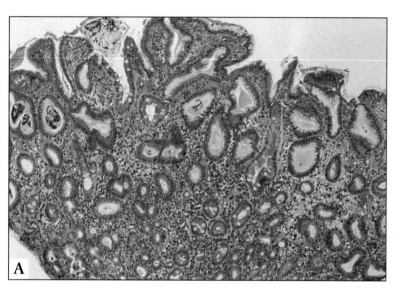

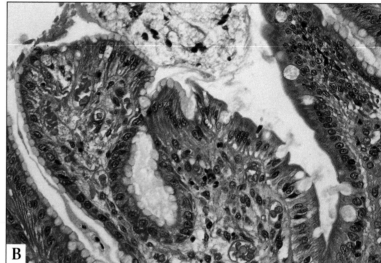

FIGURE 10-31.

A, Intestinal metaplasia of the gastric mucosa. Intestinal type epithelium with columnar absorptive cells and goblet mucus cells replacing foveolar epithelium (hematoxylin and eosin stain; original magnification × 100). **B,** Same view as seen in *A,* although at a different magnification (hematoxylin and eosin stain; original magnification × 200).

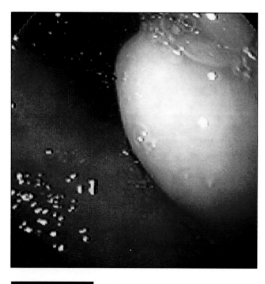

FIGURE 10-32.

Gastric lipoma. Lipomas of the stomach tend to occur in the antrum, are rare, and are often distinguished endoscopically by a "cushion sign."

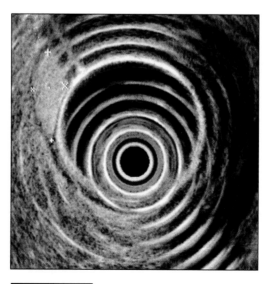

FIGURE 10-33.

Use of endoscopic ultrasound confirms the submucosal nature of the lesion. The lesion is confined to the third layer and is mildly hyperechoic. The experience with endoscopic ultrasound and the examination of liposarcomas are really limited because of the rare occurrence of the lesion. Thus far, it remains impossible to distinguish between lipomas and liposarcomas using endoscopic ultrasonography.

CARCINOID TUMOR

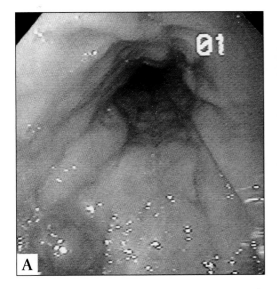

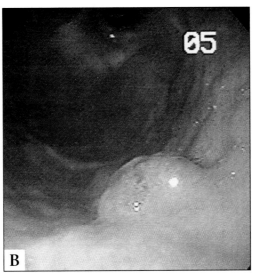

FIGURE 10-34.

A and **B**, Carcinoid tumor. Gastric carcinoids are rare tumors arising from enterochromaffin cells and are thought to be promoted by achlorhydria alone or combined with hypergastrinemia. They are rarely seen, even in persons on potent acid-inhibiting medication. This image shows multiple gastric carcinoids in a patient with chronic pernicious anemia.

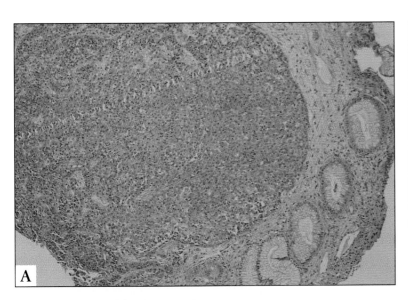

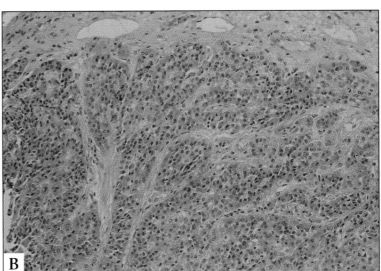

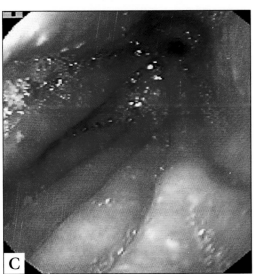

FIGURE 10-35.

A, Gastric carcinoid tumor composed of small uniform cells arranged in nests. Tumor cells form irregular anastomosing ribbons as well as some acinar formation (hemotoxylin and eosin stain; original magnification × 40). **B**, Same view as in *A*, although at a different magnification (hematoxylin and eosin stain; original magnification × 100). **C**, The patient is alive and well 5 years after a local resection and antrectomy. Gastrin levels, which were previously elevated, continue to be low.

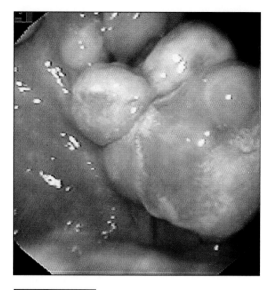

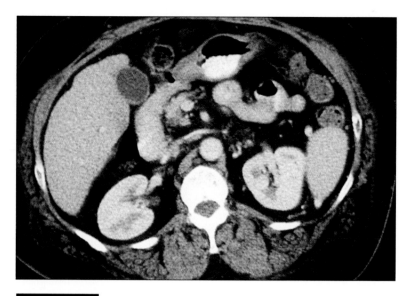

FIGURE 10-36.

Duodenal carcinoid tumor. Endoscopic image of multiple duodenal carcinoids in a 48-year-old woman who presented with gastrointestinal bleeding. These lesions may originate from anywhere in the gastrointestinal tract or in the bronchopulmonary tree. After they have a metastatic effect to the liver, these tumors can cause symptoms of the carcinoid syndrome [5].

FIGURE 10-37.

Image from computed tomographic scan surprisingly shows a normal duodenum and no evidence of metastatic disease in this patient with the duodenal carcinoid tumors as already noted in Figure 10-36.

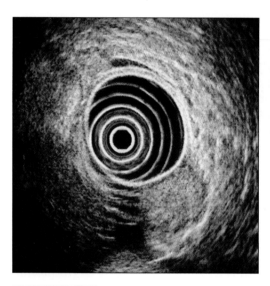

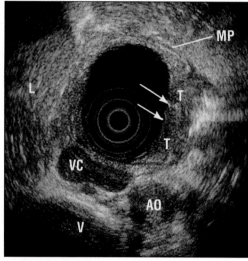

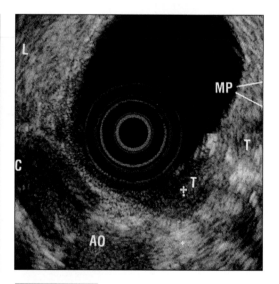

FIGURE 10-38.

Endoscopic ultrasound view of the same lesions noted in Figure 10-37. Note the presence of hypoechoic tumor 1.5 × 2.0 cm at the 5 o'clock position. Results of testing and extensive metastatic workup were negative.

FIGURE 10-39.

A 40-year-old man with a primary duodenal carcinoma found endoscopically was referred for staging. Endoscopic ultrasound reveals a diffuse, hypoechoic tumor (T) with exophytic margins (*arrows*). AO—aorta; L—right lobe of the liver; MP—muscularis propria; V—vertebral body; VC—vena cava. (*From* Tio [4]; with permission.)

FIGURE 10-40.

Another transverse section shows a deeply penetrating carcinoma (T) with minimal penetration into the subserosa. AO—aorta; L—right lobe of the liver; MP—muscularis propria, VC—vena cava. (*From* Tio [4]; with permission.)

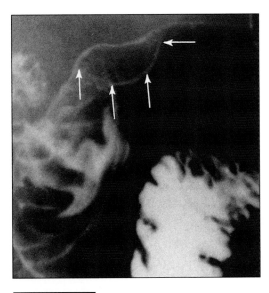

FIGURE 10-41.

Barium swallow shows a polypoid tumor (arrows) positioned in the distal part of the second portion of the duodenum. (*From* Tio [4]; with permission.)

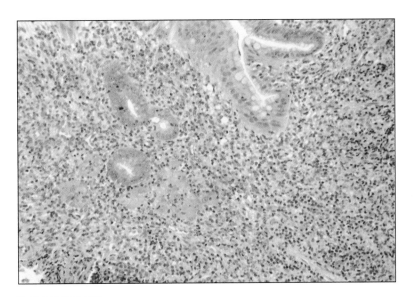

FIGURE 10-42.

Gastric mucosa showing diffuse infiltration and expansion of the lamina propria by small atypical lymphocytes. Infiltration and destruction of gastric glands form the so-called lymphoepithelial lesions (hematoxylin and eosin stain; original magnification × 100).

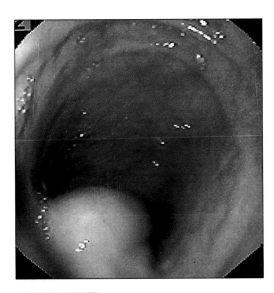

FIGURE 10-43.

Duodenal lipoma. Endoscopic view of a submucosal mass in the duodenum of a patient who presented with refractory nausea.

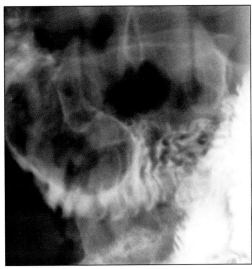

FIGURE 10-44.

Upper gastrointestinal series shows a lesion to be located in the third portion of the duodenum.

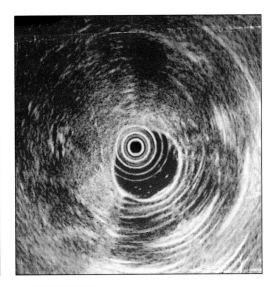

FIGURE 10-45.

Ultrasonography cannot reliably demonstrate or differentiate lipoma from liposarcoma. However, there is no evidence of metastatic disease in this patient. Furthermore, liposarcomas remain exceedingly rare.

ACKNOWLEDGMENT

The author wishes to thank Dr. Richard Meyer for his assistance with the histologic figures.

REFERENCES AND RECOMMENDED READING

1. Rösch T, Classen M: *Gastroenterologic Endosonography.* New York: Thieme; 1992; 71–105.

2. Davis GR: Neoplasms of the stomach. In *Gastrointestinal Disease.* Edited by Sleisenger MH and Fordtran JS: Philadelphia: WB Saunders; 1993:763–789.

3. Avuncluk C, Hampf F, Coughlin B: Endoscopic sonography of the stomach: Findings in benign and malignant lesions. *Am J Radiol* 1994, 163:591–595.

4. Tio TL: *Gastrointestinal TNM cancer staging by endosonography.* New York: Igaku-Shoin; 1995.

5. Merrell DE, Mansbach C, Garbutt JT: Carcinoid tumors of the duodenum: Endoscopic diagnosis of two cases. *Gastrointest Endosc* 31:269–271.

Chapter 11

Surgery of the Stomach and Duodenum

NEAL E. SEYMOUR

Surgical treatment of gastroduodenal diseases has evolved over the past 20 years. Before this era of change, the vast majority of procedures performed on the foregut involved the management of peptic ulcer disease. Except in a small subgroup of patients, this no longer holds true. Developments in minimally invasive surgery, however, have prompted a reexamination of surgical treatments of selected acid-peptic problems such as gastroesophageal reflux. The surgical treatment of gastroduodenal neoplasms and trauma remains a challenge of critical interest to the general surgeon. The physiology of the foregut must be well understood by any physician who is managing patients undergoing gastroduodenal procedures. A review of the pertinent physiology is beyond the scope of this chapter, but it must be appreciated that surgical alterations of gastric innervation, pyloric function, and gastric capacitance may have profound effects on nutrition and quality of life. These must be carefully explained to patients before beginning treatment as well as managed when necessary after the surgical procedure.

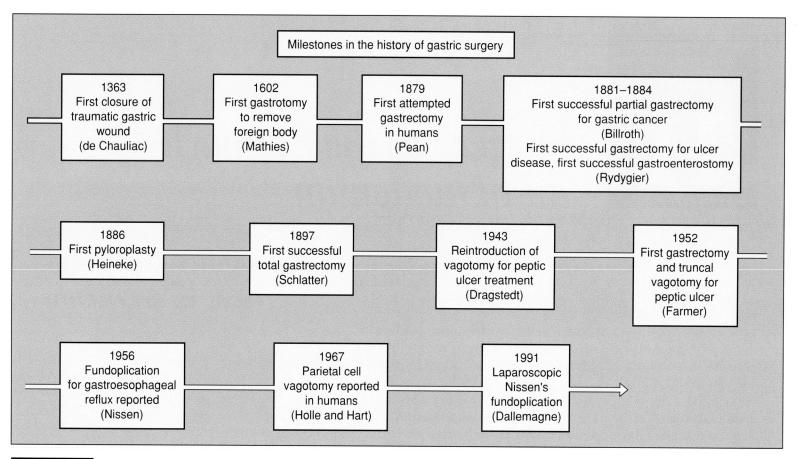

FIGURE 11-1.

Milestones in the history of gastric surgery. With a newly acquired understanding of the principles of anesthesia and asepsis, late 19th century surgeons ushered in the modern era of gastric surgery. Theodor Billroth (1829–1894) in Vienna was the single greatest pioneer in the development of surgical techniques that permitted safe gastric resection and reconstruction. Among Billroth's pupils were Czerny, Mikulicz-Radecki, Löfler, and Eiselberg, all of whom made important contributions to the practice of gastroduodenal surgery. By careful laboratory investigation and clinical study, Lester Dragstedt (1893–1975) established vagotomy as an essential component of peptic ulcer surgery in the mid-20th century. Current technologic advances permit a variety of minimally invasive procedures to be performed on the foregut, and the range of procedures that may be performed by this method continues to grow.

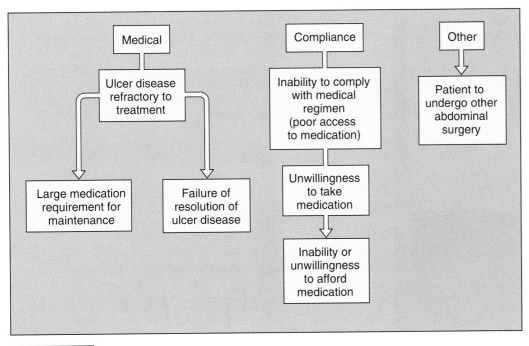

FIGURE 11-2.

Indications for elective operative treatment of peptic ulcer disease (PUD). Until the 1970s, treatment of benign ulcers of the stomach and duodenum comprised an enormous bulk of general surgical practice. Since the advent of effective antisecretory medica-

tions and now the recognition and eradication of *Helicobacter pylori*, surgery for PUD has been relegated to a secondary role, most often in a more complicated disease state. Indications for elective surgery remain but are far more circumscribed than they were in the past. Refractoriness to treatment occurs very rarely in the case of duodenal ulcers, but large maintenance medication requirements or intolerance of treatment are occasional indications for surgery. The possibility of carcinoma in gastric ulcers that fail to heal necessitates surgery even if endoscopic biopsies are negative. Patients undergoing other abdominal surgery can be considered for highly selective vagotomy depending on the magnitude of the primary procedure. With the advent of laparoscopic antiulcer surgery, straightforward procedures, such as cholecystectomy, have been combined with laparoscopic vagotomy in selected patients with concurrent symptomatic gallstone and PUD [1]. Data examining such combined operations should be available in the near future.

FIGURE 11-3.

Highly selective vagotomy (HSV). **A,** Selective denervation of the parietal cell mass is the most widely accepted elective procedure for management of duodenal ulcers. It is highly effective, with ulcer recurrence rates between 9% and 14% [2–5] and is virtually free of the risk of postsurgical dumping syndrome and postvagotomy diarrhea. It must be performed with great attention to technical concerns such as sufficient periesophageal dissection to ensure division of very high vagal branches. **B,** An "extended" HSV has been proposed that also addresses greater curvature vagal contributions to the parietal cell mass by dividing the gastroepiploic vessels at the junction of the gastric body and antrum [6].

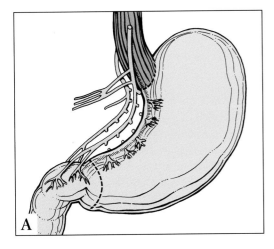

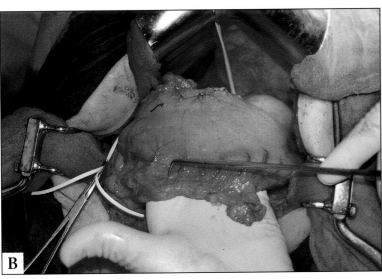

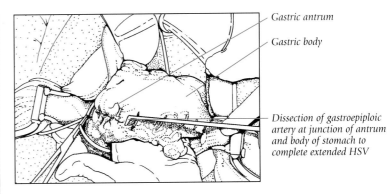

Gastric antrum

Gastric body

Dissection of gastroepiploic artery at junction of antrum and body of stomach to complete extended HSV

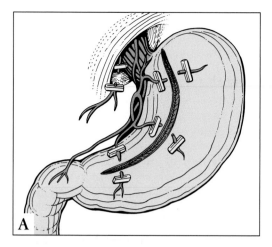

FIGURE 11-4.

Laparoscopic posterior truncal and anterior seromyotomy. **A,** Laparoscopic posterior truncal and anterior seromyotomy, an accepted open procedure [7], is gaining acceptance in Europe and Asia and more slowly in the United States. Long-term results of this approach are unavailable to compare with those of conventional open highly selective vagotomy (HSV) [8]. Despite the division of the posterior vagal trunk (dissection shown in **B**), the incidence of gastroparesis is approximately the same after this operation as after HSV. Concerns regarding recurrent ulceration include the possibility of gastric reinnervation or failure to completely denervate the parietal cell mass as a consequence of limited access to minor vagal branches. (*From* Katkhouda and Mouiel [9]; with permission.)

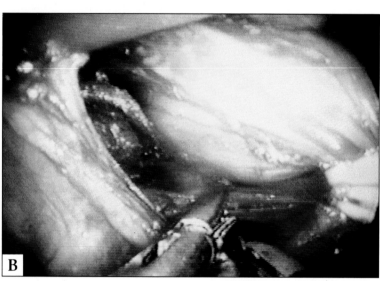

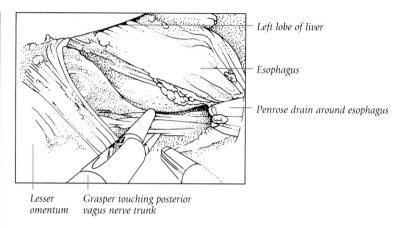

Left lobe of liver

Esophagus

Penrose drain around esophagus

Lesser omentum Grasper touching posterior vagus nerve trunk

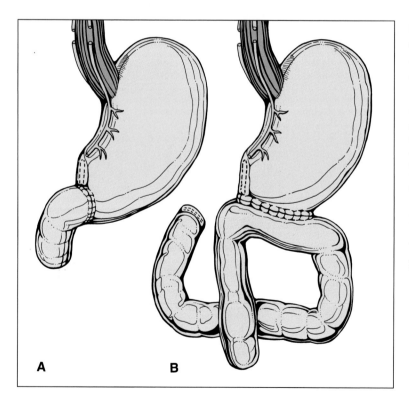

FIGURE 11-5.

Truncal vagotomy and antrectomy with either gastroduodenostomy or gastrojejunostomy. Extended gastric resection for peptic ulcer disease has largely been abandoned in favor of antrectomy combined with truncal vagotomy. This operation is extremely effective in preventing future duodenal ulcers and avoiding the complications of severely restricting the size of the gastric reservoir. **A,** Reconstruction by gastroduodenostomy (Billroth I) prevents problems associated with a closed duodenal stump (*see* Fig. 11-6). **B,** Frequently gastroduodenostomy is impossible because of deformation of the duodenal bulb and gastrojejunostomy (Billroth II) is required. This gastrojejunostomy can be performed either in a retrocolic (through the transverse mesocolon) or antecolic (anterior to the transverse colon) fashion. The jejunal loop can be brought to the gastric wall in an isoperistaltic or antiperistaltic fashion.

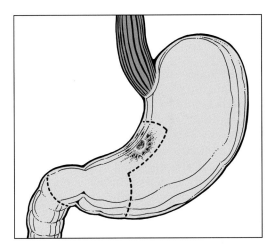

FIGURE 11-6.

Antrectomy for gastric ulcer (Pauchet's procedure). Antrectomy is the appropriate treatment for the majority of gastric ulcers (angularis, Type I) [10] without additional benefit conferred by vagotomy unless duodenal or prepyloric ulcers are also present (Type II and III, respectively). The ulcer should be resected with the specimen when possible. If the ulcer lies higher on the lesser curvature, it can be resected within a tongue of tissue extending proximally from the antrum (Pauchet's procedure is shown).

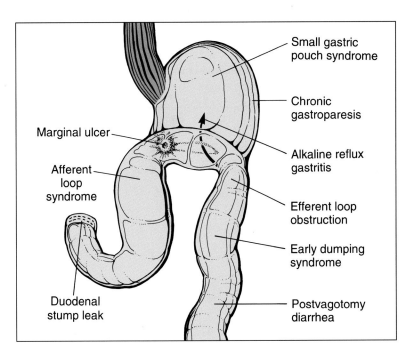

FIGURE 11-7.

Complications of gastric resection and vagotomy. Many potential complications of gastric surgery exist. Problems peculiar to Billroth II-type reconstructions include duodenal stump leak and afferent loop obstruction. These difficulties may be minimized by constructing the afferent limb to be as short as possible and ensuring that, upon completion, the gastrojejunostomy is positioned without twisting or angulation in either limb. Duodenal stump leak is a potentially lethal problem, but previously reported mortality rates of 40% to 50% are much improved as a consequence of better nutritional and antibiotic care. Up to 50% of patients will experience some symptoms of early dumping syndrome such as dizziness, sweating, palpitations, nausea, or flushing. These are generally mild and responsive to minor dietary alterations, but 1% may have severe dumping for extended periods. Between 5% and 10% of patients may experience postvagotomy diarrhea. This is generally episodic and treated effectively using antidiarrheal agents. (*From* Jordan [11]; with permission.)

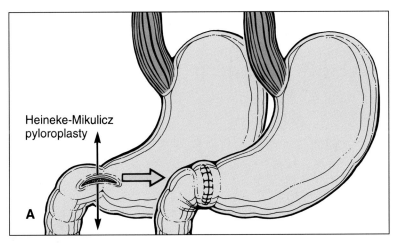

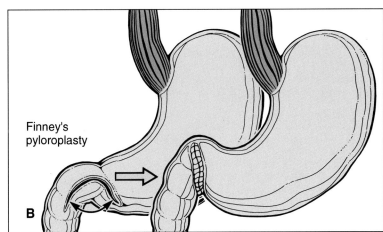

FIGURE 11-8.

Methods of gastric drainage. Bypass or destruction of the normal pyloric mechanism by pyloroplasty, gastroduodenostomy, or gastrojejunostomy is performed in conjunction with truncal vagotomy to facilitate gastric emptying. **A,** The Heineke-Mikulicz pyloroplasty is the most widely used method of drainage. The Finney's pyloroplasty (**B**), Jaboulay's gastroduodenostomy (**C**), and gastrojejunostomy (**D**) are useful alternatives in the presence of a deformed duodenal

(Continued on next page)

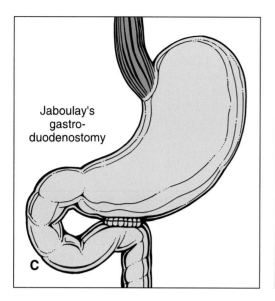

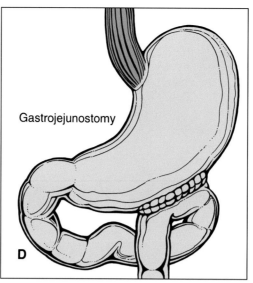

FIGURE 11-8. (*CONTINUED*)

bulb. The incidence of postoperative dumping after drainage procedures is comparable with the following antrectomy and far greater than that after highly selective vagotomy. The advantages of truncal vagotomy and pyloroplasty are that the combination is technically uncomplicated and can be performed quickly, characteristics that make it particularly suitable in patients with bleeding duodenal ulcers who require an incision across the pylorus for local control of hemorrhage.

TABLE 11-1. ULCER RECURRENCE RATES FOLLOWING SURGICAL PROCEDURES

OPERATION	RECURRENCE RATE, %	REMARKS
Gastric resection	2–5	Varies according to amount resected 75% Optimal
Vagotomy and drainage	10–15	Pyloroplasty most frequent drainage procedure
Vagotomy and antrectomy	0–2	Lowest recurrence rates
Parietal cell vagotomy [4,5]	10–17	Operator dependent

TABLE 11-1.

Ulcer recurrence rates following surgical procedures. Ulcer recurrence rates after operations for peptic ulcer disease (PUD) vary according to the nature of the procedure, the pathophysiology of the underlying disease, as well as operator skill. Gastric resection alone, although cited for historical purposes, is rarely undertaken for peptic ulcer management. The standard surgical criterion for PUD is vagotomy and antrectomy if protection from recurrent ulcers is taken as the major goal of treatment. Technical pitfalls associated with this procedure include incomplete vagotomy and retained antrum or residual antral mucosa left on the duodenal stump, which can produce hypergastrinemia and recurrent ulcer after restoring foregut continuity by gastrojejunostomy. Although unsuspected gastrinoma must be considered in any patient with marginal ulcer after vagotomy and antrectomy, routine serum gastrin testing before elective surgery has made this situation rare. Most surgeons and patients are willing to accept the slightly higher risk of recurrent ulcers with highly selective vagotomy to avoid postgastrectomy and postvagatomy complications. (*Adapted from* McFadden and Zinner [12]; with permission.)

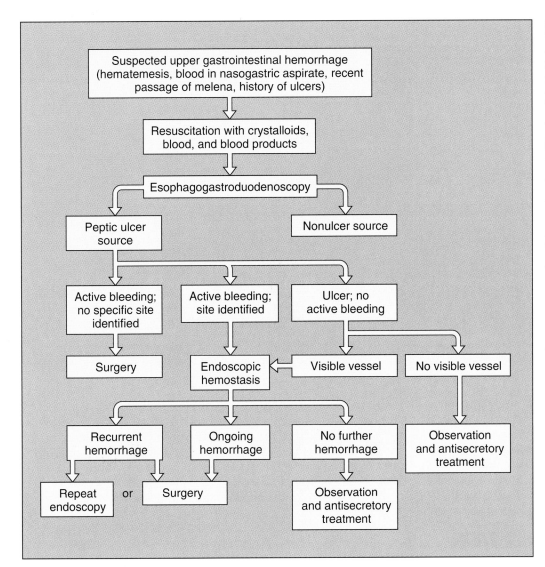

Figure 11-9.

Management of bleeding peptic ulcers. Bleeding from duodenal and gastric ulcers is among the most immediately life-threatening sequelae of peptic ulcer disease (PUD) and requires prompt but carefully planned treatment. Early identification of the bleeding source requires esophagogastroduodenoscopy. Endoscopic bipolar cautery, heater probe, or injection treatment is the most efficacious immediate method of halting ongoing bleeding and minimizing the risk of rebleeding from ulcer disease. These therapeutic measures lessen the need for emergency abdominal surgery in often direly ill patients [13,14] and are thought to lessen morbidity and mortality. Approximately 5% of patients with transfusion-requiring upper gastrointestinal (UGI) hemorrhage secondary to PUD will come to surgical treatment. These patients are separated from those not requiring surgery at fairly well-defined branch points in the management decision tree. Visible, ongoing hemorrhage not amenable to endoscopic treatment requires immediate operation. Inability to treat endoscopically may be caused by ulcer location, rapidity of bleeding, or inability to identify a sufficiently localized bleeding point within the ulcer. Patients who undergo successful endoscopic management have a 10% to 40% chance of rebleeding before they are discharged from the hospital. There are significant benefits in minimizing transfusion requirements [15,16] and prompt surgical treatment to address bleeding after one or two unsuccessful endoscopic attempts remains a highly definitive management strategy.

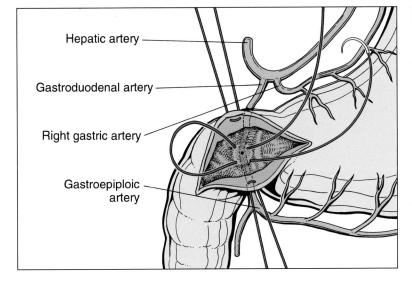

Figure 11-10.

Gastroduodenotomy and suture control of bleeding from the gastroduodenal artery. Irrespective of the choice of operation for bleeding ulcers of the first portion of the duodenum, immediate local control of bleeding must be secured. Longitudinal incision as shown, across the pylorus and proximal duodenum, exposes the point of erosion into the gastroduodenal artery or branch vessel in the posterior wall of the duodenal bulb. This incision is best managed by direct suture, undersewing the blood vessel on either side of the bleeding. The gastroduodenotomy can be closed transversely as a Heineke-Mikulicz pyloroplasty. Adding truncal vagotomy is widely accepted in this setting [17], although highly selective vagotomy with precise reconstruction of the duodenotomy and pylorus have also been advocated [18,19]. Bleeding gastric ulcers must be exposed by appropriately placed gastrotomies. Bleeding may be managed by antrectomy with ulcer excision, ulcer excision alone, or simple oversew of bleeding sites if the patient is unstable.

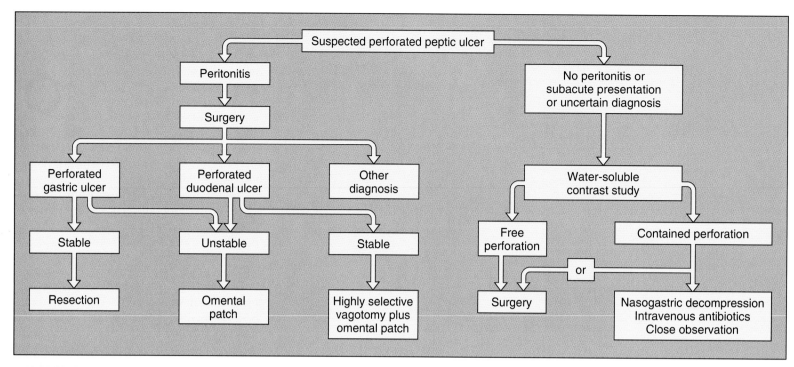

FIGURE 11-11.

Management of perforated peptic ulcers. Clinical suspicion of perforated duodenal ulcer may be prompted by abdominal pain sufficiently acute in onset that the patient recalls its precise moment of occurrence. The presentation may also be nonclassical, and this diagnosis must be considered in any patient with peritonitis requiring abdominal exploration. Pneumoperitoneum evident on upright chest or left lateral decubitus radiographs may be seen but no

gastric insufflation should be attempted to aid in the diagnosis. Nonoperative management of selected patients with contained perforations demonstrated by water-soluble contrast study is possible in conjunction with nasogastric drainage and antibiotics [20,21]. This approach has not gained popularity in the United States, and prompt laparotomy is generally undertaken to minimize the degree of local inflammation as well as the risk of sepsis.

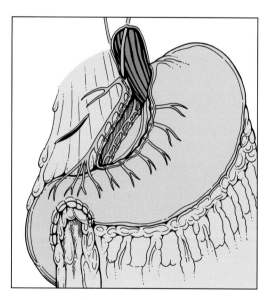

FIGURE 11-12.

Omental patch and highly selective vagotomy. Historically, perforations of duodenal ulcers have been patched with pedicles of greater omentum. Direct suture closure has a high risk of failure and is unnecessary if an omental patch is used. Some reports have demonstrated that omental patch placement is possible laparoscopically [22]. If the patient is stable and local inflammation is not severe, a highly selective vagotomy can be performed, conferring the benefits of a definitive antiulcer procedure without opening and closing the gastrointestinal tract and subjecting the patient to the risk of suture line breakdown in the presence of peritonitis [23,24]. Although gastric ulcer perforations may also be repaired by omental patch, gastric resection inclusive of the ulcer is preferred to lessen the risk of recurrent ulcer. Risk factors for mortality in gastric and duodenal ulcer perforations include advanced age, pulmonary disease, perforation of more than 24 hours' duration, and steroid use [25]. (*From* Sawyers [26]; with permission.)

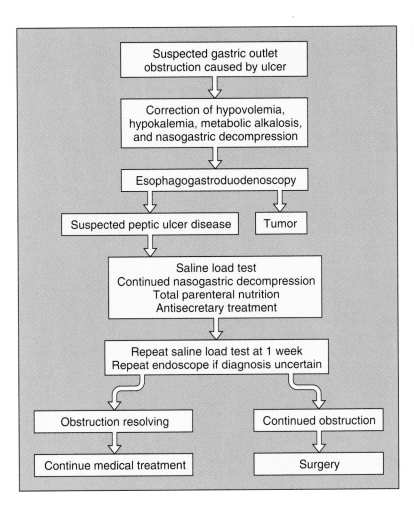

FIGURE 11-13.

Management of obstructing duodenal ulcers. Deformation and scarring of the duodenal bulb and pylorus can cause gastric outlet obstruction. If obstruction is not corrected by treatment of any acute inflammatory changes, surgery provides the most definitive means of returning the patient to a normal diet. Patients who present after a prolonged course of vomiting may have significant hypovolemia, alkalosis, and hypokalemia, which must be carefully corrected. The saline load test is a simple functional means to assess obstruction and should be performed early during the hospitalization. After a 1-week course of total parenteral nutrition, nasogastric decompression, and antisecretory treatment, the saline load test is repeated. If conservative treatment has improved pyloric edema and spasm, saline recovery may decrease. After instilling 700 mL of saline, however, a return of more than 350 mL indicates that obstruction is unlikely to resolve with additional conservative management. Surgical options include vagotomy and antrectomy, vagotomy and drainage, and highly selective vagotomy (HSV) and drainage. Concerns regarding denervation of an enlarged, paretic stomach have recently prompted careful examination of HSV. A prospective comparison showed that HSV plus gastrojejunostomy performed for obstruction produced nutritional results superior to vagotomy and antrectomy as well as to vagotomy and pyloroplasty [27].

SURGERY FOR GASTROESOPHAGEAL REFLUX DISEASE

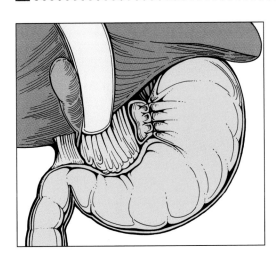

FIGURE 11-14.

Nissen's fundoplication. The surgical treatment of gastroesophageal reflux disease entered the modern era in 1956 with Nissen's report of a 360° fundoplication preventing pathologic reflux [28]. This operation affords excellent protection of the esophagus and airway from refluxed gastric contents and came into wide use during the 1960s. It rapidly became clear that Nissen's fundoplication was not without complications. Too long or too tight a wrap can result in permanent dysphagia and severe gas bloat with an inability to belch and vomit. Because of this potential to replace one set of symptoms with another, sometimes equally distressing one, modifications to the procedure emphasizing "looseness" have been introduced [29]. Laparoscopic Nissen's fundoplication is currently becoming the preferred method of surgical treatment of pathologic reflux. (*From* Donahue *et al.* [30]; with permission.)

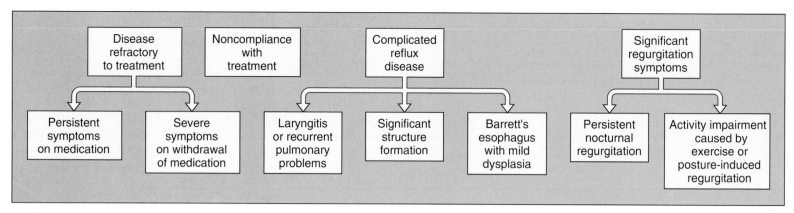

FIGURE 11-15.

Indications for surgical treatment of gastroesophageal reflux disease (GERD). Surgical treatment is generally reserved for those patients with severe or complicated GERD. At present, safety concerns regarding the long-term omeprazole treatment are unsubstantiated, but avoidance of prolonged and perhaps lifetime reliance on medication may offer an economic advantage that remains to be verified. Refractoriness to treatment can result from persistence of symptoms with proton pump inhibition or from relapse of symptoms with termination of medication. Noncompliance with an appropriate medical regimen continues to be an occasional indication for surgery. Complications of GERD such as refractory laryngitis, recurrent pulmonary disease, and stricture, in selected patients, are accepted indications for surgery. Barrett's esophagus is not itself an indication or contraindication for any specific treatment, but when taken with mild dysplasia or persistent symptoms, may present a more compelling case for surgical treatment.

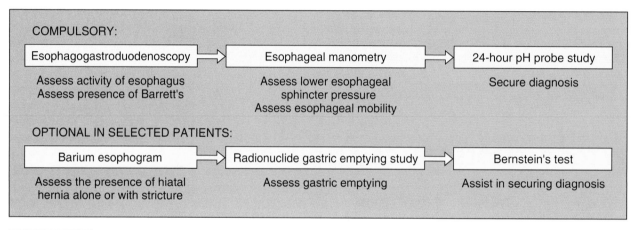

FIGURE 11-16.

Preoperative evaluation of patients with gastroesophageal reflux disease (GERD). The major goals of preoperative evaluation of patients with GERD are to secure the diagnosis firmly, to assess the degree of esophagitis and the presence or absence of Barrett's esophagus, and to rule out other problems that might interfere with a good surgical outcome. To these ends all patients undergo esophagogastroduodenoscopy with biopsy, 24-hour pH monitoring, and esophageal manometry. Manometry is vital to document the lower esophageal sphincter pressure and to determine if abnormal motility exists, which might contribute to the patients symptoms. Generally, some feature of the patient's presentation suggests a motility difficulty, and although antireflux surgery is not contraindicated in these patients, the chances of a good surgical outcome are less. Barium esophogram, Bernstein's test, and radionuclide gastric emptying studies are of use in selected patients but do not provide sufficient additional information to justify their routine use.

TABLE 11-2. COMPLIANCE TO TECHNICAL PRINCIPLES OF A NISSEN FUNDOPLICATION

TECHNICAL PRINCIPLE	NUMBER	COMPLIANCE, %
Right vagus identified	52/54*	96
Left vagus identified	49/54	91
Hepatic branch preserved	41/54	75
Cardioesophageal fat pad removed	49/54	91
Gastric fundus mobilized by division of short gastrics	50/54	93
Closure of crura	49/54	91
Wrap placed between right vagus and esophagus	38/54	70
Pledgets used	35/54	65
Bougie used to quantitate wrap size	54/54	100
Length of wrap ≤ 2 cm	49/54	90

*Data for adherence to technical principles are available for 54 of 58 patients

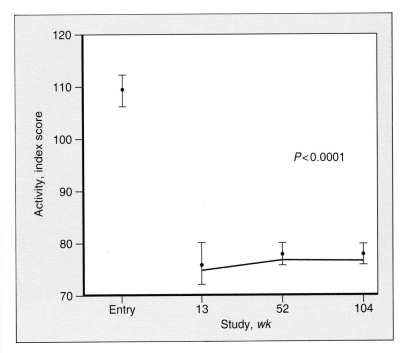

TABLE 11-2 AND FIGURE 11-17.

Postoperative results of Nissen's fundoplication. Consistently, the best results of antireflux surgery have been obtained from single-institution, single-surgeon studies, with symptomatic relief being obtained in more than 90% of patients [29,31,32]. A recent report of 58 patients managed in eight Veteran's Administration hospitals by several surgeons emphasized adherence to 10 prospectively determined technical principals with compliances between 65% and 100% and evaluation of GERD severity by a validated disease activity index (Table 11-2) [31]. This index graded disease magnitude according to the degree of heartburn, patient-perceived general severity, swallowing difficulties, and episodes of symptomatic nocturnal reflux [33]. Symptoms were relived in 93% of patients with improvement in activity index from 109 to 78 (Figure 11-17). (*From* Dunnington and DeMeester [31]; with permission.).

TABLE 11-3. LONG-TERM RESULTS OF NISSEN FUNDOPLICATION

STUDY		PATIENTS, n	FOLLOWUP, y	IMPROVED, %	DYSPHAGIA, %	GAS BLOAT, %
Dunnington and DeMeester [31]	1993	58	2	93	14	28
Luostarinen and coworkers [35]	1992	25	20	88	16	16
Schirazi and coworkers [34]	1987	350	2–20	95	3	6
Demeester and coworkers [32]	1986	100	10	91	14	15
Donahue and coworkers [29]	1985	77	1–8	100	0	2
Negre and coworkers [36]	1983	60	10	81	43*	33*

TABLE 11-3.

Long-term results of Nissen's fundoplication. The goals of surgical treatment of gastroesophageal reflux disease (GERD) are to provide 1) good relief of symptoms and prevention of further esophagitis; 2) freedom from the need to take further medication; and 3) avoidance of postfundoplication sequelae such as gas bloat and dysphagia. In recent reports, the ability of a loosely constructed 360° wrap to control reflux has been clearly demonstrated [29,31,32,34]. Those studies examining patients at 5 years and more after antireflux surgery generally indicate that long-term relief of symptoms can also be expected. However, Luostarinen and coworkers [35] reported that up to 29% of wraps were defective (slipped or disrupted) after a 20-year median follow-up and that half of these patients had recurrent symptoms. Other investigators, emphasizing technical features of the surgery, have achieved far lower rates of wrap failure (0% to 2%). Because it is uncertain that a fundoplication is ever completely free of the risk of disruption, reports of antireflux surgery should be carefully scrutinized for a period of follow-up. Postfundoplication dysphagia and gas bloat are encountered in 5% to 30% of patients. No standardized method of assessing these complaints exists and their presence is not indicative of a bad outcome unless they were clearly not present before the surgery and the patient finds them more distressing than the original esophagitis symptoms. Although the high rates (*asterisks*) reported by Negre and coworkers [36] may suggest a poor outcome, according to the authors, all were mild cases of no serious distress to the patients. The most serious post-wrap complaint is dysphagia. Dilation may be required in up to 14% of patients with excellent relief and a low rate of repeat dilation [31].

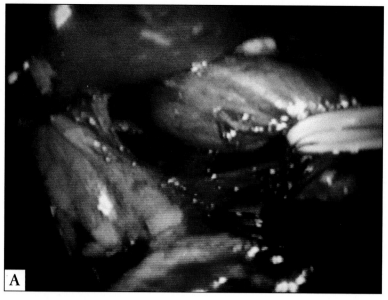

A

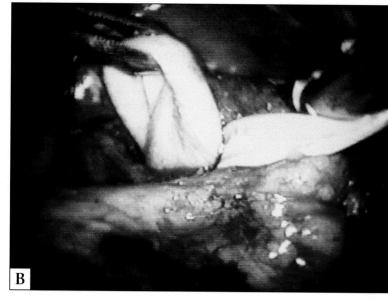

B

Esophagus
Left lateral segment of liver
Penrose drain around esophagus
Stomach
Grasper pointing to posterior vagus trunk and dissected hiatus behind esophagus and gastric cardia

Left lobe of liver
Esophagus
Fundus pulled behind esophagus
Penrose drain wound esophagus
Stomach

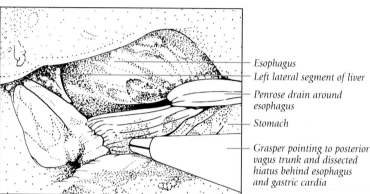

C

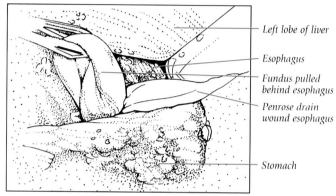

Left lobe of liver

Three sutures securing short, loose 360° wrap of gastric fundus

Stomach

FIGURE 11-18.

Laparoscopic Nissen's fundoplication. Antireflux surgery lends itself well to the minimally invasive approach because of superior visualization of the gastroesophageal junction, adaptability of the open procedure to laparoscopic technique and gastroesophageal junction, adaptability of the open procedure to laparoscopic technique, and the benefits of avoiding a large abdominal incision. The procedure is performed through 5 abdominal ports and calls for expertise in laparoscopic suturing and knot tying as well as facility with 30° telescopes. Complete mobilization of the esophagus, cardia, and fundus (**A**) creates an adequate space to bring a mobile tongue of fundus behind the esophagus (**B**), leaving an adequate amount anteriorly to permit tensionless suturing (**C**). This procedure frequently requires dividing the highest one or two short gastric vessels. A short, loose 360° wrap is performed over an esophageal bougie of between 50 and 60F size.

TABLE 11-4. RESULTS OF LAPAROSCOPIC NISSEN FUNDOPLICATION

STUDY		PATIENTS, *n*	IMPROVED, %	DYSPHAGIA, %	GAS BLOAT, %
Dallemagne and Weert [37]	1991	12	100	NA	NA
Geaga [42]	1991	10	100	0	NA
Bagnato [43]	1992	16	100	0	NA
McKernan and Laws [39]	1993	28	95	18	NA
Cadière and coworkers [41]	1993	80	100	0	0
Weerts and coworkers [38]	1993	132	99	5.4	0
Bittner and coworkers [40]	1994	35	96	5.4	50*

* at 3 wks

TABLE 11-4.

Results of laparoscopic Nissen's fundoplication. Dallemagne and Weerts [37] reported the first 360° laparoscopic fundoplication for gastroesophageal reflux disease in 1991, and since then the results of several series have been published, albeit with limited periods of follow-up [38–43]. Early experience with this procedure is favorable with results comparable with those obtained with the open procedure in terms of relief of reflux symptoms and incidence of dysphagia and gas bloat. Hospital stay is significantly shortened as compared with the open procedure, as is the delay to return to normal function and work. Preliminary data suggest that the rate of splenic injury is far lower than that reported for the open procedure. NA—not available.

■ SURGICAL TREATMENT OF GASTRODUODENAL MALIGNANCIES

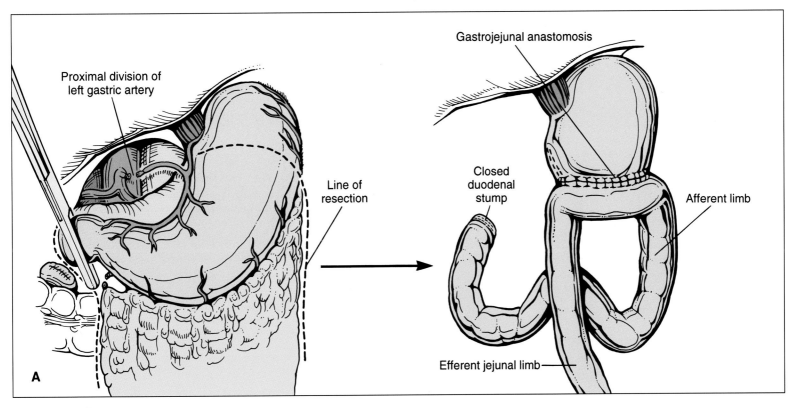

FIGURE 11-19.

Operations for gastric carcinoma. At the present time, surgical extirpation is the only method of cure for invasive gastric cancer. In the United States, however, 10% to 15% of patients with gastric carcinoma will prove to be resectable for possible cure (removal of all gross disease with microscopic margins free of tumor) at operation. Of these, only a subgroup of patients with early disease by careful staging have a good chance of 5-year survival. Although the operations offered to patients for gastric cancer vary in their technical aspects related to lymph node dissection, distal subtotal gastrectomy (**A**) and total gastrectomy (**B**) remain the operations of

(Continued on next page)

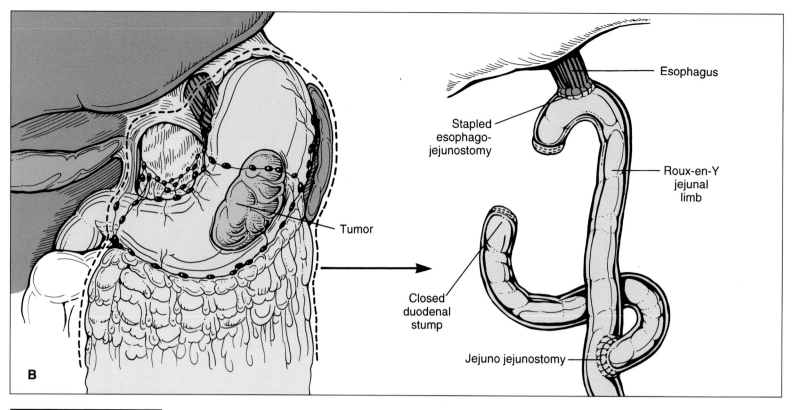

Labels (right diagram):
- Esophagus
- Stapled esophago-jejunostomy
- Roux-en-Y jejunal limb
- Closed duodenal stump
- Jejuno jejunostomy

Label (left diagram):
- Tumor
- B

FIGURE 11-19. (CONTINUED)

choice in treating resectable gastric cancers with the exception of those involving the gastric cardia. This latter group is managed by esophagogastrectomy. The distal stomach can be brought up to either the midesophagus in the right chest or to the cervical esophagus after transhiatal esophagectomy [44]. (*From* Scott *et al.* [45]; with permission.)

FIGURE 11-20.

Overall survival of operation for gastric cancer. In a recent review of multiple surgeons' practices in Great Britain between 1980 and 1985, the operative treatments and results in terms of survival were summarized in this graph [46]. The percentage of surviving patients levels off 2 years after potentially curative resection but continues to fall unabated in the palliatively treated group. Although it was disappointing that only 15% of patients who had surgical operations were deemed to have had potentially curative procedures, this figure appears to be on the rise in Great Britain, a finding recently attributed to more aggressive use of endoscopy to investigate gastrointestinal complaints [47]. The best hope of a good outcome in gastric cancer treatment lies in early diagnosis of disease. In Japan, where aggressive screening occurs, up to 30% of gastric carcinoma is diagnosed before its invasion of muscularis propria. (*From* McCulloch [46]; with permission.)

Chart legend:
- Curative resection
- Palliative resection
- No resection

Y-axis: Survival rate, %
X-axis: Time, d

Number of patients at risk

Curative	31	17	14	13	11
Paliative	56	41	33	20	12
No resection	119	26	10	4	4

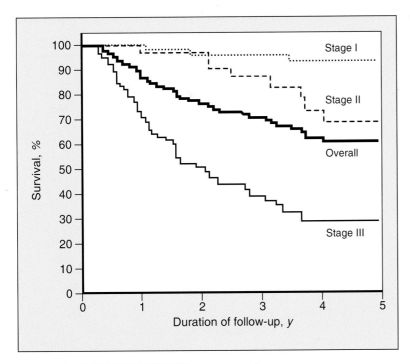

FIGURE 11-21 AND TABLE 11-5.

TABLE 11-5. 1987 UNIFIED INTERNATIONAL TUMOR, NODE, METASTASES STAGING OF GASTRIC CANCER

STAGE OF DISEASE	TNM		
I	T1N0M0	T1N1M0	T2N0M0
II	T1N2M0	T2N1M0	T3N0M0
IIIa	T2N2M0	T3N1M0	T4N0M0
IIIb	T3N2M0	T4N1M0	

T1=confined to mucosa/submucosa
T2=invading muscularis propria to subserosa
T3=through serosa
T4=through serosa with involvement of contiguous structures
N0=no nodal involvement
N1=affected nodes < 3 cm from tumor
N2=affected nodes > 3 cm from tumor
M0=no distant metastases

Survival after operation for gastric cancer by tumor stage. In a recent study of gastric cancer in England, 42% (207 of 493) of treated patients were able to undergo potentially curative resection. Survival results after potentially curative treatment are shown here by stage of disease (Figure 11-21) along with the Unified International Tumor, Node, Metastasis (UICC TNM) staging system for gastric cancer (Table 11-5) [48]. UICC TNM stage I and II patients had generally good results, and although they were the smallest group of patients overall (24%), they constituted 58% of potentially curative treatments. Stage III disease, as in other studies, fared considerably worse than patients staged earlier and were the single largest group receiving potentially curative treatment (42%). This experience was felt to reflect an increase in the incidence of curable cases being detected. (*Adapted from* Sue-Ling *et al.* [47]; with permission.)

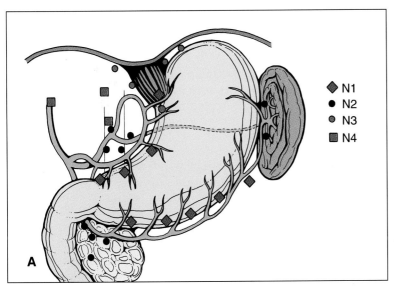

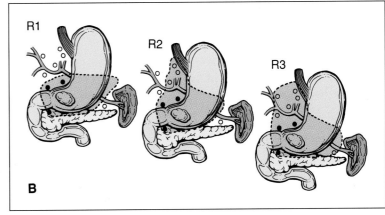

FIGURE 11-22.

Level of lymph node dissection. Data from several series suggest that the level of lymph node dissection accompanying gastrectomy for gastric cancer can influence survival. The lymphadenectomies that have come into use are classified according to the specific echelon of nodes removed and may differ depending on tumor location. **A,** Tiers of nodes from perigastric (N1) to para-aortic (N4) are shown. **B,** Removal of the primary draining lymph nodes (N1) shown as *closed circles* in with greater and lesser omenta is an R1 dissection and constitutes the minimal acceptable operation for gastric cancer. R2 dissection requires secondary lymph node excision (N2) in the celiac and hepatic regions, as well as splenic hilar nodes when the tumor involves the adjacent stomach. Splenectomy is controversial as a means to remove the latter nodes. More extensive dissections (R3) of tertiary nodes and the lining of the lesser sac are rarely performed because of their greater morbidity and unclear benefits. (**A,** *From* Jeyasingham [48]; with permission.) (**B,** *Adapted from* Shui *et al.* [49]; with permission.)

TABLE 11-6. SURVIVAL AFTER RESECTION FOR GASTRIC CANCER ANALYZED BY LYMPH NODE STATUS

		5-YEAR SURVIVAL RATE, %				
INVESTIGATIONS	PATIENTS, *n*	N0	N1	N2	N3	N4
Noguchi [50]	3145	80	53	26	10	3
Maruyama [51]	3176	85	61	31	10	2
Bozetti [91]	361	57	43	43	43	43
Hermanek [53]	977	74	36	20	10	
Shiu [54]	246	67	32	9		

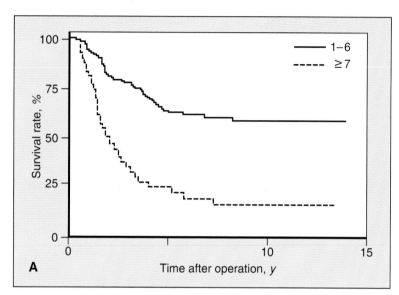

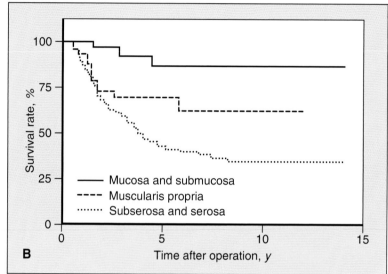

TABLE 11-6 AND FIGURE 11-23.

Prognostic significance of positive lymph nodes in gastric cancer. Recent reports from Japan, Europe, and the United States indicate that involvement of N2 and N3 nodes significantly lessens 5-year survival [50–54] (Table 11-6). N1 nodal involvement in early (mucosal or submucosal) gastric cancers did not preclude a good outcome in Japanese series, and 5-year survival rates of 61% to 85% have been reported after radical treatment [52,56]. Survival curves with regard to the number of positive lymph nodes (A) depth of tumor invasion (B) are shown [56]. Multivariate analysis indicated that the number of lymph nodes, depth of invasion, and histologic type (well-differentiated versus poorly differentiated) correlated independently with survival, but that the total number of positive nodes was the most significant prognostic factor in patients with node-positive disease. More than six positive lymph nodes decreased 11-year survival from 62% to 28%, and 10 or more positive nodes were associated with a 11-year survival rate of 10%. (*Adapted from* Alexander *et al.* [57] and Adachi *et al.* [58]; with permission.)

TABLE 11-7. RESULTS OF A PROSPECTIVE RANDOMIZED TRIAL COMPARING R1 AND R2 RESECTIONS FOR POTENTIALLY CURABLE GASTRIC CARCINOMA

STANDARDS FOR COMPARISON	R1	R2	*P* VALUE
n	22	21	—
Operating time (h ± SEM)	1.7 ± 0.6	2.33 ± 0.7	< 0.005
Transfusions (units/group)	4	25	< 0.005
3-year survival (log rank test)	0.78	0.76	< 0.77

TABLE 11-7.

R1 versus R2 lymph node dissection for potentially curable gastric cancer. Recent data on survival rates in retrospective cohort studies and prospective nonrandomized studies have favored R2 dissections over R1 for tumor, node, metastasis (TNM) stage II and III gastric cancers [51,53, 56,59,60]. Although R2 lymphadenectomy is performed routinely with minimal morbidity in Japan, it is not as widely accepted in the United States. The only randomized prospective comparison of R1 versus R2 dissections failed to reveal a difference in survival outcomes between the two procedures [61]. Operating time and transfusion requirements for the more radical procedure were significantly greater, and overall morbidity was much increased. Although the question of efficacy of R2 dissection has not been fully explored, the apparent success reported by Japanese investigators has led many clinicians to conclude that when the operation can be performed with low morbidity, removal of second echelon lymph nodes should be performed with the goal of improving survival. (*From* Alexander *et al.* [57]; with permission.)

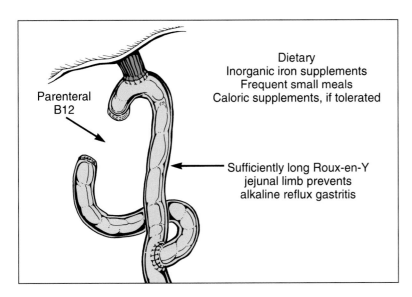

Parenteral
B12

Dietary
Inorganic iron supplements
Frequent small meals
Caloric supplements, if tolerated

Sufficiently long Roux-en-Y
jejunal limb prevents
alkaline reflux gastritis

FIGURE 11-24.

Management of patients after total gastrectomy. Potential problems following total gastrectomy for gastric cancer can be classified as relating to the primary disease (tumor recurrence), nutrition, as well as to mechanical and functional aspects of the patient's reconstruction. Vitamin B12 deficiency resulting from loss of intrinsic factor can lead to anemia if not supplemented parenterally at least 1 to 2 times per year. Malabsorption of organic iron is corrected by inorganic iron supplements. Caloric malnutrition and weight loss are addressed by frequent (up to 8) small meals per day and caloric supplements if their use does not produce dumping symptoms. With aggressive monitoring and treatment, weight loss can be kept below 15%. The ability to tolerate larger meals generally increases with time. Postsurgical dumping and alkaline reflux esophagitis are extremely difficult problems to treat when severe. Dumping is usually responsive to dietary manipulation. Alkaline reflux is best avoided by constructing a jejunal Roux-en-Y limb of adequate length at the time of the original procedure (45 to 60 cm).

TABLE 11-8. SURGICAL TREATMENT OF GASTRIC LYMPHOMA BY ANN ARBOR STAGE

SERIES	PATIENTS, *n*	SURVIVAL I & II, %	SURVIVAL III, %
Shiu and coworkers [63]*	46	90/66	NA
Hockey and coworkers [64]†	155	44	39
Rosen and coworkers [65]†	84	68/43	14
Jones and coworkers [66]*	28	40	NA
Schutze and Halpern [67]*	21	65	NA

*Modality treatment (adjuvant chemotherapy±radiotherapy
†Adjuvant radiotherapy in selected patients

TABLE 11-8.

Surgical treatment of gastric lymphoma by Ann Arbor stage. Surgical procedures offered to patients with primary gastric lymphoma are similar to those used in treating gastric adenocarcinoma to the N1 echelon of nodes (R1 dissection). Chemotherapeutic agents used in the treatment of non-Hodgkin's lymphoma in nongastrointestinal sites, as well as radiation therapy, have been used as adjuvant therapies, and although results are improved as compared with historical controls and nonrandomized cohorts, clear benefit in prospective trials has not been shown. Surgical debulking has been advocated to facilitate subsequent chemotherapy in advanced gastrointestinal lymphoma [62], however, this facilitation is not commonly accepted as sufficient justification to surgically treat Ann Arbor stage III and IV disease involving the stomach. Surgical treatment of stage Ie gastric lymphoma (single site) and IIe (positive regional nodes) when all gross disease is removed, is associated with a 5-year survival rate of 40% to 65% with variably applied adjuvant treatments [63–67]. Most studies indicate that tumor size, depth of invasion, and lymph node involvement have a negative impact on survival rates. Early stage I disease (no muscularis propria or serosal involvement) may be treated surgically without further measures; however, more advanced stage I or IIe disease is felt to warrant systemic chemotherapy because of higher expected failure rates. Although the surgical treatment of stage Ie and IIe primary gastric lymphomas is widely accepted, good results have also been reported with nonsurgical treatment alone [67]. NA—not available.

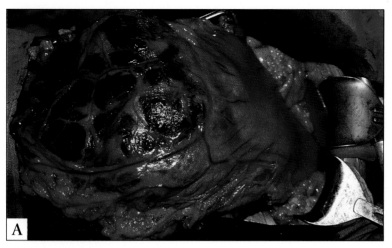

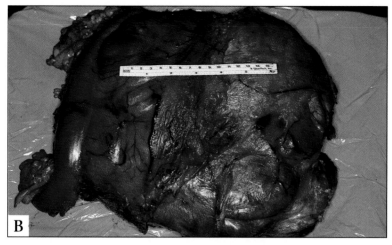

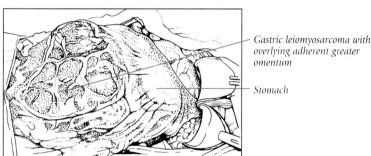
Gastric leiomyosarcoma with overlying adherent greater omentum

Stomach

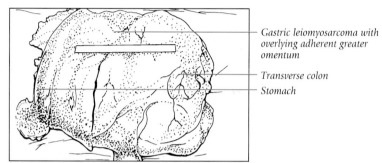
Gastric leiomyosarcoma with overlying adherent greater omentum

Transverse colon
Stomach

Other malignant gastric tumors. Gastric leiomyosarcomas and carcinoid tumors comprise the bulk of the remainder of gastric cancers. The former have a pattern of radial growth from the gastric wall and can become extremely bulky before diagnosis, as shown in **A** and **B**. Involvement of adjacent organs such as transverse colon (as in this case) occurs in up to 34% [68]. Resection results in 5-year survival rates of 25% to 56% [68,69], although local recurrence rates are as high as 46% [69]. Increasing tumor size and histologic grade correlate closely with diminished survival. Shiu and coworkers [68] reported a 100% 5-year survival rate for lesions up to 6 cm in size, but only 67% for larger tumors and 14% if adjacent structures were involved. Interestingly, survival rates and disease-free survival rates were similar after wedge resection and gastrectomy for smaller tumors. Gastric carcinoids are associated with the malignant carcinoid syndrome in less than 10% of cases. These lesions can be treated by excision if small (<1 cm) or gastrectomy, with an expected overall 5-year survival rate of 52% [70].

TABLE 11-9. RESULTS OF POTENTIALLY CURATIVE RESECTION IN ZES

Series	Year	Explored	Resected*	Cure rate, %[†]	Follow-up, mo
Thompson and coworkers [72]	1983	26	NA	12	Mean:45
Malagelada and coworkers [73]	1983	44	7	16	7–59
Richardson and coworkers [74]	1985	21	6	20	1–60
Norton and coworkers [75]	1986	32	12	22	6–40
Ellison and coworkers [76]	1987	30	18	30	24–72
Howard and coworkers [77]	1990	11	10	82	2–72
Norton and coworkers [78]	1992	37	34	62	3–6

*Those cases in which all visible tumor was removed
[†]Percentage of patients explored with resolution of acid hypersecretion and hypergastrinemia

Results of surgical treatment of the Zollinger-Ellison syndrome (ZES). With extremely effective antisecretory medication available, elective operation is generally undertaken in patients with ZES to resect tumor for cure. In 40 cases accumulated over 30 years, Zollinger *et al.* [71] reported that 71% of deaths resulted from progression of tumor, underscoring the neoplastic aspect of this disease. The surgical treatment of gastrin-secreting tumors has been examined recently by several investigators [72–78]. Overall biochemical cure rates with resection of gastrinoma at all sites ranges from 20% to 82% with limited periods of follow-up. Ellison and coworkers [76] reported a 2 to 6 year follow-up and a "cure" rate of 30%, which is a reasonable expectation after exploration by an experienced surgeon. Whether aggressive surgical management results in improved survival rates remains to be determined. (*From* Seymour and Andersen [79]; with permission.)

TABLE 11-10. LOCATION OF PRIMARY TUMORS IN 73 PATIENTS WITH ZES

LOCATION	NUMBER OF TUMORS, %
Pancreas	23 (32)
Duodenum	20 (27)
Lymph nodes	13 (18)
Ovary	1 (1)
No tumor found	16 (22)

TABLE 11-10.

Location of primary tumors in Zollinger-Ellison syndrome. In a carefully studied population of patients at the National Institutes of Health, tumors were found to be equally distributed between the duodenum and pancreas, although together these comprised only 59% of gastrinomas. Of these, 22% were not found despite comprehensive preoperative and operative efforts which included computed tomography and transhepatic portal venous sampling for gastrin levels [78]. Duodenal microgastrinomas are an increasingly recognized source of gastrin secretion which, if resected, can be associated with biochemical cure rates of up to 100% in small series [80]. Furthermore, these duodenal lesions are far less likely to be associated with hepatic metastases than pancreatic gastrinomas, despite a high incidence of regional lymph node metastases [81,82]. (*From* Norton *et al.* [78]; with permission.)

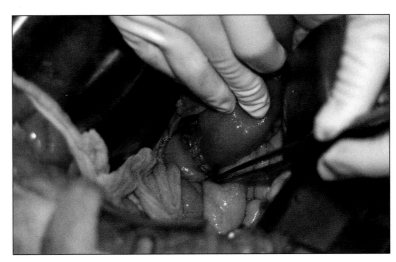

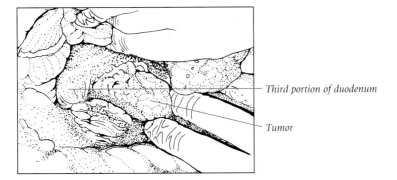

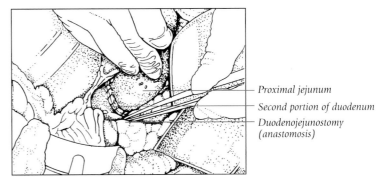

FIGURE 11-26.

Localization of duodenal microgastrinomas. Operative localization of gastrinomas requires pancreatic mobilization and careful palpation, as well as familiarity with intraoperative ultrasound techniques. The examination of the duodenum presents special challenges because tumors there tend to be small (*ie*, below 2 cm), difficult to palpate, and not detectable with ultrasound. A long duodenotomy permits the placement of a finger in the duodenal lumen and careful palpation of the duodenal wall between the thumb and forefinger [80]. Alternatively, duodenal transillumination, as shown here, has been demonstrated to be an effective means of identifying even small lesions [83].

FIGURE 11-27.

Duodenal adenocarcinoma. These tumors occur with roughly equal frequency throughout the duodenum. The typical presentation is with bleeding or obstruction, although patients with tumors in the periampullary region may present with obstructive jaundice. With few exceptions, cancers of the first and second portions of the duodenum are treated by pancreatoduodenectomy. More distal carcinomas can be treated by segmental resection. The mobilized third and fourth portions of the duodenum are shown with a 4-cm tumor, which proved amenable to segmental resection and primary anastomosis. Approximately 50% to 60% of patients explored for duodenal cancers will prove to have disease amenable to resection [84–86]. Prognosis depends on extent of local disease, lymph node involvement, and history. Five-year survival rates range from 33% to 60% after potentially curative resection.

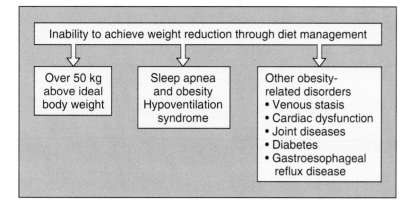

FIGURE 11-28.

Indications for surgical treatment of morbid obesity. Gastric surgery for morbid obesity is undertaken because of the generally unsatisfactory long-term results of dieting as well as the potential severity of systemic diseases associated with uncorrected obesity. Candidates are usually more than 50 kg over ideal body weight, without excessive operative risk caused by comorbidities.

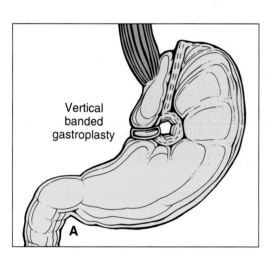

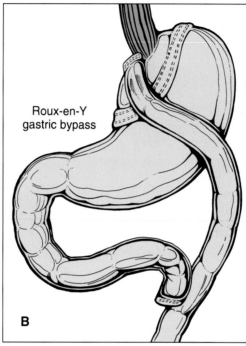

FIGURE 11-29.

Vertical banded gastroplasty and Roux-en-Y gastric bypass. Gastric procedures designed to reduce weight involve partitioning the stomach with drainage of the proximal compartment through a severely restricted orifice into the remainder of the stomach (vertical banded gastroplasty) (**A**) or a gastrojejunostomy (gastric bypass) (**B**). Sustained weight loss has been achieved after both procedures with maximum weight loss being observed 12 to 18 months postoperatively [87,88]. Problems associated with these procedures include wound infection, deep venous thrombosis and pulmonary embolism, gastric leak, gastric outlet obstruction, and protein-calorie malnutrition. Despite of technically adequate initial surgery, up to 15% of patients will fail to lose weight. Although this failure may result from disruption of a gastric band or stapled partition, more typically no such problem is identified. (*From* Sugarman *et al.* [88]; with permission.)

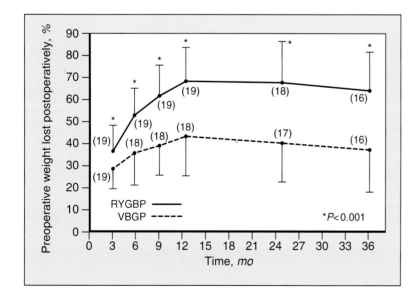

FIGURE 11-30.

Results of vertical banded gastroplasty (VBGP) and Roux-en-Y gastric bypass (RYGBP). The percentage of preoperative weight lost at 3 to 36 months after randomization to VBGP and RYGBP is shown. Sustained weight loss is feasible after both procedures, although bypass resulted in significantly greater weight loss at all time points after 6 months [88]. Patients eating sweets tended to respond less well after gastroplasty than after bypass, a difference attributed to dumping symptoms that resulted from ingestion of high-sugar foods. (*From* Sugarman *et al.* [88]; with permission.)

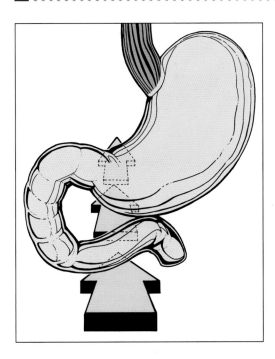

FIGURE 11-31.

Mechanism of duodenal injuries. Whereas gastric trauma results almost exclusively from penetrating injuries and can generally be managed by simple closure, duodenal injuries pose far more challenging problems to the surgeon. Penetrating injuries result from knife and gunshot wounds. Blunt injuries occur more frequently and usually result from compression of the duodenum against the vertebral column after either a direct blow, rapid deceleration, or a combination of the two (*ie*, steering column injury).

TABLE 11-11. CLASSIFICATION OF DUODENAL INJURIES

TYPE	DESCRIPTION
1	Serosal tears, significant hematoma without perforation
2	Full thickness injuries of duodenal wall, including perforation or transection; no pancreatic injury
3	Combined pancreatic and duodenal injuries
3A	Combined contusion and hematoma, or singly
3B	Perforation, laceration, or transection of either duodenum or pancreas with contusion or hematoma of the other
4	Perforation, laceration, or transection of duodenum with disruption of pancreas, ampulla, or common bile duct

TABLE 11-11.

Classification of duodenal injuries. The extent of the injury as well as the promptness of recognition and treatment dictate how individual duodenal injuries are managed. Adkins and Keyser [89] have proposed a scheme for duodenal injuries based on severity and involvement of the ampulla and pancreas.

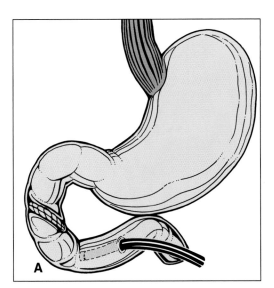

A

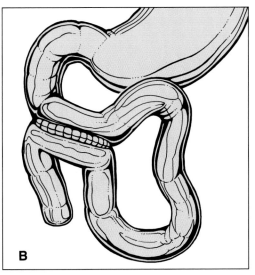

B

FIGURE 11-32.

Repair of duodenal injuries. **A** and **B**, Simple injuries (Type II) may be repaired primarily, although some surgeons advocate a protective decompressive duodenostomy tube for larger injuries or transections.

(Continued on next page)

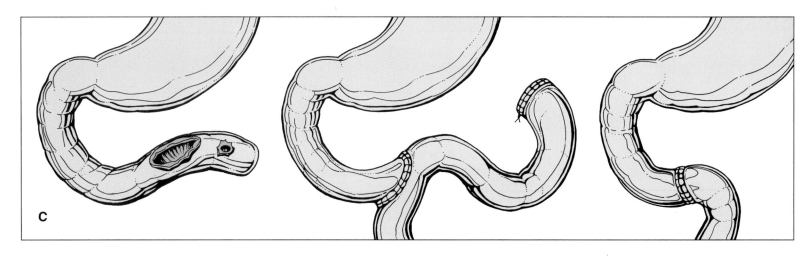

C

FIGURE 11-32. (CONTINUED)

C, More complex injuries can be addressed by jejunal patch or segmental resection. D, Severe type III or type IV injuries, especially those detected after a delay in diagnosis, may be managed by pyloric exclusion. E, The mortality of type IV injuries may be as high as 60% and in selected cases, may require pancreatoduodenectomy for management. (*From* Jordan [90]; with permission.)

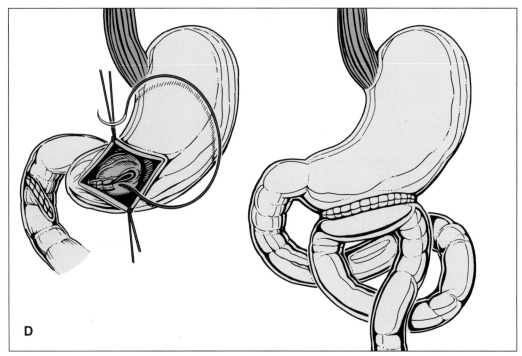

D

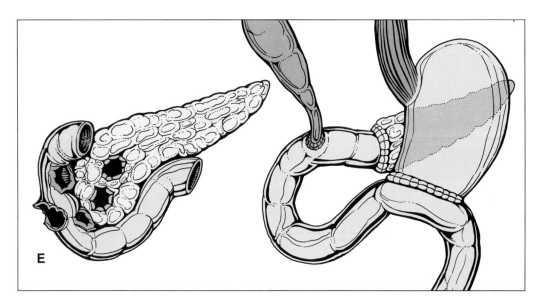

E

■ REFERENCES AND RECOMMENDED READING

1. Bailey RW, Flowers JL, Graham SM: Combined laparoscopic cholecystectomy and selective vagotomy. *Surg Laparosc Endosc* 1991, 1:45–49.

2. Blackett RL, Johnston D: Recurrent ulceration after highly selective vagotomy for duodenal ulcer. *Br J Surg* 1981, 68:705–710.

3. Enskog L, Rudberg B, Adami HO, *et al.*: Clinical results 1–10 years after highly selected vagotomy in 306 patients with prepyloric and duodenal ulcer disease. *Br J Surg* 1986, 73:357–370.

4. Byrne DJ, Brock BM, Morgan AG, *et al.*: Highly selective vagotomy: A 14-year experience. *Br J Surg* 1988, 75:869–872.

5. Jordan PH: Indications for parietal cell vagotomy without drainage in gastrointestinal surgery. *Ann Surg* 1989, 210:29–41.

6. Donahue PE, Richter HM, Liu KJM, *et al.*: Experimental basis and clinical application of extended highly selective vagotomy for duodenal ulcer. *Surg Gynecol Obstet* 1993, 176:39–48.

7. Taylor TV, Lythgoe JP, McFarland JB, *et al.*: Anterior lesser curve seromyotomy and posterior truncal vagotomy versus vagotomy and pyloroplasty in the treatment of chronic duodenal ulcer. *Br J Surg* 1990, 77:1007–1009.

8. Katkhouda N, Mouiel J: A new technique of surgical treatment of chronic duodenal ulcer without laparotomy by videocoelioscopy. *Am J Surg* 1991, 161:361–363.

9. Katkhouda H, Mouiel J: Laparascopic treatment of peptic ulcer disease. In *Minimally Invasive Surgery*. Edited by Hunter JG, Sackler JM. New York: McGraw-Hill; 1993: 123–130.

10. Johnson HD: Gastric ulcers: Classification, blood group characteristics, secretion patterns and pathogenesis. *Ann Surg* 1965, 162:996–1004.

11. Jordan PH Jr: Stomach and duodenum. In *Hardy's Textbook of Surgery*, edn 2. Edited by Hardy JD. Philadelphia: JB Lippincott; 1988:514–539.

12. McFadden DW, Zinner MJ: Reoperation for recurrent peptic ulcer disease. *Surg Clin North Am* 1991, 71:77–92.

13. Laine L: Multipolar electrocoagulation in the treatment of peptic ulcers with nonbleeding visible vessels. A prospective, controlled trial. *Ann Intern Med* 1989, 110:510–514.

14. Lin HJ, Lee FY, Kang WM, *et al.*: A controlled study of therapeutic endoscopy for peptic ulcer with non-bleeding visible vessel. *Gastrointest Endosc* 1990, 36:241–246.

15. Branicki FJ, Boey J, Fok JP, *et al.*: Bleeding duodenal ulcer. A prospective evaluation of risk factors for rebleeding and death. *Ann Surg* 1990, 211:411–418.

16. Larsen DE, Schmidt T, Gott J, *et al.*: Upper gastrointestinal bleeding: Predictors of outcome. *Surgery* 1986, 100:765–773.

17. Herrington JL, Davidson J, III: Bleeding gastroduodenal ulcers: Choice of operations. *World J Surg* 1987, 11:304–314.

18. Johnston D: Division and repair of the sphincter mechanism at the gastric outlet in emergency operations for bleeding peptic ulcer. *Ann Surg* 1977, 186:723–729.

19. Hoffmann J, Devantier A, Koelle T, Jensen HE: Parietal cell vagotomy as an emergency procedure for bleeding peptic ulcer. *Ann Surg* 1987, 206:583–585.

20. Taylor H: The non-surgical treatment of perforated peptic ulcer. *Gastroenterology* 1957, 33:353–368.

21. Berne TV, Donovan AJ: Nonoperative treatment of perforated duodenal ulcer. *Arch Surg* 1989, 124:830–832.

22. Nathanson LK, Easter DW, Cuschieri A: Laparoscopic repair: Peritoneal toilet of perforated duodenal ulcer. *Surg Endosc* 1990, 4:232–233.

23. Jordan PH, Morrow C: Perforated peptic ulcer. *Surg Clin North Am* 1988, 68:315–329.

24. Boey J, Braniki FJ, Alagaratnam TT, *et al.*: Proximal gastric vagotomy. The preferred operation for perforations in acute duodenal ulcer. *Ann Surg* 1988, 208:169–174.

25. Hamby LS, Zweng TN, Strodel WE: Perforated gastric and duodenal ulcer: An analysis of prognostic factors. *Am Surg* 1993, 59:319–324.

26. Sawyers JL: Acute perforation of peptic ulcer. In *Surgery of the Stomach, Duodenum and Small Intestine*. Edited by Scott HW, Sawyers JL. Boston: Blackwell; 1992:566–572.

27. Csendes A, Maluenda F, Braghetto I, *et al.*: Prospective randomized study comparing three surgical techniques for the treatment of gastric outlet obstruction secondary to duodenal ulcer. *Am J Surg* 1993, 166:45–49.

28. Nissen R: Eine einfache Operation zur Beeinflussung der Refluxösophagitis *Schweiz Med Wochenschr* 1956, 86:590–592.

29. Donahue PE, Samelson S, Nyhus LM, *et al.*: The floppy Nissen fundoplication-effective long-term control of pathologic reflux. *Arch Surg* 1985, 120:721–730.

30. Donahue PE, Bombeck CT, Nyhus LM: Antireflux procedures. In *Operative Surgery: Principles and Techniques*, edn 3. Edited by Nova PF. Philadelphia: WB Saunders; 1990:537–544.

31. Dunnington GL, DeMeester TR: Outcome effect of adherence to operative principles of Nissen fundoplication by multiple surgeons. *Am J Surg* 1993, 166:654–659.

32. Demeester TR, Bonavina L, Albertolucci M: Nissen fundoplication for gastroesophageal reflux disease. *Ann Surg* 1986, 204:9–20.

33. Spechler SJ, Williford WO, Krol WF, *et al.*: Development and validation of a Gastroesophageal Reflux disease Activity Index (GRACI) [Abstract]. *Gastroenterology* 1992, 98:A130.

34. Schirazi SS, Schulze K, Soper RT: Long-term follow-up for treatment of complicated chronic reflux esophagitis. *Arch Surg* 1987, 122:548–552.

35. Luostarinen M, Isolauri J, Koskinen M, *et al.*: Fate of Nissen fundoplication after 20 years. A clinical, endoscopical, and functional analysis. *Gut* 1993, 34:1015–1020.

36. Negre JB, Markkula HT, Keyrilainen O, *et al.*: Nissen fundoplication. Results at 10 year follow-up. *Am J Surg* 1983, 146:635–638.

37. Dallemagne B, Weerts JM: Laparoscopic Nissen fundoplication: A preliminary report. *Surg Laparosc Endosc* 1991, 1:138–143.

38. Weerts JM, Dallemagne B, Hamoir E, *et al.*: Laparoscopic Nissen fundoplication: Detailed analysis of 132 patients. *Surg Laparosc Endosc* 1993, 3:359–364.

39. McKernan JB, Laws HL: Laparoscopic Nissen fundoplication for the treatment of gastroesophageal reflux disease. *Am Surg* 1993, 60:87–93.

40. Bittner HB, Meyers WC, Brazer SR, *et al.*: Laparoscopic Nissen fundoplication: Operative results and short-term follow-up. *Am J Surg* 1994, 167:193–200.

41. Cadiere GB, Houben JJ, Bruyns J, *et al.*: Laparoscopic Nissen fundoplication: Technique and preliminary results. *Br J Surg* 1994, 81:400–403.

42. Gaega T: Laparoscopic Nissen fundoplication: Preliminary report on ten cases. *Surg Endosc* 1991, 5:170–173.

43. Bagnato VJ: Laparoscopic Nissen fundoplication. *Surg Laparosc Endosc* 1992, 2:188–190.

44. Goldfaden D, Orringer MB, Appelman HD, *et al*: Adenocarcinoma of the distal esophagus and gastric cardia: Comparison of results of transhiatal esophagectomy and thoracoabdominal esophagogastrectomy. *J Thorac Cardiovasc Surg* 1986, 91:242–247.

45. Scott HW, Longmire WP, Gray GF Jr: Carcinoma of the stomach. In *Surgery of the Stomach, Duodenum, and Small Intestine*. Edited by Scott HW, Sawyers JL. Boston: Blackwell Scientific; 1992:333–360.

46. McCulloch P: Should general surgeons treat gastric carcinoma? An audit of practice and results, 1980–1985. *Br J Surg* 1994, 81:417–420.

47. Sue-Ling HM, Johnston D, Martin IG, *et al.*: Gastric cancer: A curable disease in Britain. *BMJ* 1993, 307:591–596.

48. Jeyasingham K: Oesophageal and gastric carcinoma. In *Operative Surgery and Management*, edn 2. Edited by Keen G. New York: Macmillan; 1987:71.

49. Shui MH, Moore E, Sanders M, *et al.*: Influence of the extent of resection on survival after curative treatment of gastric carcinoma: A retrospective multivariate analysis. *Arch Surg* 1987, 122:1347–1351.

50. Noguchi Y, Imada T, Matsumoto A, *et al.*: Radical surgery for gastric cancer: A review of the Japanese experience. *Cancer* 1989, 64:2053–2062.

51. Maruyama K, Okabayashi K, Kinoshita T: Progress in gastric cancer surgery in Japan and its limits of radicality. *World J Surg* 1987, 11:418–425.

52. Scott HW Jr, Adkins RB, Sawyers JL: Results of an aggressive surgical approach of gastric carcinoma during a twenty-three year period. *Surgery* 1985, 97:55–59.

53. Hermanek P: Prognostic factors in stomach cancer surgery. *Eur J Surg Oncol* 1986, 12:241–246.

54. Shui MH, Moore E, Sanders M, *et al.*: Influence of the extent of resection on survival after curative treatment of gastric carcinoma. *Arch Surg* 1987, 122:1347–1351.

55. Kitaoka H, Yoshikawa K, Hirota T, Itabashi M: Surgical treatment of early gastric cancer. *Jpn J Clin Oncol* 1984, 14:283–293.

56. Adachi Y, Kamakura T, Mori M, *et al.*: Prognostic significance of the number of positive lymph nodes in gastric carcinoma. *Br J Surg* 1994, 81:414–416.

57. Alexander HR, Kelsen DP, Tepper JE: Cancer of the stomach. In *Cancer: Principles and Practice of Oncology*, edn 4. Edited by DeVita VT, Hellman S, Rosenberg SA. Philadelphia: JB Lippincott; 1993:818–848.

58. Adachi Y, Kamakura T, Mori M, *et al.*: Prognostic significance of the number of positive lymph nodes in gastric carcinoma. *Br J Surg* 1994, 81:414–416.

59. Siewert JR, Böttcher K, Roder JD, *et al.*: Prognostic relevance of systematic lymph node dissection in gastric carcinoma. *Br J Surg* 1993, 80:1015–1018.

60. Maruyama K, Gunvén P, Okabayashi K, *et al.*: Lymph node metastases of gastric cancer. *Ann Surg* 1989, 210:596–602.

61. Dent DM, Madden MV, Price SK: Randomized comparison of R-1 and R-2 gastrectomy for gastric carcinoma. *Br J Surg* 1988, 75:110–112.

62. Romaguera JE, Velasquez WS, Silvermintz KB, *et al.*: Surgical debulking is associated with improved survival in stage I-II diffuse large cell lymphoma. *Cancer* 1990, 66:267–272.

63. Shiu MH, Nisce LZ, Pinna A, *et al.*: Recent results of multimodal therapy of gastric lymphoma. *Cancer* 1986, 58:1389–1399.

64. Hockey MS, Powell J, Crocker J, *et al.*: Primary gastric lymphoma. *Br J Surg* 1987, 74:483–487.

65. Rosen CB, Van Heerden MB, Martin JK, *et al.*: Is an aggressive surgical approach to the patient with gastric lymphoma warranted? *Ann Surg* 1987, 205:634–640.

66. Jones RE, Willis S, Innes DJ, *et al.*: Primary gastric lymphoma. Problems in diagnosis and management. *Am J Surg* 1988, 155:118–123.

67. Schutze WP, Halpern NB: Gastric lymphoma. *Surg Gynecol Obstet* 1991, 172:33–38.

68. Shiu MH, Farr GH, Papachristou DN, *et al.*: Myosarcomas of the stomach. Natural history, prognostic factors and management. *Cancer* 1982, 49:177–187.

69. Bedikian AY, Khankhanian N, Heilbrun LK, *et al.*: Primary lymphomas and sarcomas of the stomach. *South Med J* 1980, 73:21–24.

70. Godwin JD: Carcinoid tumors. An analysis of 2837 cases. *Cancer* 1975, 36:550–569.

71. Zollinger RM, Ellison EC, Fabri PJ, *et al.*: Primary peptic ulcerations of the jejunum associated with islet cell tumors. Twenty-five year appraial. *Ann Surg* 1980, 192:422–430.

72. Thompson JC, Lewis BG, Wiener I, Townsend CM: The role of surgery in the Zollinger-Ellison Syndrome. *Ann Surg* 1983, 197:594–607.

73. Malagelada JR, Edis AJ, Adson MA, *et al.*: Medical and surgical options in the management of patients with gastrinoma. *Gastroenterology* 1983, 84:1524–1532.

74. Richardson CT, Peters MN, Feldman M, *et al.*: Treatment of Zollinger-Ellison syndrome with exploratory laparotomy, proximal gastric vagotomy, and H2-receptor antagonists. A prospective study. *Gastroenterology* 1985, 89:357–367.

75. Norton J, Collin M, Gardiner J, *et al.*: Prospective study of gastrinoma localization and resection in patients with Zollinger-Ellison syndrome. *Ann Surg* 1986, 204:468–479.

76. Ellison EC, Carey LC, Sparks J, *et al.*: Early surgical treatment of gastrinoma. *Am J Med* 1987, 82(suppl 5B):17–24.

77. Howard TJ, Zinner MJ, Stabile BE, Passaro EP Jr: Gastrinoma excision for cure: A prospective analysis. *Ann Surg* 1990, 211:9–14.

78. Norton JA, Doppman JL, Jensen RT: Curative resection in Zollinger-Ellison syndrome. *Ann Surg* 1992, 215:8–18.

79. Seymour NE, Andersen DK: Endocrine lesions of the pancreas. In *Surgical Disease of the Biliary Tract and Pancreas: Multidisciplinary Management*. Edited by Braasch JW, Tompkins RK. St. Louis: Mosby-Year Book; 1994:605-625.

80. Thompson NW, Vinik AI, Eckhauser FE: Microgastrinomas of the duodenum, a cause of failed operations for the Zollinger-Ellison syndrome. *Ann Surg* 1989, 209:396–404.

81. Oberhelman HA Jr: Excisional therapy for ulcerogenic tumors of the duodenum: Long-term results. *Arch Surg* 1972, 104:447–453.

82. Imamura M, Kanda M, Takahashi K, *et al.*: Clinicopathological characteristics of duodenal microgastrinomas. *World J Surg* 1992, 16:703–710.

83. Frucht H, Norton JA, London JF, *et al.*: Detection of duodenal gastrinomas by operative endoscopic transillumination, a prospective study. *Gastroenterology* 1990, 99:1622–1627.

84. Joesting DR, Beart RW, van Heerden JA, *et al*: Improving survival in adenocarcinoma of the duodenum. *Am J Surg* 1981, 141:228–231.

85. Awlmark A, Andersson A, Larsson A: Primary carcinoma of the duodenum. *Ann Surg* 1980, 191:13–18.

86. Brennan MF: Duodenal cancer. *Asian J Surg* 1990, 13:204–209.

87. Mason EE: Vertical banded gastroplasty for obesity. *Arch Surg* 1982, 117:701–706.

88. Sugerman HJ, Starkey J, Birkenhauer R: A randomized prospective trial of gastric bypass versus vertical banded gastroplasty for morbid obesity and their effects on sweets versus non-sweets eaters. *Ann Surg* 1987, 205:613–614.

89. Adkins RB, Keyser JE: Recent experiences with duodenal trauma. *Am Surg* 1985, 51:121–131.

90. Jordan GL Jr: Injury to the pancreas and duodenum. In *Trauma*. Edited by Mattox KL, Moore EE, Feliciano DV. Norwalk: Appleton and Lange; 1988:473–494.

91. Bozetti F, Bonfanti G, Morabito A, *et al*: A multifaceted approach for the prognosis of patients with carcinoma of the stomach after curative resection. *Surg Gynecol Obstet* 1986, 162:229–234.

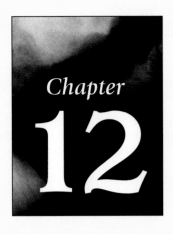

Chapter 12

The Skin and Gastrointestinal System

AMIT G. PANDYA

Diseases of the skin may be associated with various gastrointestinal abnormalities, and conversely, gastrointestinal diseases may present with changes in the skin, hair, and nails. Evaluation of a patient with a gastrointestinal disease should include an examination of the skin; a simple, efficient, inexpensive procedure that may yield valuable information. Skin signs may precede gastrointestinal signs and symptoms. Cutaneous changes may also allow the clinician to monitor the patient's disease and response to therapy, as in vasculitis. Mucosal disease may be an extension of skin disease, as in erythema multiforme. On the other hand, skin changes may be a sign of more serious internal disease, such as a metastasis from a carcinoma of the colon.

CUTANEOUS MANIFESTATIONS OF GASTROINTESTINAL TRACT POLYPOSIS SYNDROMES

TABLE 12-1. CUTANEOUS MANIFESTATIONS OF GASTROINTESTINAL TRACT POLYPOSIS SYNDROMES

FAMILIAL ADENOMATOUS POLYPOSIS AND GARDNER'S SYNDROME
Epidermoid cysts
Desmoid tumors
Pigmented lesions

PEUTZ-JEGHERS SYNDROME
Mucocutaneous pigmentation

MULTIPLE HAMARTOMA SYNDROME (COWDEN'S DISEASE)
Trichilemmomas
Oral mucosal papillomatosis
Cowden's fibroma
Acral keratoses

MUIR-TORRE SYNDROME
Sebaceous hyperplasia
Sebaceous adenomas
Sebaceous epithelioma
Sebaceous carcinoma
Multiple keratoacanthomas

TABLE 12-1.
Several syndromes present with multiple gastrointestinal polyps as well as cutaneous changes. These skin manifestations may serve as important clues to their diagnosis. Gastrointestinal malignancy may develop in these patients, and early diagnosis of the syndrome may be followed by closer monitoring of the gastrointestinal tract and occasionally prophylactic surgery to remove the affected bowel segment. These procedures may have a significant impact on patient morbidity and mortality. Inheritance of these syndromes is autosomal dominant with variable expressivity.

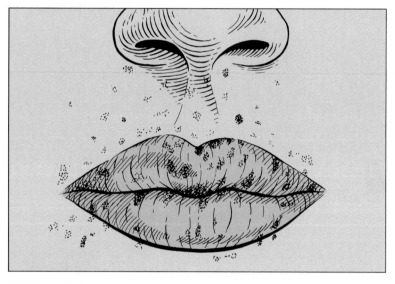

FIGURE 12-1.
Peutz-Jeghers syndrome is an autosomal dominant disorder in which multiple pigmented macules arise on the lips and buccal mucosa, beginning in childhood. Patients have polyps in the jejunum and ileum, which may present with intussusception or bleeding. Adenomatous and carcinomatous changes may also occur in the polyps. The diagnosis is usually suspected when brown macules resembling freckles or lentigos develop on the lips in patients with a positive family history of such lesions, as seen in this patient.

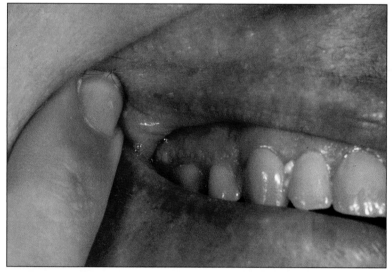

FIGURE 12-2.
Multiple hamartoma syndrome, or Cowden's disease, presents with flesh colored papules on the oral mucosa, representing benign fibromata. These lesions coalesce to form a cobblestone appearance on the gingival, palatal, lingual, and labial surfaces. Patients usually have cutaneous trichilemmomas, which are flat-topped or verrucous papules around the mouth, nose, and eyes. (*Courtesy of* D. Whiting, Dallas, TX)

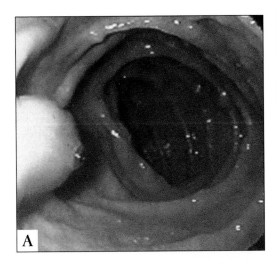

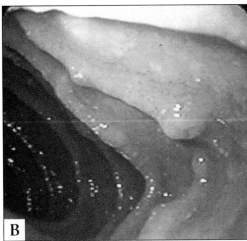

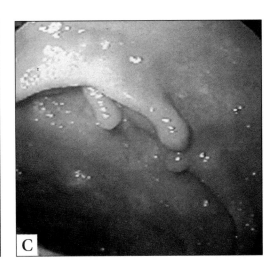

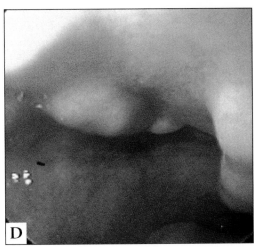

FIGURE 12-3.

A–D, Endoscopic view of duodenum showing multiple polyps in a patient with Cowden's syndrome. The polyps are hamartomas and are not thought to be premalignant. They are most commonly found in the rectosigmoid area. Cowden's syndrome is associated with increased incidence of malignancies in women, particularly breast and thyroid carcinomas. (*Courtesy of* D. Whiting, Dallas, TX)

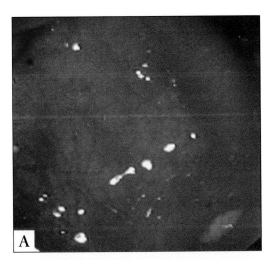

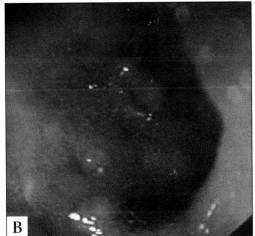

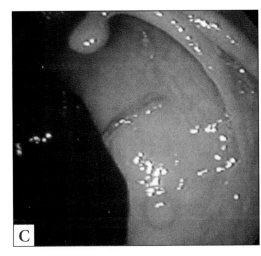

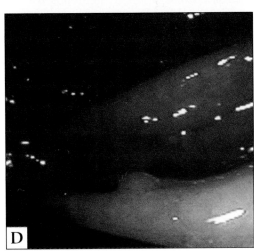

FIGURE 12-4.

A–D, Endoscopic view of the colon in the same patient depicted in Figure 12-3, demonstrating polyps in this location as well. Benign tumors of the breast, such as fibrocystic disease, are also common in Cowden's syndrome. Thyroid adenomas and goiters have been described in more than 50% of affected patients. (*Courtesy of* D. Whiting, Dallas, TX)

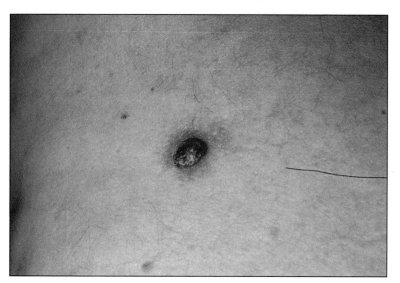

FIGURE 12-5.

A sebaceous epithelioma in a patient with multiple similar lesions. The patient had a colon carcinoma and an autosomal dominant inheritance pattern of similar cutaneous lesions found in other family members, giving the diagnosis of Muir-Torre syndrome. Sebaceous adenoma is the most common sebaceous neoplasm associated with this syndrome and is most specific for diagnosis. Sebaceous neoplasms may be yellow, flesh-colored, erythematous, or have a serous or hemorrhagic crust and require a biopsy for diagnosis. Visceral malignancies, especially of the gastrointestinal tract, develop in many patients with Muir-Torre syndrome. Adenomatous polyposis is often present, from which colonic carcinoma may arise. Other reported malignancies include non-Hodgkin's lymphoma and tumors of the larynx, duodenum, ileum, ampulla of Vater, stomach, kidney, ureter, ovary, and uterus. Such malignancies are not usually aggressive in their behavior. (*Courtesy of* P. Eichhorn, Dallas, TX)

CUTANEOUS MANIFESTATIONS OF GASTROINTESTINAL TRACT MALIGNANCY

TABLE 12-2. CUTANEOUS MANIFESTATIONS OF GASTROINTESTINAL TRACT MALIGNANCY

PARANEOPLASTIC

Malignant acanthosis nigricans—gastric adenocarcinoma

Acrokeratosis paraneoplastica (Basex syndrome)—carcinoma of upper respiratory tract, lung, tongue, or esophagus

Necrolytic migratory erythema—glucagonoma

Superficial migratory thrombophlebitis—pancreatic carcinoma

Carcinoid syndrome—gastrointestinal carcinoid tumor

METASTATIC

Sister Mary Joseph's nodule—gastric carcinoma

Cutaneous nodules from colon cancer

TABLE 12-2.

Gastrointestinal tract malignancy may lead to a paraneoplastic phenomenon with skin manifestations or direct metastases to the skin. Recognition of these skin changes may lead to early diagnosis of the tumor.

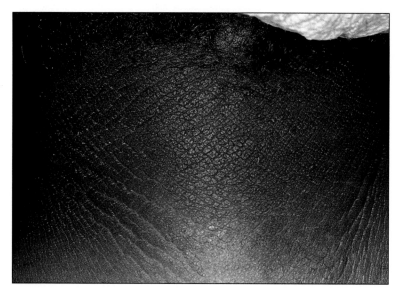

FIGURE 12-6.

Acanthosis nigricans is a disorder in which dark brown to black velvety plaques appear in flexural areas. The most common locations are the neck (as seen in this patient), axilla, and groin. Although usually associated with gastrointestinal cancer, this lesion is also generally associated with obesity and insulin resistance.

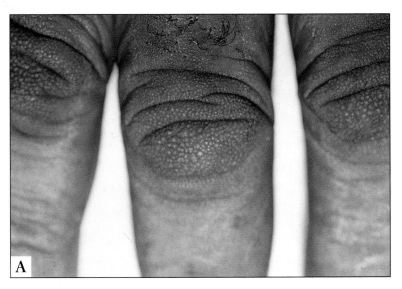

A

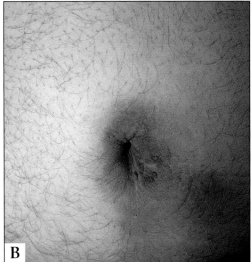

B

FIGURE 12-7.

Malignant acanthosis nigricans is a disorder of sudden onset that appears in unusual locations, such as the hands (**A**) and umbilicus (**B**) in addition to other more common locations. This disorder is frequently caused by a tumor, with gastric carcinoma as the associated malignancy in two-thirds of patients.

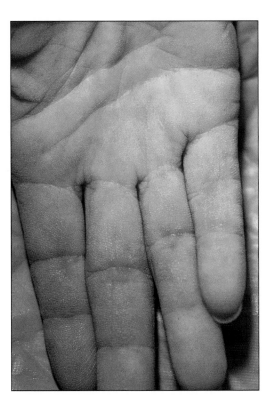

FIGURE 12-8.

"Tripe hands" in a patient with esophageal carcinoma. Acanthosis nigricans of the palmar surface resembles the lining of the stomach. Patients with malignant acanthosis nigricans usually have well-established internal tumors by the time cutaneous changes are diagnosed. (*Courtesy of* P. Eichhorn, Dallas, TX)

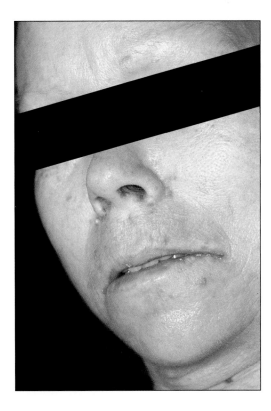

FIGURE 12-9.

Glucagonoma syndrome in a patient with a glucagon-secreting tumor of the pancreas. Necrolytic migratory erythema begins as erythematous scaly plaques in periorificial areas and flexures. The plaques may become blisters, followed by erosions, crusting, and desquamation, which occur in 1 to 2 week cycles. The skin changes may precede diagnosis of the tumor by several years. Angular cheilitis may occur, as in this patient, who also has involvement of the perinasal skin.

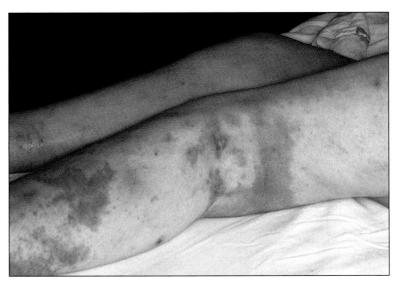

FIGURE 12-10.

Erythematous, scaly plaques seen in glucagonoma syndrome. Glucagon levels are elevated, due to a glucagon-secreting tumor. The skin changes improve with resection of the tumor. Associated symptoms are weight loss, diarrhea, anemia, hypoaminoacidemia, and zinc deficiency.

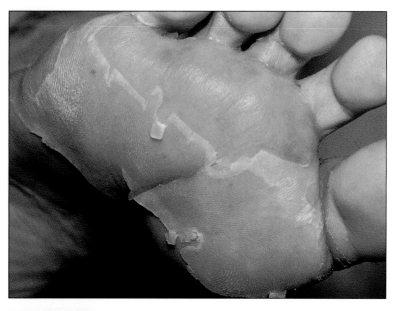

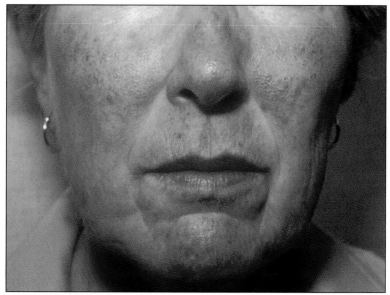

FIGURE 12-11.

Desquamation of the fingers, toes, hands, and feet may be seen in necrolytic migratory erythema. The eruption is similar to that seen with zinc deficiency, essential fatty acid deficiency, and hypoaminoacidemia.

FIGURE 12-12.

A patient with carcinoid syndrome demonstrating facial telangiectasias and flushing. Other skin manifestations include pruritus, rhinophyma, xerosis, and angular cheilitis. Gastrointestinal changes, such as diarrheal malabsorption, abdominal pain, and small bowel obstruction, may precede or coexist with the syndrome. (*Courtesy of* D. Whiting, Dallas, TX)

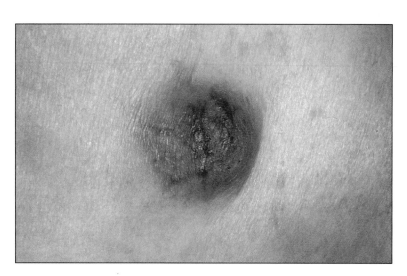

FIGURE 12-13.

Metastatic adenocarcinomas of the colon. A firm nodule, fixed to the underlying tissue, with several overlying large telangiectasias is seen here on the abdomen. The abdominal skin is the most common location for gastrointestinal tract metastases. Colonic adenocarcinomas are the most common cause, followed by gastric carcinomas. The lesions are usually nontender and may range from flesh colored to plum colored. They usually occur in advanced disease states.

CUTANEOUS MANIFESTATIONS OF INFLAMMATORY BOWEL DISEASE

TABLE 12-3. CUTANEOUS MANIFESTATIONS OF INFLAMMATORY BOWEL DISEASE

ULCERATIVE COLITIS	CROHN'S DISEASE
Erythema nodosum	Oral lesions from Crohn's disease
Pyoderma gangrenosum	Cutaneous lesions from Crohn's disease
Aphthous ulcers	Erythema nodosum
Pyoderma vegetans	Pyoderma gangrenosum
	Fissures and fistulas

TABLE 12-3.

Ulcerative colitis and Crohn's disease may present with a wide variety of skin lesions. The lesions may be caused by specific involvement of the skin by the same disease process that affects the gastrointestinal tract or a reactive process, secondary to the underlying inflammatory bowel disease.

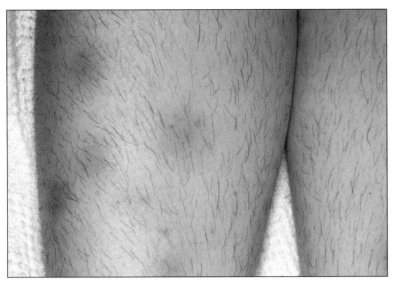

FIGURE 12-14.

Red nodules of erythema nodosum in the pretibial area. Lesions are usually tender, poorly circumscribed, and located deep within the subcutaneous fat. Their appearance is usually accompanied by an exacerbation in the underlying inflammatory bowel disease. Erythema nodosum occurs in about 4% of patients with ulcerative colitis and in 2% of patients with Crohn's disease. Treatment includes bed rest, systemic or intralesional steroids, nonsteroidal anti-inflammatory agents, potassium iodide, colchicine, and dapsone.

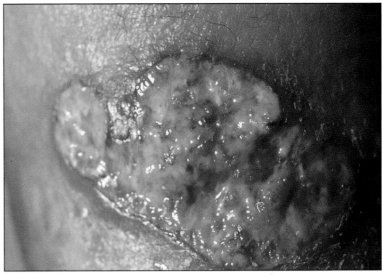

FIGURE 12-15.

Pyoderma gangrenosum first presents as erythematous papules, which rapidly form pustules and vesicles. These lesions coalesce to form large hemorrhagic bullae with dusky, raised edges. The bullae then rupture, leaving behind an enlarging, indurated ulcer with raised edges and a yellowish exudate as seen in this patient. The lesions are most common on the legs but may occur anywhere. Trauma may give rise to a lesion. Ulcerative colitis is the most common underlying cause of pyoderma gangrenosum and is present in 50% of all patients with these lesions. Although Crohn's disease may be associated with this condition, it is much less common. Therapy involves corticosteroids, with or without other immunosuppressive drugs.

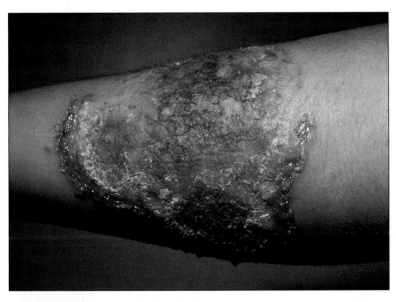

FIGURE 12-16.

Pyoderma vegetans may occur in patients with ulcerative colitis. It may represent an incomplete form of pyoderma gangrenosum. Vegetating plaques occur with vesicopustules which coalesce to form larger lesions. Intertriginous and mucosal sites may also be involved.

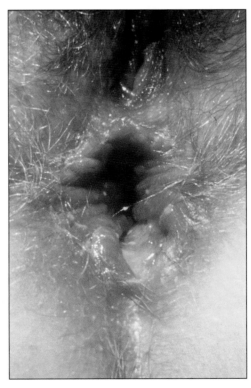

FIGURE 12-17.

Crohn's disease of the anus with an ulcer visible on the inferior aspect. Biopsy of the ulcer will typically show noncaseating granulomas. Granulomas may also be present in the mouth, on the vulva, and at colostomy and ileostomy sites. Metastatic Crohn's disease, a rare finding, presents as nodules, plaques, or ulcers at sites distant from gastrointestinal tract lesions of Crohn's disease. (*Courtesy of* D. Whiting, Dallas, TX)

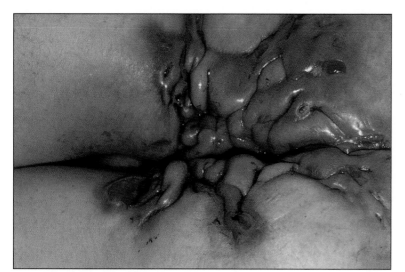

FIGURE 12-18.
Multiple fissures and fistulas in a patient with long-standing Crohn's disease. Chronic abscesses and draining sinuses are commonly seen in the perineal and perianal areas.

CUTANEOUS MANIFESTATIONS OF VASCULAR DISORDERS OF THE GASTROINTESTINAL TRACT

TABLE 12-4. CUTANEOUS MANIFESTATIONS OF VASCULAR DISORDERS OF THE GASTROINTESTINAL TRACT

Hereditary hemorrhagic telangiectasia (Osler-Weber-Rendu syndrome)	Kaposi's sarcoma
	Henoch-Schönlein purpura
Blue rubber bleb bevus syndrome	Pseudoxanthoma elasticum

TABLE 12-4.

Vascular disorders of the gastrointestinal tract are important to recognize in order to identify patients at risk of gastrointestinal hemorrhage. Cutaneous lesions can be helpful in making a diagnosis of a vascular disorder. Patients can be warned to seek prompt medical attention if any indication of an internal hemorrhage exists.

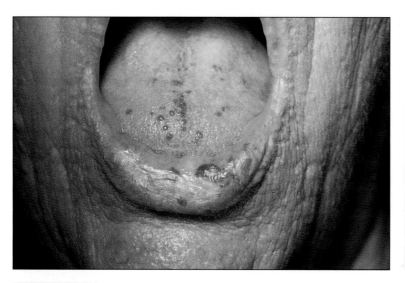

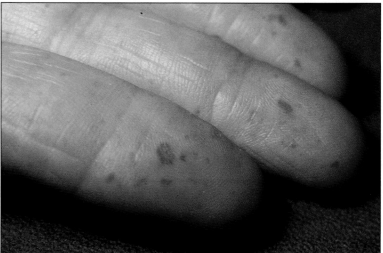

FIGURE 12-19.

A patient with Rendu-Osler-Weber syndrome, demonstrating multiple telangiectasias on the tongue and lips. The lesions usually begin as flat macules, then slowly enlarge to form papules. They commonly occur on the face, lips, tongue, palate, ears, hands, chest, and feet. Arteriovenous malformations and aneurysms may develop throughout the body, causing epistaxis and gastrointestinal tract bleeding. Although the syndrome is autosomal dominant, up to 46% of patients develop the syndrome without a positive family history.

FIGURE 12-20.

Multiple, flat, matlike telangiectasias on the fingers in a patient with Osler-Weber-Rendu syndrome. Nodular angiomas may be present in the stomach and duodenum, which may lead to gastrointestinal hemorrhage. Lesions are usually treated with electrosurgery or with laser therapy.

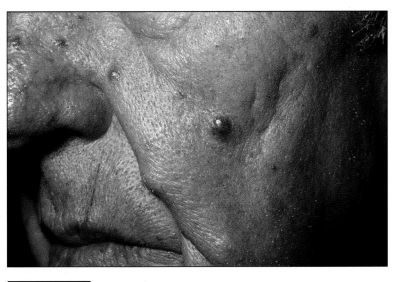

FIGURE 12-21.

A patient with multiple, soft, rubbery, bluish nodules on the nose and cheek caused by the blue rubber bleb nevus syndrome. This syndrome usually occurs sporadically, although autosomal dominant forms have been reported. Cutaneous lesions may be soft and compressible or punctate, flat, and painful. The bluish color is characteristic of this condition. Gastrointestinal lesions in this syndrome consist of cavernous hemangiomas and can be found throughout the gastrointestinal tract, although the large and small intestines are the most common locations.

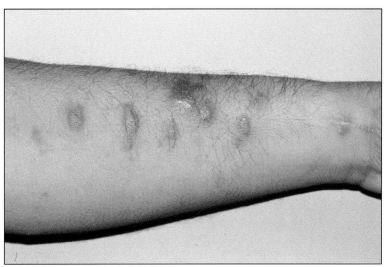

FIGURE 12-22.

Multiple firm, purple nodules on the arm resulting from Kaposi's sarcoma in a patient with AIDS. Most patients with Kaposi's sarcoma lesions, especially those of the mucous membranes, will have gastrointestinal tract lesions. The cutaneous lesions begin as brown or purple macules, which enlarge to form firm papules and nodules. Multiple lesions are common, and they may occur anywhere on the skin. Treatment includes local and systemic chemotherapy, radiation, cryotherapy, and interferon.

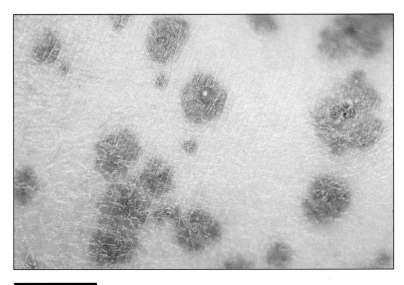

FIGURE 12-23.

Leukocytoclastic vasculitis may produce palpable purpuric lesions on the skin, caused by inflammation and extravasation of erythrocytes from blood vessels. Henoch-Schönlein purpura presents with leukocytoclastic vasculitis, most commonly in children, distributed on the buttocks and legs. Children often have accompanying abdominal pain, musculoskeletal pain, and hematuria. Bowel involvement may be present, resulting in crampy abdominal pain. Gastrointestinal tract bleeding, usually occult, occurs in 40% to 60% of patients, and intussusception and perforation may occur. A skin biopsy of a lesion will often show immunoglobulin A deposited in the vessel walls.

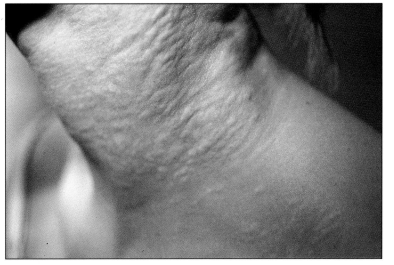

FIGURE 12-24.

Yellowish papules along the side of the neck in a patient with pseudoxanthoma elasticum giving a "plucked chicken" appearance. Gastrointestinal hemorrhage may occur, usually in the upper tract. Endoscopy reveals yellow cobblestone-like lesions similar to those seen on the skin. Cutaneous lesions arise in flexures, as well as the lips, buccal mucosa, and soft palate. Involvement of arteries may lead to hypertension and blood vessel obstruction.

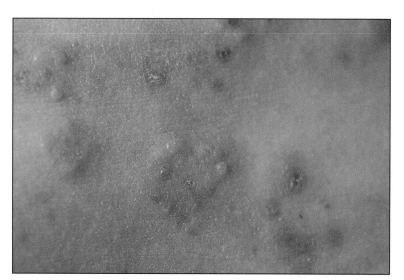

FIGURE 12-25.

Dermatitis herpetiformis presents as grouped papules and vesicles, usually with excoriations, caused by extreme pruritus of the lesions. Clinically evident celiac disease is present in 20% of these patients, whereas 80% have histologic or endoscopic evidence of celiac disease in the jejunum. Weight loss, diarrhea, steatorrhea, and other manifestations of malabsorption are present in patients with symptomatic gastrointestinal disease. Skin lesions usually appear on extensor surfaces as well as on the scalp and lower back. Granular deposition of immunoglobulin A is seen at the dermoepidermal junction. A gluten-free diet can greatly improve skin and gastrointestinal manifestations. Dapsone and sulfapyridine are also effective.

SKIN ABNORMALITIES ASSOCIATED WITH DYSPHAGIA

TABLE 12-5. SKIN ABNORMALITIES ASSOCIATED WITH DYSPHAGIA

Epidermolysis bullosa	Behçet's disease
Cicatricial pemphigoid	Systemic lupus erythematosus
Pemphigus	Scleroderma
Stevens-Johnson syndrome	Dermatomyositis

TABLE 12-5.

Several blistering skin disorders are associated with mucous membrane lesions which may extend into the oropharynx and esophagus, leading to dysphagia. The internal lesions usually develop parallel to the cutaneous lesions, although they may occur independently of one another. Connective tissue diseases may be associated with dysphagia caused by abnormalities in muscles associated with swallowing, including the esophagus.

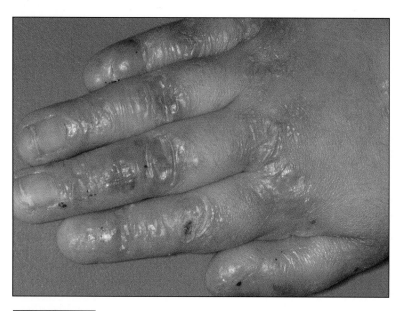

FIGURE 12-26.

Epidermolysis bullosa is a congenital blistering disease with a variety of subtypes, classified according to the depth of the blistering process. Recurrent blistering occurs on cutaneous surfaces, often leaving scars and loss of nails, as seen in this patient with lesions on the hands. Mucous membrane involvement may lead to loss of teeth. Esophageal involvement manifests itself as blisters and erosions, which may lead to strictures.

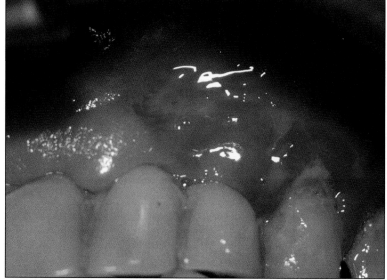

FIGURE 12-27.

Superficial erosions of the gums caused by cicatricial pemphigoid. Cicatricial pemphigoid is an autoimmune disease in which antibodies bind to the dermoepidermal junction of mucous membranes, leading to erosions and scarring. Although extra mucosal lesions may occur, blistering and erosions are most severe on mucous membranes. Scarring and esophageal stenosis may require dilatation of strictures. (*Courtesy of* P. Eichhorn, Dallas, TX)

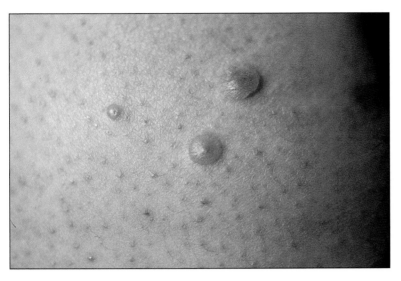

FIGURE 12-28.

Early lesions of pemphigus vulgaris present as easily ruptured blisters that leave superficial erosions. This autoimmune blistering disease is caused by immunoglobulin G antibodies that bind to the desmosomal junction between keratinocytes, leading to this dissolution and superficial blistering. Blisters may occur anywhere on the body, although the head, trunk, proximal extremities, and mucous membranes are the most common locations.

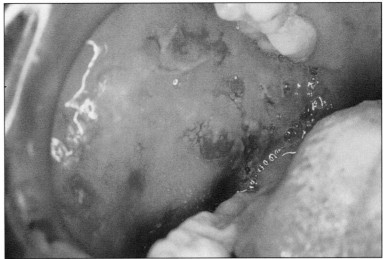

FIGURE 12-29.

Pemphigus vulgaris of the oral mucosa. Diagnosis is confirmed with a biopsy of the edge of the blister, which shows the characteristic split in the epidermis, and immunoglobulin G deposition around the keratinocytes. Before the advent of steroids, most of these afflicted patients died, usually because of protein loss through the skin and because of secondary infection.

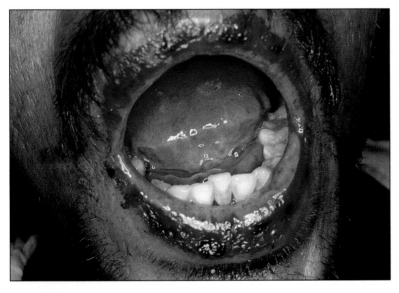

FIGURE 12-30.

Stevens-Johnson syndrome presents with erosions of the oral, conjunctival, and genital mucosa, along with lesions of erythema multiforme on cutaneous surfaces. This patient has erosions of the lips and tongue caused by Stevens-Johnson syndrome secondary to the use of a prescribed medication. Lesions often extend to the esophagus, where they cause dysphagia.

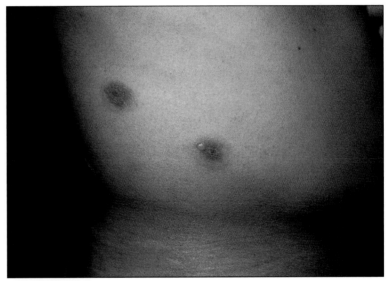

FIGURE 12-31.

Typical target lesions of erythema multiforme. Erythema multiforme major, or Stevens-Johnson syndrome, includes cutaneous lesions along with involvement of two or more mucous membranes. Skin lesions may present as erythematous macules, papules, plaques, vesicles, bullae, or erosions; thus the descriptive name *multiforme*.

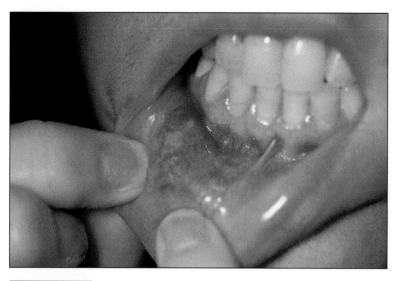

FIGURE 12-32.

Behçet's disease presents with oral and genital ulcers, as well as with eye disease. Esophageal lesions may cause dysphagia. Oral lesions usually appear as punched-out ulcers, similar to those seen with aphthous stomatitis. Colitis may also be present. (*Courtesy of* P. Eichhorn, Dallas, TX)

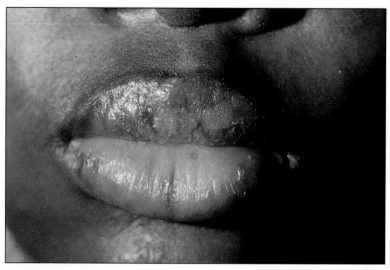

FIGURE 12-33.

Lupus erythematosus frequently presents with oral ulcers, which usually parallel the development of cutaneous and systemic disease. Ulcers may occur in the oropharynx and produce dysphagia. Oral ulcers are associated with the systemic form of the disease, but are less common in subacute cutaneous or discoid lupus erythematosus. This patient demonstrates erosions on the lips associated with a flare of systemic lupus erythematosus.

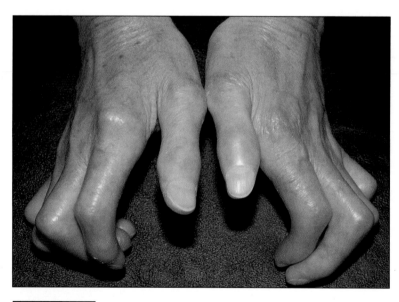

FIGURE 12-34.

Scleroderma, or progressive systemic sclerosis, is characterized by sclerodactyly as seen in this patient. The skin is shiny, thickened, firm, and bound down on the hands, arms, face, and shoulders. Gastroesophageal reflux diseases resulting from loss of lower esophageal sphincter function and reduced or absent peristalsis leads to esophagitis and stricture formation. Dysphagia may result from stricture or from esophageal dysmotility.

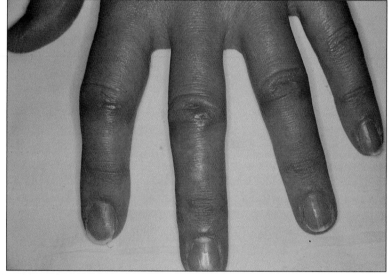

FIGURE 12-35.

The musculature of the oropharynx and upper esophagus may be involved in dermatomyositis, leading to dysphagia. Characteristic cutaneous signs include Gottron's sign, in which a violaceous, scaly erythema appears on the skin over the tendons of the hands, particularly over the knuckles, as seen in this patient. Papules occurring in this location are referred to as *Gottron's papules*. Pruritic, erythematous plaques may be present over the elbows, knees, posterior neck, buttocks, and other extensor surfaces. Edema and erythema of the eyelids may occur, producing the characteristic "heliotrope rash."

SKIN CHANGES OF MALABSORPTION

TABLE 12-6. SKIN CHANGES OF MALABSORPTION

NONSPECIFIC	SPECIFIC
Ichthyosis	Acrodermatitis enteropathica
Pruritus	Scurvy
Brittle hair and nails	Pellagra
Hyperpigmentation	

TABLE 12-6.

Both specific and nonspecific skin changes are associated with malabsorption. Severe dryness of the skin is also a common finding. Dryness can be severe enough to form ichthyotic or fish-like scales. Essential fatty acid deficiency plays a role in the development of dry skin. Hyperpigmentation is usually diffuse, as in Addison's disease.

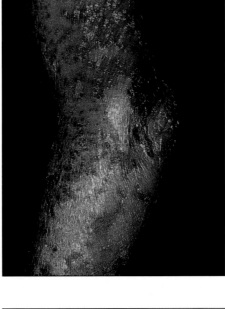

FIGURE 12-36.

A patient with malabsorption and wasting, demonstrating hyperpigmentation, xerosis, and flaking of the skin. Pruritus is very common and eczematous or psoriasiform lesions may develop. Nails and hair are weak, brittle, and slow-growing.

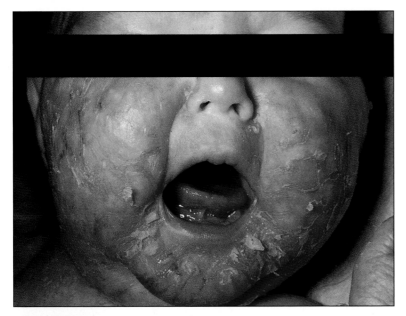

FIGURE 12-37.

Acrodermatitis enteropathica is a dermatitis that occurs at the time of weaning and is a manifestation of zinc deficiency. Blistering and erosions occur around the mouth and anus, followed by erythema and scale, as seen in this infant. Large doses of zinc are usually sufficient to reverse these cutaneous changes. Zinc is thought to be chelated in the bowel of the patients by an abnormal ligand, leading to zinc deficiency.

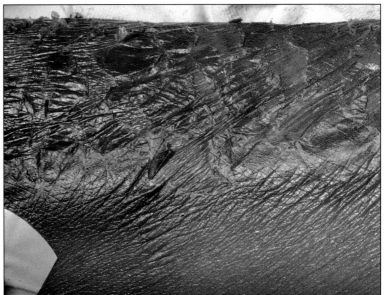

FIGURE 12-38.

Deficiency of the B-complex vitamin niacin may lead to pellagra; the symptoms include diarrhea, dementia, and dermatitis. A diet based predominantly on corn is thought to contribute to the development of pellagra. The skin becomes pigmented, scaly, cracked, and brittle, as seen in this patient. The most common sites are the dorsa of the hands, giving a glovelike pigmentation. There is often a well-circumscribed collar around the neck, known as Casal's necklace. Oral administration of niacinamide is usually curative.

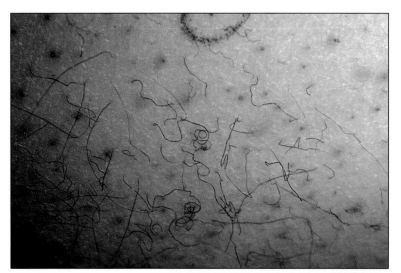

FIGURE 12-39.

A patient with scurvy, demonstrating purpuric macules and papules in a perifollicular location. This disease, which results from a vitamin C deficiency, causes abnormalities of the hair follicle, leading to the development of *corkscrew hairs*, as seen in this patient. The most common location for these changes are the legs, buttocks, and arms. Gingivitis and aphthous ulcers may occur on mucous membranes.

SKIN SIGNS OF HEPATOBILIARY DISEASE

TABLE 12-7. SKIN SIGNS OF HEPATOBILIARY DISEASE

DIFFUSE HYPERPIGMENTATION
Cirrhosis
Primary biliary cirrhosis
Hemochromatosis

VASCULAR CHANGES
Spider telangiectasias
Palmar erythema
Dilated abdominal veins caused by portal hypertension

HORMONE-INDUCED CHANGES
Striae distensae
Gynecomastia
Dupuytren's contractures
Parotid swelling

PORPHYRIA CUTANEA TARDA
Bullae
Hypertrichosis
Milia

HEPATITIS-ASSOCIATED SKIN CHANGES
Leukocytoclastic vasculitis resulting from cryoglobulinemia
Polyarteritis nodosa
Lichen planus
Papular acrodermatitis of childhood (Gianotti-Crosti syndrome)

NAIL CHANGES
White nails (Terry's nails)
Azure lunules (Wilson's disease)
Clubbing

TABLE 12-7.
Many cutaneous changes may be seen in association with liver disease. Jaundice, itching, and pigmentary changes are commonly seen with many types of liver disease. Other changes, however, are specific for a particular type of liver disease, such as azure lunules of nails as seen with Wilson's disease.

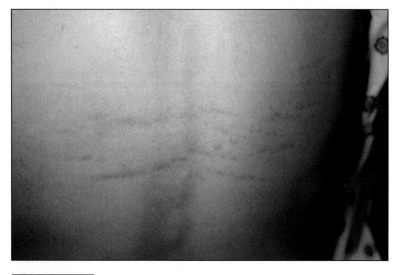

FIGURE 12-40.

Striae distensae occur frequently in chronic liver disease. They usually appear on the abdomen and thighs. Occasionally they can be more extensive, as they are in this patient with striae on the back.

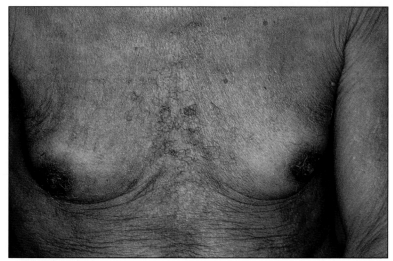

FIGURE 12-41.

Gynecomastia is a hormone-induced change seen frequently with cirrhosis, along with Dupuytren's contractures and parotid swelling. Although hyperestrogenism is thought to play a role in the development of gynecomastia, the exact mechanism remains unknown.

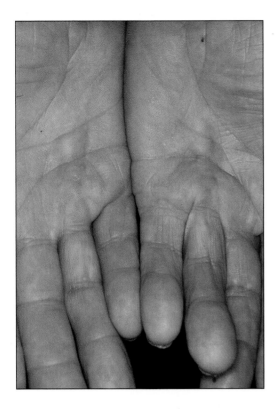

FIGURE 12-42.

Dupuytren's contractures in a patient with liver disease. Chronic cirrhosis may lead to the development of these contractures, which involve the flexor tendons of the hands. The contractures are often painful and usually require surgical correction to restore the hands to normal.

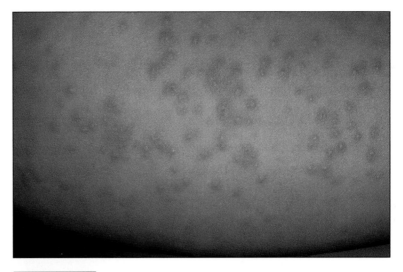

FIGURE 12-43.

A patient with papular acrodermatitis of childhood, or Gianotti-Crosti syndrome, demonstrating multiple erythematous papules on the leg. This eruption usually occurs in childhood, with most of the lesions on the face and extremities. Acute, nonicteric hepatitis and adenopathy is associated with the eruption, which lasts 2 to 3 weeks. Hepatitis is usually caused by the hepatitis B virus.

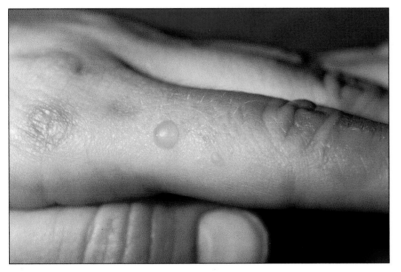

FIGURE 12-44.

Tense vesicles filled with clear fluid, atrophic scarring, and milia formation on the lateral aspect of the finger in a patient with porphyria cutanea tarda. Other common cutaneous features of this disorder include hypertrichosis (especially of the face) and photosensitivity. Patients with porphyrias have defects in the control of the porphyrin-heme biosynthetic pathway, usually as a result of deficient activity of specific enzymes. Hepatic iron stores are usually elevated and serum transaminase levels may also be high.

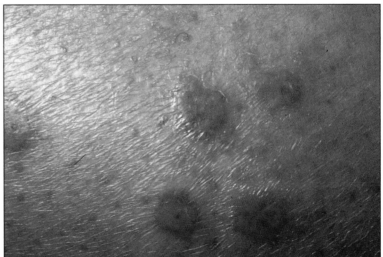

FIGURE 12-45.

Lichen planus presents as multiple, polygonal, violaceous, flat-topped papules on the wrists, ankles, shins, neck, thighs, and lower back. A lacy white scale can sometimes be seen on the lesions, known as Wickham's striae. Genital and oral involvement is most common, although many variations in presentation exist. Liver disease has been reported in association with lichen planus, including chronic active hepatitis and primary biliary cirrhosis.

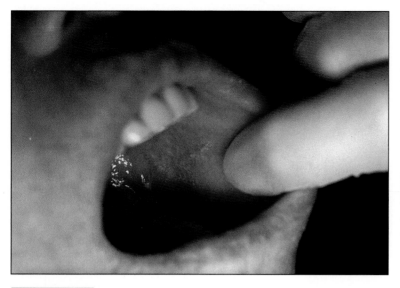

FIGURE 12-46.

Lacy white lesions on the buccal mucosa in a patient with lichen planus. The lips, gingiva, and tongue are other common sites of involvement. A wide variety of drugs, including gold, antimalarial medications, captopril, and thiazide diuretics may induce a lichen planus-like reaction.

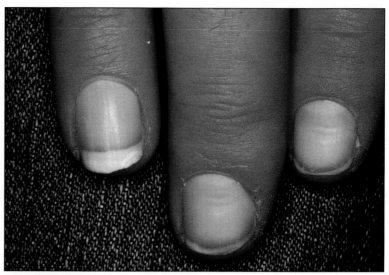

FIGURE 12-47.

Intensely white nails, also called Terry's nails, are a sign of cirrhosis. The white color is not in the nail plate but rather in the nail bed itself. There is often a thin zone of pink nail bed at the distal edge of the nail. Decreased blood flow to the nail bed because of increased connective tissue between the nail and the underlying bone is thought to be the cause of this abnormality. Up to 82% of patients with cirrhosis may have Terry's nails.

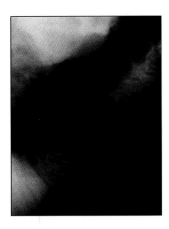

Index

Page numbers followed by *t* or *f* indicate tables or figures, respectively.

Gianotti-Crosti syndrome, 12.15f
Glucagon, properties, 2.3t
Glucagonoma syndrome, 12.5f
Glutathione, in mucosal defense, 4.2, 4.10f, 4.11f
Goiter, in Cowden's syndrome, 12.3f
Gottron's papules, 12.12f
Granuloma(s), gastric, 5.10f
   associated diseases, 5.10f, 5.10t
   formation, 5.10f
Growth hormone-releasing factor, tumor producing, 8.17f
Gynecomastia, in cirrhosis, 12.14f

H

Heat shock proteins, and ethanol-induced gastric
       mucosal injury, 4.2, 4.10f
Heineke-Mikulicz pyloroplasty, 11.5f
Helicobacter pylori, 6.1–6.16
   adherence to gastric epithelium, 6.2f
   antritis, and somatostatin cell function, 7.4f
   contact angle and, 4.1, 4.3f
   culture, 6.7t
   cytokine induction by, 3.13f
   eradication
      effect on gastric acid secretion, 7.6f
      effect on serum gastrin, 7.6f
      effect on ulcer healing, 7.16f
      effect on ulcer recurrence, 6.11f, 6.12f, 7.17f
      mucosa-associated lymphoid tissue lymphoma
         regression with, 6.16t
      treatment regimens for, 1.8f, 1.9f, 6.12t
   gastritis, 5.5f, 5.5t, 5.6f, 5.8f, 6.7f, 6.7t, 6.8f
      pathogenesis, 3.13f
      and secondary G-cell hyperplasia, 2.16t
      serum pepsinogens in, 5.9f
   glycocalyx, 6.2f
   histology, 6.7t
   induction of IL-8, pathway for, 3.13f
   infection
      antibiotic therapy for, 6.12t, 6.16t
      antral (type B) gastritis and, 6.8f
      chronic active gastritis and, 6.7f, 6.7t
      clustering in family groups, 6.4f
      diagnosis, 6.6–6.12
      diseases associated with, 6.1, 6.7t
      duodenal ulcer and, 6.7t, 7.16f
      effect on mucosal defense, 4.1, 4.3f, 4.4f
      epidemiology, 6.1, 6.3–6.4
      and gastric cancer, 6.7t, 6.13–6.14
      and gastric metaplasia, 6.9f, 6.10f
      and gastric non-Hodgkin's lymphoma, 6.7t, 6.14t
      gastric ulcer and, 6.7t
      and gastrointestinal disease, 3.2, 3.3
      histologic staining of, 6.5f
      lymphoepithelial lesions and, 6.15f
      mucosal inflammation in, 6.8f
      mucosal lymphoid follicles with, 6.9f
      mucosal ulceration caused by, pathogenesis, 3.13f
      in peptic ulcer, prevalence, 7.6f
      and peptic ulcer disease, 6.10f, 6.11f, 7.1, 7.2, 7.16f, 7.17f
      in peptic ulcer disease vs. Zollinger-Ellison syndrome, 8.4t

prevalence, 6.3f, 6.4f
   and primary G-cell hyperplasia, 2.16t
   serum gastrin concentration in, 6.11f, 7.6f
   tests for, 6.6f, 6.7t
   urease test for, 6.6f, 6.7t
   ingestion of gastric mucosal surfactant, 4.1, 4.4f
   mode of transmission, 6.3f, 6.4f
   morphology, 6.2f
   and mucosa-associated lymphoid tissue, 6.15–6.16
   mucosa-associated lymphoid tissue lymphoma and,
      6.15f, 6.16t
   rapid urease assay for, 6.6f, 6.7t
   serology, 6.7t
   taxonomy, 6.2f
   urea breath test for, 6.6f, 6.7t
Henoch-Schönlein purpura, 12.9f
Hepatitis, cutaneous manifestations, 12.15f
Hepatobiliary disease, cutaneous manifestations, 12.14–12.16
Hepatoid adenocarcinoma, gastric, 10.2f
Hereditary hemorrhagic telangiectasia.
      See Osler-Weber-Rendu syndrome
Histamine, 2.13–2.15
   gastric, cell sources, 2.13t
   in gastric acid secretion, 1.2f, 1.3f, 1.4f, 7.3f
   interactions with other gastric hormones, 2.15f
   properties, 2.3t
   structure, 2.14f
Histamine H_2-receptor antagonists, 1.4t, 1.5f, 8.2f
   duration of action, 8.8f
   gastric acid control and, 1.8f
   long-term maintenance therapy, effects on ulcer
      recurrence, 7.17f
   for peptic ulcer disease, 7.2, 7.2f–7.3f
   structure, 2.14f
   ulcer healing rates with, 7.16f
   for Zollinger-Ellison syndrome, 8.7f, 8.9f
Histamine H_3-receptor, in gastric acid secretion, 1.3f
Histidine decarboxylase, in gastric acid secretion, 1.2f
Histoplasmosis, gastric, 5.11f
Hormone(s), 2.2f. *See also specific hormone*
   gut, 2.3t
Host defense. *See also* Mucosal defense
   compromise, and gastrointestinal disease, 3.2
   of gut, 3.3f
Hydrochloric acid, penetration of gastric mucus, 4.2, 4.6f
Hydrophobicity, 4.1, 4.3f
Hyperpigmentation
   with hepatobiliary disease, 12.14t
   in malabsorption, 12.13f
Hypertrophic gastropathy, idiopathic, differential
      diagnosis, 10.5f

I

Imidazopyridines, 1.8f
Immune tolerance, oral. *See* Oral tolerance
Immunoglobulin A
   polymeric, 3.2, 3.6f
   response to antigen stimulus, 3.7f, 3.8f, 3.9f
   secretory, 3.2, 3.6f, 3.8f
      absence of or decrease in, 3.9f

S

T

U